Caring *and* Compassionate

THE MATER CHILDREN'S HOSPITAL

1931 to 2014

Caring *and* Compassionate

The Mater Children's Hospital
1931 to 2014

Helen Gregory

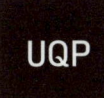

First published 2015 by University of Queensland Press
PO Box 6042, St Lucia, Queensland 4067, Australia

uqp.com.au
uqp@uqp.uq.edu.au

© Mater Health Services 2015

This book is copyright. Except for private study, research, criticism or reviews, as permitted under the Copyright Act, no part of this book may be reproduced, stored in a retrieval system or transmitted in any form or by any means without prior written permission. Enquiries should be made to the publisher.

Project Manager: Stan Lamond
Designer: Stan Lamond
Editor: Janet Parker
Proofreader: Kate Etherington

Printed in Australia by McPherson's Printing Group, Melbourne

Cataloguing-in-Publication Data
National Library of Australia
Cataloguing-in-publication data is available at http://catalogue.nla.gov.au

ISBN 978 0 7022 5389 8

University of Queensland Press uses papers that are natural, renewable and recyclable products made from wood grown in sustainable forests. The logging and manufacturing processes conform to the environmental regulations of the country of origin.

Contents

Introduction vi

Part One 1931 to 1950s 1
    Chapter 1   A Pressing Need 2
    Chapter 2   Realising the Dream 12
    Chapter 3   Broader Horizons 28

Part Two 1960s to 1970s 41
    Chapter 4   Growth and Pressure. 42
    Chapter 5   Transition .54
    Chapter 6   Phoenix Rising 63
    Chapter 7   Future Visions 78

Part Three 1980s to 1990s 91
    Chapter 8   Celebration and Construction 92
    Chapter 9   Dealing with Damage 106
    Chapter 10   We Shall Not Be Moved 118
    Chapter 11   Making Do 136
    Chapter 12   Reaching Out 149
    Chapter 13   Plans and Preparations 161

Part Four The 2000s 173
    Chapter 14   The Sparkling New Hospital in Stanley Street . . . 174
    Chapter 15   Transition: The Queensland Children's Hospital . 188
    Chapter 16   Changing Childhoods Forever 206

Vale Mater Children's Hospital 211

Acknowledgments 214
Endnotes 216
Brisbane Hospitals 256
Index 257

Introduction

Mater values are me now, and will go with me wherever I go.
Anna Price, ORMIS Administrator, 2014[1]

The Mater Children's Hospital opened its doors in 1931. Throughout its 83-year history, tens of thousands of 'Mater children' have experienced Mater care – high-quality clinical treatment blended with compassion and delivered with commitment to the best possible outcome for every patient.

These hallmarks of the Mater Children's Hospital – indeed all the Mater hospitals – derive from the values and philosophy of the Sisters of Mercy. The Sisters integrated their dedication to the poor, the sick and the uneducated with a very practical approach to the world and its needs. They created hospitals from dreams and expanded them through clever financial management.

In 1931, at the depths of the Great Depression, only half of the planned Mater Children's Hospital became reality, setting a pattern of mending, 'making do' and growing, even when not a spare inch of space or a single cent seemed available.

A distinctive Mater culture – never diminished by the constant need to adapt to changing circumstances – grew out of the Mercy way of doing things: warmth, humour, friendliness and 'family' feeling enlivening dedication, hard work, clinical expertise and aspiration. The Mater Children's Hospital developed a distinctive 'feel', enveloping patients and their parents – those who left with medical problems resolved; those whose conditions could only be managed, rather than cured; and those who found compassion and empathy when, sadly, death intervened.

Introduction

The hospital itself passed through many troubled and difficult times. Pressures came from every side: developments in paediatrics; new technologies, invariably expensive, as well as exciting; staff shortages; changes in governmental health policies and funding packages. As a privately owned hospital admitting patients free of charge, Brisbane's Mater hospitals – the Mater Children's Hospital among them – often trod a shaky tightrope between maintaining independent decision-making and needing government support.

Mercy philosophy seemed capable of endless adaptation to accommodate the enormous changes at the core of the Mater Children's Hospital story. The Sisters, in their immaculate white habits, ceded their primacy in the wards to nurses educated in the secular tradition, wards expanded and shrank, buildings adapted to changing modes of paediatric care, new ones appeared and, in 2001, an entirely new Mater Children's Hospital opened on the opposite side of the large Mater campus, dedicated to intimate, family-centred care, while sharing high-level technical services with other Mater hospitals.

Buildings, no matter how sophisticated, do not make a hospital. Its people – the patients, their families and the staff – define its essential character. Yet, in the early twenty-first century, the people of the Mater Children's Hospital faced great change – the closure of their hospital, with its services incorporated into the Lady Cilento Children's Hospital, Queensland's enormous, new, tertiary children's hospital. Long an ambition of paediatricians, the single children's hospital will be capable of delivering the most advanced tertiary clinical services under one roof.

Loss can never be borne without grief. Grieving the loss of jobs, as not everyone could be placed at the new hospital, and grieving the loss of the Mater Children's Hospital, a sentiment echoed on the other side of the river with the closure of the Royal Children's Hospital, reflect the strength of each hospital's distinctive culture. Yet values learnt and constantly practised are never lost – they remain alive and well inside Mater Children's Hospital people: the patients, the families and the staff who have cared for them.

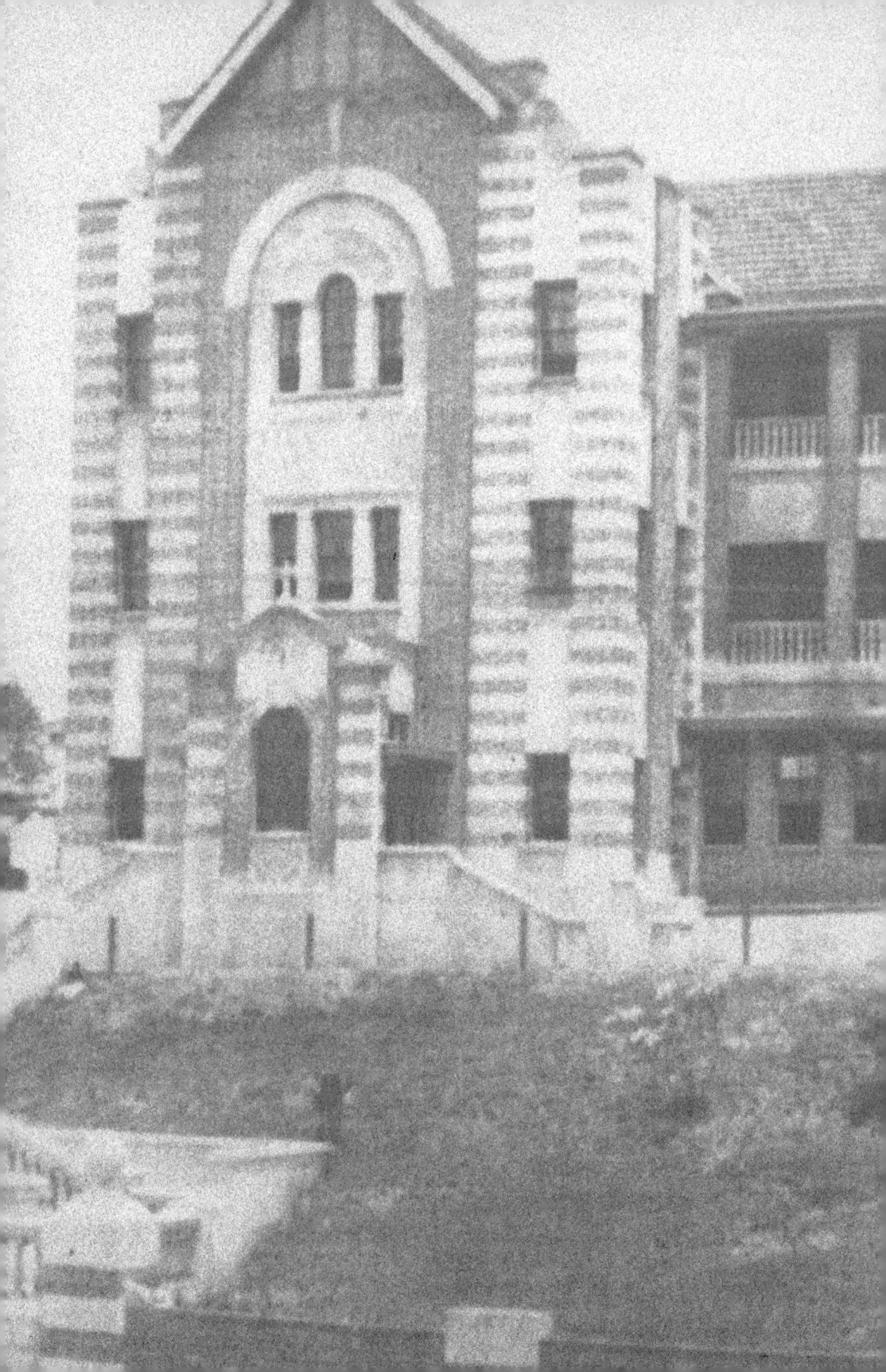

Part One
1931 to 1950s

Chapter 1

A Pressing Need

Owing to the rapid growth of Brisbane, and the enormous increase in city traffic, many problems are presenting themselves for solution, not the least of these is the pressing need for a Children's Hospital at the south side of the city.

The *Brisbane Courier*, 14 November 1925[1]

The year 1925 was an exciting one for Brisbane. The cities of North Brisbane and South Brisbane joined the shires and towns scattered across the metropolitan area to form one sprawling city, Greater Brisbane. The population was indeed growing. Between 1891, at the depths of the 1890s Depression, and 1921, three years after the end of the First World War, metropolitan Brisbane's population doubled to almost 211,000. Population was highest on the northern side of the river at 137,442, overshadowing the 73,388 on the southern side. A population spurt in the comparatively affluent early 1920s increased Brisbane's population to 263,711 in December 1925.[2]

The density of population in the inner city was falling, but the suburbs were growing. Earlier in 1925, the population of the city core was 86,279, a further 107,739 people lived in the inner suburbs and 59,202 in the outer suburbs.[3] Public transport networks were developing. Train and tram services linked inner suburbs on the north side to the city and, on the south side, tramlines were spreading outwards.[4] There was, however, no rail bridge and only one road bridge across the wide Brisbane River, which separated the southern side of Brisbane from the central business district on the north bank.

The river remained a 'great divide' in Brisbane for decades; the south side was regarded – financially, politically and socially – as the 'poor cousin' of the north side. Despite the scepticism that doctors would not bother to cross the river to treat patients in any large hospital on the south side, the Sisters of Mercy established a private hospital – where patients paid a fee – at South Brisbane in 1910, and, in 1911, a hospital for those who couldn't afford to pay. Both hospitals were very busy and, indeed, the city's leading medical practitioners treated patients in both hospitals.[5]

Brisbane's only children's hospital, the Hospital for Sick Children, as the Royal Children's Hospital was then known, was situated at Herston, a few kilometres north-west of the city centre, close to the public adult hospital, the Brisbane Hospital (now the Royal Brisbane and Women's Hospital). The children's hospital was groaning under the strain. In 1923, it had treated 3,542 in-patients and a further 6,000 children in its out-patient department.[6] The need for a new children's hospital was not lost on the Mater's honorary medical staff. In September 1925, Dr ED Ahern, chairman of the Mater's medical board, said that a 'strong recommendation' should be made to the Sisters for 'the establishment of a Children's Department as soon as convenient'. He continued:

> Apart from the urgency and great necessity for a children's hospital in South Brisbane, the Board considers that such an establishment would be of the greatest assistance in the training of nurses and Resident Medical Officers ...[7]

Dr Ahern's belief that the government would assist generously was based more on optimism than experience. He may, however, have been relying on a statement made by the Acting Premier, WN Gillies, at the Mater in 1924:

> It has been said that the real test of good government in any country is the high percentage of happy, healthy men, women and children ... The test of whether a people are highly civilised or have a right to call themselves Christian ... depends on how they care for the sick and suffering, the aged, and the helpless little children. If higher forms of education do not develop a social conscience among the people, so as to ensure that this [the Mater] and kindred institutions caring for the sufferers shall never want for funds, then we are not advancing.[8]

Despite these fine sentiments, the Hospital for Sick Children had always fought hard for financial support and government attention. The hospital was founded in 1878 by a Scottish-born philanthropist, Mary McConnel, wife of a pioneering pastoralist. Mary McConnel, familiar with the children's hospital in Edinburgh, which had been established in 1860, was appalled that sick children in Brisbane were admitted to adult wards at the Brisbane Hospital, if their parents could not afford a private doctor to treat them at home. The Hospital for Sick Children was a 'voluntary' hospital managed by a committee of women, with limited government support.[9]

Voluntary hospitals in the British tradition had been founded in towns and cities across Australia. They were established by philanthropically minded people and maintained by subscribers who contributed towards their running costs. In the nineteenth century – particularly before the era of professional nurse training – public hospitals were patronised mainly by those who could not afford treatment in their homes by private doctors. Fear that hospitals were death traps was not irrational. Private doctors attended poor patients in the voluntary hospitals on an honorary basis, but subscribers could rarely keep pace with rising costs and, consequently, many hospitals languished. Governments stepped in with grants of various kinds, but this assistance was rarely sufficient, particularly in hospitals rapidly becoming overcrowded in growing societies such as Queensland.

Immigrants had been attracted to Queensland for decades by governments desperate to increase population in order to develop a large, sparsely peopled colony. Promises of land, employment, good housing and a warm, sunny climate were used to entice new settlers. Brisbane was not, however, a place of unalloyed joy as far as either immigrant or Queensland-born children were concerned. Gastrointestinal diseases plagued the city before clean water and sanitation became available and diphtheria exacted a high death toll among infants and small children in Brisbane, as it did all over the world. Repeated outbreaks of typhoid fever and diarrhoea from contaminated milk were common. Quite apart from the tragedy that infant and child deaths inflicted on families, this was not at all the image of a safe, healthy settler colony that Queensland governments were anxious to promote.

The Queensland government had also taken steps to improve on infant mortality rates as high as 120 per 1,000 live births in 1903.[10] Alfred Jefferis Turner, a paediatrician at the Hospital for Sick Children, was heavily involved in the infant welfare movement and established Queensland's first infant welfare clinic in 1909; in 1918, the government opened four baby clinics. Turner had campaigned for the *Infant Life Protection Act 1905*, which mandated the registration of 'nursing homes' – a euphemism for baby farms where, for a fee, babies could be left, supposedly with a wet nurse. Often, however, babies were artificially fed, frequently with contaminated milk and inappropriate solid food. As a precaution against infanticide, the reporting of the births and deaths of illegitimate children was made compulsory.[11]

Some diseases had local origins. Nephritis and eyesight deficits from lead poisoning and chronic anaemia from hookworm affected Queensland children at an alarming rate. Penetrating investigations by Brisbane doctors at the Hospital for Sick Children identified lead in paint as the culprit in the lead poisoning epidemic and, for the first time in the world, identified hookworm as a parasite that could affect children as well as underground workers, its more recognised victims.[12] In the early 1890s, Turner, one of the doctors involved in both the lead poisoning and hookworm investigations, began to use anti-toxin to treat diphtheria at the Hospital for Sick Children. He was one of the first doctors in the world to use this method developed by Ehrlich and von Behring in Robert Koch's laboratory in Germany, where he had studied.[13]

Advances in medical science and improvements in public health through clean water and sanitation gradually changed the pattern of diseases affecting Queensland children. New problems arose. Poliomyelitis, often called infantile paralysis, emerged in the late nineteenth century as a terrifying disease threatening children and, to a lesser extent, adults. This viral infection was not usually fatal, but could leave a terrible legacy of physical disability.

Although the virus probably affected children from ancient times, epidemics did not attract serious medical attention until the late eighteenth century.[14] In 1789, a British physician, Michael Underwood, compiled the first clinical description of an illness that caused 'debility of the lower extremities'.[15] A German physician, Jacob Heine, described the clinical features of the disease in 1840, and noted that its symptoms suggested the involvement of the spinal cord.[16] Two Austrian physicians, Landsteiner and Popper, identified and described the infective agent in 1908.

The first major outbreak in the United States – some 132 cases – occurred in Vermont in the summer of 1894. Epidemics every few years produced a larger and larger toll of children with disabilities ranging from inability to breathe – the infamous 'iron lung' appeared during the 1920s – to paralysis of limbs, to no apparent long-term effects at the mild end of the spectrum.[17] In Queensland, the Commissioner for Public Health, Dr Burnett Ham, reported in 1905 that infantile paralysis, 'a new and rare disease', had occurred in Queensland.[18]

Ironically, cleaner living conditions – sanitation and pure water – emerged as a factor in the increasing incidence of polio. Young children had fewer opportunities to encounter the virus, delaying exposure until late childhood or adulthood, when it was more likely to take the paralytic form. Polio became recognised as a disease of cleanliness.

Polio epidemics were reported in Queensland every few years after 1905, adding to the strain at the Hospital for Sick Children. Many children remained in hospital for a year or longer, putting immense pressure on hospital beds. Other childhood illnesses could also mean long-term hospitalisation: chest infections and chronic osteomyelitis before the era of antibiotics, asthma before effective treatment became available in the 1960s, the after-effects of diphtheria, and congenital hip, limb and spinal abnormalities.[19] Accidents of many kinds – including road and horse accidents – and child abuse also hospitalised Queensland children.[20]

The Hospital for Sick Children struggled on as a voluntary hospital, but the writing was on the wall. Voluntary hospitals could not carry on relying only on subscriptions and meagre government grants. The *Hospitals Act 1923* created the Brisbane and South Coast Hospitals Board to manage public hospitals in Brisbane and as far south as Coolangatta on the New South Wales border. Existence as a government hospital did not eliminate either the chronic overcrowding at Queensland's only children's hospital or its struggle for adequate funding.

The Sisters of Mercy's Mater Misericordiae Adult Hospital at South Brisbane did not come under the government's umbrella. It was Queensland's only privately owned hospital treating patients free of charge. The Sisters of Mercy began in Dublin in 1824 – a time of political and economic distress in Ireland – as a group of laywomen devoted to service to the poor.[21] They soon added visits to the sick in their homes and in two Dublin hospitals to their work in education and in caring for orphans.

The founder, Catherine McAuley, was persuaded that the group living at her House of Mercy in Baggot Street had taken on the characteristics of a religious order. The Institute of the Sisters of Mercy was formally established in 1831. The practical service emphasis of the original group did not change and the Sisters of Mercy, like Mary Aikenhead's Sisters of Charity, continued as 'walking nuns', out in the world of poverty, illness and ignorance, rather than enclosed as a contemplative order devoted to prayer, then the more usual model of a religious order.[22] The Sisters' work in health care was recognised when the Dublin Board of Health appealed to them for help during a cholera epidemic in 1832. The Sisters' work slashed the death rate at the Townsend Street hospital in Dublin.

Seriously minded laywomen in Britain and Europe also worked with poor and disadvantaged communities. Throughout the nineteenth century, women of the growing middle class, often led by charismatic leaders like Catherine McAuley, reformed prisons, cared for 'fallen' women and single girls, promoted education and established hospitals. The women who established the Hospital for Sick Children, the Lady Bowen maternity hospital and other social service organisations in Brisbane belonged to this tradition.[23]

Catherine McAuley died in 1841. Sister Mary Vincent Whitty, who had worked closely with Catherine, was elected Superior in 1849 and stretched Mercy work to include a home for unmarried mothers and an industrial school. Yet she kept her eye firmly on the McAuley vision of providing health care to the poor. Health care at that time was better in Europe than in Britain or Ireland. European religious orders, particularly the Order of the Visitation of Holy Mary and the Daughters of Charity of St Vincent de Paul, had been working since the seventeenth century to establish hospitals and to improve health care for the poor. The Irish Sisters of Charity followed the French model when they established St Vincent's Hospital in Dublin in 1834.[24]

In Dublin, the Sisters of Mercy were managing the nursing at the Jervis Street Charitable Infirmary when a surprising opportunity came their way. In 1854, the British government, embarrassed by high death rates among wounded and sick soldiers during the Crimean War, asked for their help.[25] Nuns ran the French military hospitals, where death rates were lower. Mother Vincent sent Sisters to care for some 10,000 Irish soldiers fighting in the British army. This was the Sisters' chance to demonstrate that the Mercy mission to the sick extended to people of all religious faiths in all situations. Despite the Sisters' contribution, nineteenth-century bigotry against the Roman Catholic church ensured that Florence Nightingale, the English advocate of trained nursing, who had studied the nursing methods of religious orders, accrued most of the credit for improving the military hospitals.

Mother Vincent did not serve in the Crimea, but joined another Mercy venture abroad.[26] During the 1840s, visiting Bishops persuaded her to send Sisters overseas, even though continuing distress in Ireland during the 1840s famine stretched their resources. The church was struggling in new societies in North America and the southern hemisphere; hordes of refugees had fled starvation and poverty in Ireland. Among the first Sisters to come to Australia were Sister Ursula Frayne RSM, who arrived in Western Australia in 1845, and Mother Mary Xavier Maguire RSM, who started work in Melbourne in 1859.[27]

Although one of her greatest ambitions, the new Mater hospital in Dublin, was coming to reality, James Quinn, first Bishop of Brisbane, persuaded Mother Vincent to join his pioneering work in the small, struggling city of Brisbane.[28] On 10 May 1861, Mother Vincent, two Sisters, one novice and two postulants arrived in Brisbane aboard the coastal steamer *Wonga Wonga*, which they had boarded in Sydney after the long voyage from Ireland. They were only a few of the crowds of immigrants pouring into Brisbane, attracted by a government program of assisted immigration designed to boost population in the first decade of Queensland's existence as a separate, self-governing colony. Many immigrants existed in poor living conditions and the Sisters made their first sick calls within days of their arrival.

The first Sisters in Brisbane never lost sight of their aim to care for the sick. Within a month of their arrival, the Sisters visited patients in the Brisbane Hospital. Education was, however, a more urgent priority for the diocese.[29] By 1863, the Sisters' work had extended to the nearby town of Ipswich. They managed a flourishing school and were so well received on their visits to the local hospital that Mother Vincent held high hopes that the Ipswich hospital 'will be yet under nuns', but this was not to be.

In the first 40 years of their work in the Brisbane diocese, the Sisters opened St Vincent's Orphanage and created an ever-expanding network of parish schools and Queensland's first secondary school for girls, All Hallows' School in Ann Street, which grew up around Adderton, the Sisters' main convent.[30] The fees paid by parents for their daughters' education at All Hallows' helped to subsidise less affluent parish schools, a method the Sisters used later when, at last, their mission could be extended to health care.

When Mother Vincent died in 1892, more than 200 Sisters were working in Brisbane and regional Queensland managing 26 schools with 7,000 pupils, a training college for teachers, a secondary girls' school, an orphanage, an industrial school, and a Magdalen asylum for unmarried mothers. Nevertheless, a hospital was one of Mother Vincent's dreams. The purchase of just over four hectares of land at South Brisbane shortly after her death laid the basis for the achievement of this goal.

The land, adjacent to St Kilian's College, a Catholic secondary school that also educated trainee teachers and seminarians, was beautifully situated high on a hill overlooking South Brisbane and Woolloongabba, clearly visible from the city side of the Brisbane River. In 1893, the year the land at South Brisbane entered the Sisters' property portfolio, huge floods devastated Brisbane and were particularly ruinous in South Brisbane, further complicating social distress due to a serious economic depression. Mother Mary Patrick Potter RSM, Mother Vincent's successor, had to postpone the construction of a hospital, but it remained high on her agenda. Mother Patrick, whose business skills were demonstrated by the catalogue of achievements during her years of leadership between 1892 and 1927, had to balance the Sisters' health-care objectives against continuing pressures to open new schools.[31]

Standards of hospital care had been improving with significant developments in surgery. Professional nursing contributed greatly to improving the image of hospitals. The first group of nurses to be trained in Brisbane were awarded their certificates at the Brisbane Hospital in 1888. Nurses came to be accepted by the community as professional people of intellectual accomplishment, ethical standing and good character.[32] Many nurses took their knowledge and skill to smaller hospitals all over Queensland; others improved the standard of care for sick people in their own homes or worked in new private hospitals, such as St Helen's Hospital on the riverbank at South Brisbane, just upstream of the Victoria Bridge.[33]

Dr Ernest Sandford Jackson, the 'father' of trained nursing at Brisbane Hospital, became the owner of St Helen's Hospital in 1901. The economic situation improved in the early years of the twentieth century, despite drought in the years immediately following the federation of the Australian colonies in 1901. St Helen's Hospital had begun in a building converted from other uses. On 4 January 1906, the Brisbane Sisters of Mercy, helped by a £500 gift from a grazier, William Naughton, opened their first 20-bed Mater Private

Hospital at Aubigny, a house at North Quay on the northern bank of the Brisbane River.[34] Before long, leading doctors, including Queensland's first woman surgeon, Dr Lilian Cooper, referred patients to the new hospital.[35]

The Sisters had a grander plan: to use the slender profits from their private hospital to support a hospital where people without financial means could receive excellent care. The city's main newspaper, the *Brisbane Courier*, helped by describing the Mater Private Hospital as 'an important addition to the hospitals of the city', which would be a 'boon to those in need of medical or surgical treatment, and of good nursing'.[36] The Mater staff was led by the Superior, Sister Mary Felix McInerney RSM, and the matron, Sister Mary Antonia Brosnan RSM, who had trained at the Brisbane General Hospital.[37] There were also two lay trained nurses, Molly Malone and Norma McLeod, and three newly professed Sisters, Francis Mary Fitzgerald RSM, Mary Edmund Stritch RSM and Mary Assissium Dunne RSM, soon joined by Sister Mary Chanel England RSM, who became one of the Mater's best-known nursing Sisters.[38]

The hospital quickly became very popular and was soon too small. In 1908, fundraising began in earnest to build a new hospital at the highest point of the Sisters' land at South Brisbane. The Brisbane press supported the appeal for funds, as they did two decades later for the Mater Children's Hospital. The new Mater Private Hospital was opened on 14 August 1910, soon followed by the Mater Adult (Public) Hospital, where treatment was free of charge, which opened six months later on 2 February 1911. Both buildings demonstrated a very high quality in design and construction. Robin Dods, one of the most distinguished architects of the era, designed the hospitals following the 'open air' philosophy of the day. Both hospitals had verandahs to take best advantage of the site and passing breezes. The Sisters' aim to care for the sick and afflicted, whether or not they had the financial means to pay for their care, was realised.

Two hospitals needed a large nursing staff. In the early days at South Brisbane, Sisters of Mercy nurse trainees staffed both hospitals under the direction of trained Sisters. It was inevitable, however, that the rapid growth of the hospitals would outstrip the Sisters' capacity to supply nurses from their own ranks. The Sisters established their own training school in 1912 and, in 1914, admitted the first 14 lay probationers to the training school. Nurse trainees lived in St Mary's Nurses Home, opened close to the Mater Adult Hospital in 1914.

The period before the First World War was very busy on Mater Hill and generally turbulent in Queensland's public hospitals. The secular public hospitals were still voluntary, community-based organisations, funded by subscribers and supplemented – more in theory than reality – by fees paid by patients who could afford to do so. To make matters worse, the Queensland government refused to contribute to the cost of maintaining patients at the Mater Adult Hospital until the 1913–14 financial year. Even then, the subsidy per occupied bed went only part of the way towards meeting costs.

The pressure on space was intense. The Mater Adult Hospital was extended within a few years of its opening, demonstrating the need for hospitals south of the river. Innovations such as installing Queensland's first 'deep X-ray therapy' machine to treat cancer and Dr James Vincent Duhig's pathology department put immense pressure on the hospital's finances. Funding was precariously balanced between insufficient government subsidy for each patient in a public bed, any profit that might flow from the private hospital, and the sturdy fundraising regime maintained by friends and supporters. In 1920, Mother Patrick was delighted that the Mater Adult Hospital would receive some of the proceeds of the government's Golden Casket Art Union on the same basis as other public hospitals, but the Mater was the last in a long list of beneficiaries.

Even though money was a constant worry, the continuing growth of Brisbane's southern suburbs increased pressure on the Mater Adult Hospital. It was often accommodating 110 patients – including some children – in wards designed for 70. Another extension in 1920 increased the number of surgical beds and added an operating theatre suited to the particular needs of ear, nose and throat surgery and eye surgery.

A beautiful building constructed in the 1920s replaced a temporary chapel in the nearby Mater Private Hospital. A new convent attached to the western end of the private hospital near the chapel eliminated the need for the Sisters to live on the top floor of the private hospital, which was also under pressure with calls to accommodate ever-increasing numbers of patients.

The work accomplished in developing the Mater hospitals in the first 15 years at South Brisbane was spectacular, but Mother Patrick was not about to consider her work complete. Even before the chapel and convent were completed, plans were being laid to add a missing piece to the Mercy health-care mission: a children's hospital.

Chapter 2

Realising the Dream

Children ... are Queensland's greatest asset ... more precious than gold or silver mines and more to be treasured than wealth or pastoral lands, and as brilliant as the sun ...

Archbishop James Duhig, May 1926[1]

In May 1926, plans for the Mater Children's Hospital were well advanced. The Sisters had received a wonderful windfall, which moved the children's hospital from the realm of dreams to the real world. Their staunch friend George Wilkie Gray, who had helped them financially in earlier times, came to the rescue posthumously.[2] The Sisters were beneficiaries of Gray's life insurances, which were valued at £2,691/12/- when he died in 1924. Gray had also transferred a property, Shalimar at Sandgate, to the Sisters and left them city land, which sold for £1,000.[3] This legacy eased the debt remaining on the two earlier hospitals.

A large photograph appeared in the *Brisbane Courier*, showing the proposed hospital as an imposing building standing on a row of terraces with gracious stairways leading from Annerley Road. There were two wings to be constructed in brick – enlivened by specially designed face bricks – with twin gables on either side of a tower topped by a Celtic cross. Each wing was three storeys high. The accompanying article assured readers that:

> All modern conveniences will be included in the building and the internal finish will be carried out in the best accepted hygienic treatment, with tiled floors, and walls, and the equipment so essential in this type of building.[4]

This original plan allocated the entire ground floor to out-patients and 'casualties', with wards on the two upper floors.

An equally grand photograph recorded the ceremony when the foundation stone was laid by the Lieutenant-Governor, William Lennon, on 23 May 1926 and blessed by Archbishop Duhig.[5] The Archbishop reiterated Mother Patrick's theme that this was 'the beginning of a long cherished wish'.[6] His hope 'that it would not be long before stone began to rise upon stone and that they might see the last one laid' could not be realised until a great deal of money had been raised: the £2,420 already allocated to the hospital was only a drop in a very deep bucket. At least £30,000 was required.[7]

A well-organised fundraising campaign had dual aims: to raise money and to place the idea of the new hospital before the people of Brisbane. The Sisters' purpose in building a new, separate hospital was at the centre of the fundraising publicity:

> There is no class of sufferers that appeals to us more touchingly than sick or afflicted children … There was a time when a children's department in the Mater Hospital might have sufficed to aid the suffering little ones but the time has arrived when neither an odd bed nor ward will suffice. … The Sisters of Mercy have determined to give South Brisbane a Children's Hospital. They feel that what they have done for the grownup sick they can do for the child sufferers.[8]

The Sisters devised a pretty gift for donors to their appeal: a miniature brick displaying a picture of a child.

Art unions, street collections, balls, concerts arranged by All Hallows' past pupils and bridge parties were organised with almost military precision. Street collections, essential to the fundraising campaign, were highly visible reminders of the Sisters' great plan. The 1925 street collection attracted an important sponsor, Lillie Jolly, wife of Brisbane's Lord Mayor, who convened meetings to organise collections in Brisbane's central business district, South Brisbane and several suburbs.[9] No opportunity was overlooked to increase the fundraising potential and publicity value of the collections. In 1926, stalls selling a variety of goods were planned at the Town Hall, Lennon's Hotel in George Street, the corner of Queen and Edward streets and Fortitude Valley. Nothing was left to chance.[10] Nurses in uniform worked as collectors.[11]

Two art unions in 1926 were equally visible and highly successful. The prizes in the first, drawn on 23 September, were very generous. A six-cylinder Chrysler motor car valued at £495 was the first prize, followed by a gentleman's gold watch valued at £63 and bedroom furniture worth £52/10/-. There were a total of 20 prizes; the last was a gentleman's armchair, upholstered in leather, valued at £5/5/-.[12] All that for a one-shilling ticket!

The second art union brought to the fore an energetic fundraiser: Esther Theodore, wife of a former Queensland Premier and Treasurer, EG Theodore, who had attracted the ire of the Hospital for Sick Children when he was reluctant to increase the government's financial assistance.[13] The first prize was a racehorse, Wee Glen, transferred to Mrs Theodore by the Chief Justice, Sir James Blair, in June 1926. The grand drawing in November revealed that £3,005/12/- had been raised in this one art union.[14] Even before the 1926 Mater Ball, funds from all sources had developed remarkably to just over £6,000.[15]

The balls became notable fundraising events, always attracting newspaper attention. Such publicity was very important in keeping the children's hospital in the public mind. Publicity for the July 1927 Mater Ball in both the prestigious *Queenslander* weekly journal and the daily *Brisbane Courier* included photographs of many of the 22 debutantes.[16] A banner headline described the ball as a 'brilliant social success'. The ballroom presented a 'gay appearance with its festoons of coloured electric lights and rows of small pennants' with a pièce de résistance, an electrically illuminated Union Jack surmounting the alcove reserved for Sir John Goodwin, the Governor, and Lady Goodwin.[17] The ball was financially successful, as was a grand two-day fete in the grounds of All Hallows' in November 1927. Building could proceed.

The growing group of Mater buildings – the private hospital, the adult hospital, St Mary's Nurses Home, the convent, the beautiful chapel – exhibited the skills of leading architects of the day. Robin Dods, a partner in the firm established by Francis Richard Hall, had designed the first two hospitals. Thomas Ramsay Hall, FR Hall's stepbrother, and his partner, George Gray Prentice, designed the Mater Children's Hospital. Hall and Prentice, who practised together from 1913, became renowned for some of the most eminent buildings in Brisbane, including the Brisbane City Hall, Tattersall's Club and Shell House in Ann Street.[18] FJ Corbett was appointed to build the new hospital and selected high-quality materials from local sources.[19]

The design of the new hospital was distinguished, the need was great, but the timing was poignant. Mother Patrick, who had led the Sisters through years of great expansion in their work in education, health and social welfare, died on 13 November 1927. Work was beginning on the site, but her dream of a modern hospital for sick children was far from fulfilled.[20] It was not long before Mater annual reports – and the newspapers – began to refer to the hospital as a memorial to Mother Patrick.[21]

Events far from the control of the Sisters impeded the complete realisation of Mother Patrick's dream, and added considerably to the multitude of challenges that were part of daily life for her successor as Superior, an Irish-born teacher, Mother Alban Salmon RSM. The pleasant, relatively prosperous period that had followed the First World War and the devastating Spanish influenza pandemic in 1919 faltered in Queensland when a severe drought in 1926 seriously affected the pastoral industries. The situation became much worse in the late 1920s when the world was plunged into a deep, persistent economic depression. Queensland was not immune from the impact of economic trouble, but was spared the worst effects by its flourishing agricultural industries, particularly sugar; the other states, relying more on heavy industry, were badly affected when manufacturing collapsed.[22]

Even with this slight buffer, Queensland suffered. Unemployment rose, businesses failed, and even the most generous supporters of worthy causes, such as the Mater Children's Hospital, were forced to re-examine their capacity to give as generously as before. Fundraising efforts continued throughout the late 1920s much as usual, but receipts declined. The Sisters also had other calls on their funds. Government grants to the adult hospital were reduced, the needs of St Vincent's Orphanage increased and all the schools continued to grow.[23]

In 1928, work on the Mater Children's Hospital site was deferred. The Sisters visited children's hospitals in southern Australia to examine the latest ideas in paediatric treatment and hospital equipment. When work resumed, the Depression had deepened. There was also an important additional issue: the need for more accommodation for student nurses. The existing number of lay nurses could not possibly stretch to cover a new hospital. An extension to St Mary's Nurses Home in 1931 was also designed by Hall and Prentice. The *Brisbane Courier* was lavish in its praise:

> In this building every consideration has been given to the comfort
> of the nurses, and each nurse is provided with individual sleeping
> quarters. Beautifully tiled bathrooms and toilet conveniences,
> recreation rooms, spacious verandas, go to the comfort of the
> nurses, while assistance in their training is also catered for by
> the introduction of the lecture hall and study.[24]

The slowing economy made a difficult decision inevitable: the whole of the planned Mater Children's Hospital could not be built. The wing closest to the adult hospital was completed with the space on the opposite side disguised by a large tree, a painful reminder of a grander vision. Nevertheless, even the construction of this smaller hospital left the Sisters with a very large debt – at least £10,000.[25] There were, however, many practical helping hands. Volunteers in the Mater's Linen Club sewed for the hospital;[26] furniture in one ward was presented as a memorial to Frank McDonnell, founder of the retail firm McDonnell & East; 11 cots were donated as memorials; and the past pupils of All Hallows' donated operating theatre equipment.[27] A donation from Archbishop Duhig and the Queensland government's £500 grant helped to ease the debt.[28]

Disappointment that only one wing of the hospital could be completed was cast aside for the blessing of the hospital by Archbishop Duhig on 9 May 1931. A huge crowd, alerted by a prominent advertisement, watched the Governor, Sir John Goodwin, open the hospital on 10 May 1931, exactly 70 years after the Sisters of Mercy had arrived in Queensland, and in the centenary year of their foundation in Dublin.[29] The Governor's address was built on the theme that 'a bright childhood is the birthright of every child'. Sir John's interest in developments at the Mater – and in health in Queensland generally – was doubtless influenced by his own background as a doctor.[30] The Governor continued: 'It was one of the primary duties of every man and woman to try to ensure that the lives of children should as far as was possible be healthy and happy'.[31]

The newspapers were generous in their praise:

> The building has been planned on the most modern and up-to-date
> lines, and is equipped throughout with the very latest appliances
> necessary for the recovery and treatment of the young inmates.[32]

A large photograph showed a dignified building with the planned grand staircase to Annerley Road, although the concrete terraces featured in the 1926 plan seem to have been casualties of the battle against declining finances. One of the decorative external features had, however, been retained; the exterior of the building was constructed in brick with cement enrichments, presenting, as the *Brisbane Courier* continued, 'a magnificent facade to Annerley Road'.

Silky oak, a beautiful Queensland native timber that had been used extensively in the earlier buildings on Mater Hill, lined the entrance hall and staircase; there was an elevator, but this was to be used mainly for 'stretcher cases'. The ground floor was devoted mainly to out-patient treatment, with an operating theatre for minor operations at the rear adjacent to a 'commodious ward for the recovery of children after such "minor" operations as tonsils, adenoids, etc.'.[33] Doors to the resident doctor's office and the consulting and examining rooms were entered from a long corridor leading to the ear, nose and throat ward. A separate entry to the left of the main reception area was provided for ambulances bringing 'casualties' to the hospital. On this level, the floors were polished terrazzo blending harmoniously with the tiled walls, which were in a 'pleasing colour scheme of light blue and mastic'.[34]

The two higher floors were devoted to medical and surgical wards. Two medical wards and a babies' ward occupied the top floor. The surgical wards were on the floor below, which also accommodated the main operating theatre and the kitchen. A large, many-ovened stove stood in the centre of the kitchen, which was also equipped with three steam boilers for 'broth, vegetables and porridge etc.'. A large steamer stood at one end and there was room for invalid cookery classes at the other.[35] Then, as now, education of parents in the appropriate care of children was a priority in children's hospitals.

The walls of the surgical wards were 'tastefully decorated in grey and dark blue' with 'a delightfully stencilled menagerie along the frieze on which Brer Rabbit, Reynard the Fox, Eeyore the Donkey, Tigger and even the Pushmepullyou may be espied by the careful observer'. Bathrooms and lavatories were installed at either end of the wards, each with its own 'sterilising chamber'.[36] The newspapers also mentioned a planned 'isolation ward', likely to have been made more urgent by the severe 1931 poliomyelitis epidemic.[37]

Ventilation was obviously a central requirement in the brief to the architects: 'The wards opened to verandahs on both sides through French doors. One feature speaks of the days before awareness that the Queensland sun could be very damaging: 'On the top floor a flat roof has been planned for the main operating theatre, which will be used for patients requiring sun treatment.'[38]

The first matron, a Queensland-born Sister, Mary Marcelline Kehoe RSM, was entrusted with the vital task of leading the new hospital.

> MARGARET ELLEN KEHOE was born on 29 December 1885 at Charlton, near Toowoomba, the fourth of 12 children of Irish-born parents. Margaret Kehoe was educated at the local state primary school and finished her formal schooling at the end of Year 6. After working in the family business, as a dressmaker in Toowoomba and in the dressmaking department of the Warwick firm GP Barnes, Margaret Kehoe decided to join the Sisters of Mercy in March 1911 when she was 25, and was received into the novitiate in January 1912, taking the religious name of Sister Mary Marcelline. After a few days' holiday at Sandgate, she was sent to the Mater to begin 53 years in nursing. At various times, Sister Mary Marcelline was appointed matron of all three hospitals: the Mater Adult, the Mater Private and the Mater Children's. A Mater surgeon remembered that, at the Mater Private Hospital, 'She looked frail but could climb the stairs and outwalk, with her great strides, any of her colleagues' and that she was always very dignified, increasing hospital discipline by her courteous, professional example.[39] Sister Mary Marcelline died on 26 October 1970, aged 84.

The staff structure at the new children's hospital was similar to arrangements at the Mater Adult Hospital. Sisters of Mercy were in charge of the wards, which were staffed by student nurses. The early Sisters at the Mater Children's Hospital included Sister Mary Audrey (Hannah Agnes) Lucy RSM, in charge of the Casualty Room, Sister Mary St Aidan (Mary Ellen) Mara RSM in the nursery and medical ward, Sister Mary Asicus (Margaret Mary) Lynch RSM and Sister Mary Edwin (Jane) Alexander RSM in the general wards, Sister Mary St Pierre (Mary Irene) McCormack RSM in the operating theatres, Sister Mary Dympna (Mary Ellen) Hoare RSM in the surgical ward and Sister Mary Venard (Margaret) Gorman RSM in charge of night duty, and who also relieved other Sisters when necessary.

These were distinguished nurses. Two – Sister Mary St Aidan and Sister Mary St Pierre – became matrons of the Mater Children's Hospital; Sister Mary Audrey Lucy RSM had owned a private hospital before entering the Sisters of Mercy and, after years at the children's hospital, became the first matron of the Mater Mothers' Hospital. Sister Mary Asicus Lynch RSM spent 25 years at the Mater Private Hospital, Sister Mary Dympna Hoare RSM was also well known as a ward sister at the Mater Private Hospital, and Sister Mary Venard Gorman RSM was an early lay trainee at the Mater before entering the Sisters of Mercy.[40]

Several of the early Sisters at the Mater Children's Hospital had additional qualifications. Both Sister Mary Audrey and Sister Mary St Aidan, for instance, had completed the Maternal and Child Welfare course and both had previously trained in midwifery.[41] However, none of the early Sisters had previous experience in paediatrics. There were hazards in becoming acquainted with paediatric care. Many nurses contracted infections from small patients, always generous with their germs. Nothing deflected the staff from the Sisters' directive: never refuse admission to any child who needed treatment.

Even though Sister Mary Marcelline had spent months stocking the hospital before it opened, some pieces of equipment were missing when the first patients arrived. An impatient resident medical officer had to make a plaster slab before a child's back splint could be obtained.[42] The operating theatre presented several challenges. Sisters used to working in the theatres at the Mater Private Hospital were accustomed to surgeons bringing their own instruments. The Mater Children's Hospital, however, was a public hospital with its own instruments and the staff had to know what to put out for each surgeon and each operation. On top of this anxiety, the hospital's administration queried the costs of running the theatres, not realising that tiny instruments, catheters, nasal tubes and needles cost more than the adult-sized instruments.[43] A great deal depended on the skill and experience of the senior honorary medical officers, assisted by first-year resident medical officers; there were no senior resident medical officers for some years.

Dr Harry 'Daddy' Windsor, the Sisters' friend and adviser, was appointed to take charge of surgery. Dr Percy Alan Earnshaw was appointed senior honorary physician.

PERCY ALAN EARNSHAW, CBE, MB, ChM, FRACP, known to his colleagues as 'PA', was born in Brisbane in 1894 and, in the era before the University of Queensland Medical School opened, studied in medicine at the University of Sydney and graduated in 1916. He was a regimental medical officer in the First World War and suffered from shrapnel wounds and the effects of poison gas. After the war, he studied at the Hospital for Sick Children at Great Ormond Street under such luminaries in paediatrics as Sir Frederic Still. PA Earnshaw returned to Brisbane in 1923 and became the first doctor in private practice to work exclusively with children. He was an out-patient physician at Brisbane's first children's hospital in the 1920s and worked with AJ Turner in the early maternal and child welfare service. PA Earnshaw was appointed honorary physician to the Mater Children's Hospital when it opened in 1931 and remained for almost 30 years. During the Second World War, he was responsible for all in-patient care. Dr Earnshaw became the first president of the Paediatric Society of Queensland in 1949 and worked for the establishment of the Australian College of Paediatrics. He was chairman of the medical committee of the Royal Flying Doctor Service, a member of the Mater's Medical Advisory Board 1946–59, and a member of the Board of the Faculty of Medicine at the University of Queensland. His influence on generations of young doctors was profound. Dr Earnshaw died on 13 January 1980.[44]

Although the era of specialist paediatrics was dawning, many of the doctors in children's hospitals in the 1930s also treated adults. For some years, the Mater Children's Hospital shared honorary medical officers in fields such as surgery, urology and radiology with the adult hospital. The first resident medical officers were also shared between the two hospitals. Dr Tom Carroll, a graduate of the University of Melbourne, was one of the residents and, after the Second World War, became the first orthopaedic registrar. Orthopaedics was developed at the children's hospital under the 'father' of Queensland orthopaedics, Arthur Vincent Meehan.

AV Meehan found an able professional colleague in John Rudolph Sergius Lahz, who consulted Meehan for treatment for chronic osteomyelitis.

ARTHUR VINCENT MEEHAN, MB, FRCS, FRACS, was born in Sydney in 1890 and graduated in medicine at the University of Sydney in 1914. After serving as a resident medical officer at Sydney Hospital, he joined the Australian Army Medical Corps for service in the First World War. He treated casualties on the Western Front and was wounded at Passchendaele in October 1917, an injury that led to the amputation of his right foot. Meehan was posted to the staff of the 2nd Australian Auxiliary Hospital, Southall, England, in March 1918 and then studied orthopaedics under Sir Robert Jones at the Royal Southern Hospital, Liverpool. In 1919, he became a Fellow of the Royal College of Surgeons, Edinburgh. After returning to Australia, Meehan – usually known as 'Paddy' – moved permanently to Brisbane in 1920 and entered private practice in Wickham Terrace. Almost immediately, he established an orthopaedic unit at Brisbane's general hospital, which he supervised until 1931, when he established orthopaedics at the Mater Children's Hospital and, in 1938, at the Mater Adult Hospital. Meehan was a guiding light in the establishment of both the Montrose Home at Corinda, and the Xavier Home at Coorparoo for children with physical disabilities. Meehan was the first doctor in Queensland to devote himself solely to orthopaedics and was instrumental in the University of Queensland accepting the Mater public hospitals as training schools for medical students. His enthusiasm and skill attracted many disciples. A mentally disturbed former patient shot and killed him on 1 December 1955 in his rooms in Wickham Terrace.[45]

JOHN RUDOLPH SERGIUS LAHZ, MB, ChM, FRCS, was born at Calcifer near Chillagoe in Far North Queensland in 1900 and educated at Nudgee College. A badly set left femur, after a car accident when he was 14, left Lahz with chronic osteomyelitis. Despite this condition, which required frequent surgery, he managed to play rugby union. He graduated with honours in medicine at the University of Sydney in 1924 and entered general practice, first at Goomeri in the Burnett district and then at South

continued overleaf

> Brisbane, where he met AV Meehan. Lahz became Meehan's assistant at the Mater Children's Hospital when the orthopaedic department was established. He became a Fellow of the Royal College of Surgeons, Edinburgh, in 1936 and, from 1941, after experience in a wartime casualty clearing station, devoted himself exclusively to orthopaedics. He became the senior honorary orthopaedic surgeon at the Mater hospitals in 1953 after Meehan moved to an honorary consultancy. Dr Lahz was well read in several languages and a connoisseur of art, food and wine. His health did not recover fully after a heart attack following a narrow escape in the 1955 shooting incident when 'Paddy' Meehan was fatally wounded. John Lahz died in 1959.[46]

Meehan and Lahz established a strong foundation for one of the most enduring strengths of the Mater Children's Hospital: orthopaedic surgery.

Specialisation in medicine was developing in this era. Several Mater doctors were studying overseas, among them AW St Ledger, an honorary assistant physician at the Mater Children's Hospital. A wide variety of illness affected their patients in the 1930s. The hospital was filled beyond its official capacity in the first year. Patients came from all over southern Queensland. The highest number in the wards on any one day reached 77 and, in 1931, there were 1,153 casualties and 7,375 out-patient appointments.[47]

Tonsillitis was responsible for by far the highest number of hospital admissions in the 1931–32 year. The ear, nose and throat surgeons, Dr Arthur Murphy and his assistant, Dr Athol Quayle, shouldered a heavy load. The total of 1,445 operations included 544 tonsils and adenoids, 15 eye operations, and 69 operations on the alimentary system.[48] Some of the old enemies of child life appeared to be waning. There were only five children admitted with diphtheria and one with typhoid fever. Despite publicity of deaths due to a contaminated batch of diphtheria serum, immunisation appeared to be winning the battle. Immunisation against typhoid began in 1920, but did not eliminate all forms of gastrointestinal illness: there were 40 cases of diarrhoea in the first year. There was, however, only one case of lead poisoning. Diseases of the 'nervous system and organs of sense' appear to have been rife with 69 admissions; 15 of these were for eye disease and

20 for ear complaints. Pneumonia affected 49 children; that there were only four deaths in these pre-antibiotic days says a great deal for the importance of skilled nursing. Kidney disease was common, with 47 patients recorded.[49] One doctor was convinced that the emphasis on lead poisoning as a factor in kidney disease had obscured the probability that the serious after-effects of scarlet fever were also responsible.[50]

Poliomyelitis headed the list of patients with infectious diseases. A statewide epidemic in the summer of 1931–32 crowded the hospitals, closed the schools and brought Sister Elizabeth Kenny's unorthodox treatment to public notice. A serum developed by Dr JV Duhig, honorary pathologist at the Mater, from people who had recovered from polio, was trialled as a treatment.[51] Despite the best efforts of public health officials to limit the epidemic and the work of doctors in treating its victims, this epidemic exacted a high toll: a 14 per cent mortality rate and hundreds of children in hospital.

Drs Meehan and Lahz also treated 30 cases of osteomyelitis in the first year. Treatment of osteomyelitis in this era was slow and unpleasant. Surgeons generally used the Winnett Orr method, cleaning out the affected bone and packing it with vaseline gauze. The dressings stayed on for weeks, always becoming malodorous and often maggoty, and were removed under general anaesthetic. This procedure was, however, the most effective before antibiotics became available.[52]

The orthopaedic surgeons also treated 28 instances of congenital malformations of limbs and joints, in addition to supervising the treatment of the patients with poliomyelitis and the after-effects of accidents. A total of 109 children were treated following accidents ranging from falls and poisonings to burns and car accidents. The work was hard and unrelenting, but there were gentler moments for weary surgeons and exhausted physicians: delicious morning and afternoon teas, often featuring small tarts with cream and jelly.[53]

Orthopaedic patients who needed to stay in hospital for months, even years, were at risk of falling far behind their contemporaries at school. Although the Sisters always hoped that 'many of these will be restored to their families as useful members of the community', they also ensured that schoolwork continued for the patients who were well enough.[54] This was not the beginning of a formal hospital school – that had to wait for years – but it filled a gap while the children were hospitalised.

Paddy Meehan and John Lahz were two of the influential doctors who founded the Queensland Society for Crippled Children, which, with the support of the Rotary Club of Brisbane and a generous benefactor, George Marchant, established Montrose Home. Children with physical disabilities needed sufficient education to enable them to join the workforce. In the early 1930s, polio epidemics coincided with the Great Depression, with worryingly high unemployment rates. The doctors were well aware that children with disabilities needed to be educated as much, if not more, than children with no such disadvantages.[55]

Accidents also added to the load for the general surgeons, Dr Harry Windsor and his assistant, Dr Alban Lynch. The first two patients in the gleaming new theatres on the second floor were Thelma Brandt and Sydney Rodgers, who needed appendectomies. Apparently, Sydney had swallowed a pin, which had lodged in his appendix.[56] The trials of modern life also intruded. Although the early Sisters did not remember many instances of child abuse, they were always aware that, when family break-ups occurred, it was necessary to take care that children went home only with their official custodial parents.[57]

The philosophy guiding practice in most children's hospitals in the Western world could be very hard on worried families. Visitors were allowed at the Mater Children's Hospital only once each week, between 3.00pm and 4.30pm on Sundays. This rigidity, applying in most children's hospitals, arose from the belief that frequent contact with parents and siblings would be unduly distressing for children, especially those who had to remain in hospital for long periods. Sister Marie (Mary Rosaire) Fitzgerald RSM and Sister Germaine Greathead RSM experienced this regime as children when their brothers were patients in the 1930s.[58]

The doctors' work in the wards and the increasingly busy out-patient department proceeded against a background of dissension at the Mater and confusion in the government hospitals.[59] Mother Alban believed that the existing system whereby the medical board made appointments to the medical staff, subject only to the Sisters' veto, was unsatisfactory. She decided that the medical board should submit recommendations to the Sisters, who would make the appointments. Even though the Sisters maintained that the possibility of rejecting the doctors' recommendations was 'very remote', the doctors were concerned that the new system might mean that the best available people might not be appointed.[60] The doctors were aware that doctors at Brisbane Hospital and the Hospital for Sick Children resented the provision of the *Hospitals Act 1923*, which effectively turned state hospitals into a section of a government department.[61] There were no doctors on the board administering Brisbane's state hospitals.

These were sensitive times. Mater doctors also knew that doctors at the state hospitals in Brisbane were opposed to the government's proposal to appoint a full-time medical staff, rather than rely on part-time specialists. The government had increased control over visiting medical officers by abolishing the 'honorary' system; instead, visiting doctors were paid a fee for each attendance at the hospital. The Mater, however, retained its honorary system.

The situation at the Mater was eased by Mother Alban's promise that there would be staff representatives on her advisory board.[62] This board would advise the Sisters on medical matters. The Sisters would nominate three members and the remaining three were to be elected by the honorary staff, two from the Mater Adult Hospital and one from the Mater Children's Hospital. The board's function would be to consider applications for appointments to the honorary staff and to make recommendations to the Sisters, much as the original medical board had done.[63]

The Sisters regarded the two hospitals as one organisation that should be guided by one advisory board. In 1937, they proposed to add one more representative to the administration – a layman – who would chair the board, which would discuss professional matters common to the adult and children's hospitals and recommend appointments; the Sisters retained the right of final selection.[64] Nevertheless, the doctors feared that a lay chairman would not be acquainted with medical priorities and unable to act in the best interests of the hospitals. Mater Adult Hospital doctors also remained steadfast in their advocacy for separate advisory boards for the two hospitals.

The Sisters were determined that there would be only one advisory board.[65] The doctors were equally determined that each hospital would have its own committee.[66] Mother Alban made the Sisters' views very clear:

> The Honorary Staff must not assume that they alone should be the judges as to what is in the best interests of the hospital … Because the Administration's responsibilities are very great, it must participate in all decisions and appointments.[67]

Mother Alban asked the honoraries if they would continue under the joint board and set a deadline for their response: 14 March 1938. Many doctors resigned.[68] Much to everyone's discomfort, the issue reached the daily press and rumbled throughout 1938.[69] Mother Alban pressed ahead and the young solicitor JP Kelly was appointed to chair the advisory board, an appointment he retained for 42 years.

Drs PA Earnshaw and R Malcolm represented the Mater Children's Hospital on the new board, which proceeded to consider applications for a raft of vacant honorary positions. Drs Meehan and Lahz were appointed to open the orthopaedic section at the Mater Adult Hospital, while retaining their responsibilities at the children's hospital. Dr Harry Windsor was appointed as a consultant to the Mater Children's Hospital to take responsibility for surgery. The doctors elected their own conjoint board to make recommendations to the advisory board. Its first chairman was AV Meehan, who was succeeded in 1944 by PA Earnshaw.[70]

Another innovation perturbed the honorary medical officers. The issue was generated in 1935 by the Queensland government's introduction of intermediate beds in public hospitals. 'Intermediate' patients paid a fee – at a lower rate than at private hospitals – for their treatment and, in return, were entitled to the doctor of their choice. Mother Alban wanted to introduce a public service contribution scheme – an early form of health insurance – to assist intermediate patients to defray the costs of hospital care. The doctors were gravely concerned that members of the contribution scheme might expect preferential treatment. This was anathema: the doctors believed that priorities for treatment should be assigned on the basis of medical need alone.[71]

The doctors suggested an alternative: that the Mater Adult and Children's hospitals should adopt a New South Wales scheme, which would require the appointment of a hospital almoner, as social workers were then known, to collect the fees.[72] Mother Alban agreed, and suggested that intermediate fees be kept 'to a low scale', which would elevate many public hospital patients to the status of intermediate patients without interfering unduly with the fees charged at the Mater Private Hospital.[73]

Organisational issues were not the only challenges of the 1930s. Money was always tight. In 1933, when the Depression was still severe, the Mater Children's Hospital was at a considerable disadvantage. Most of the government grant in the previous year had been consumed at the Mater Adult

Hospital, a matter of some concern as the adult hospital also received a grant for general purposes as well as a £10 maintenance payment for each occupied bed. The children's hospital received only a maintenance grant for occupied beds. This seemed unreasonable as the Mater Children's Hospital carried a heavy patient load, including many long-term polio patients. Publicity of this inequity moved the Minister for Health and Home Affairs, Ned Hanlon, to grant £400 from the Golden Casket fund to the Mater Children's Hospital, in addition to the allocation for occupied beds.[74]

Fundraising was as important as ever. Volunteers continued to run Mater balls, organise street collections, concerts and fetes to raise money.[75] There were also many donations of cots and cash from businesses and sporting organisations. Even after long days in the Mater Children's Hospital wards, the Sisters manufactured contributions to street stalls: 'we made sweets, cakes, fancy goods and pottery and worked well into the night'.[76] Needlework auxiliaries made uniforms, replenished hospital stocks and also presented machines to the Mater Children's Hospital sewing room.

Publicity on the radio and in the *Courier-Mail* helped to ensure that the public did not forget the Mater Children's Hospital. In 1936, the Silver Jubilee year of the Mater Adult Hospital, the Prime Minister, Joe Lyons, visited the Mater. He inspected the cancer clinic at the adult hospital and 'spent even longer in the wards of the children's section, where he chatted with the majority of the little inmates, questioning the house surgeons about their ailments and their progress'.[77] The Prime Minister was photographed with a child recovering from a craniotomy, adventurous surgery in the days before antibiotics.

The Depression, the overcrowding and a very lean financial situation did not detract in any way from the joy of Christmas. In 1932 – the first of many annual Christmas parties – gifts from listeners to the local radio station 4BH enlivened the wards. This was a Catholic hospital with spiritual values at its core. A small chapel was opened January 1933, furnished largely by the gifts of generous people.[78] Calls for the hospital's services were constant, growing and changing. In 1938, it was time for the first matron, Sister Mary Marcelline, to move to fresh challenges as matron of the Mater Adult Hospital.

Chapter 3

Broader Horizons

The children all feel very much better now.
Lola, Mater Children's Hospital patient, the *Courier-Mail*, 1941

In 1938, Sister Mary St Aidan Mara RSM succeeded Sister Mary Marcelline Kehoe RSM as matron of the Mater Children's Hospital.

> SISTER MARY ST AIDAN, like Sister Mary Marcelline, was born on the Darling Downs. After attending the Pratten State School and St Mary's in Warwick, Mary Ellen Mara completed her midwifery qualifications, entered the Sisters of Mercy in 1924, taking the religious name of Sister Mary St Aidan, and joined the staff at the Mater in 1925. She became a greatly admired nurse. PA Earnshaw was 'deeply impressed' by her sympathy with the patients and their parents: 'Many children and their mothers owe Sister Mary St Aidan a great debt – greater than they realise'.[1] Sister Mary St Aidan had a lighter side to her character. It was later said that, if she had not had a religious vocation, Sister Mary St Aidan would have been very successful on the stage. She was a born mimic and several times phoned various Sisters pretending to be their Superior. She entranced the audience as the leading lady in 'Mary Jane O'Hagan – Nurse' in the first Mater concert. Sister Mary St Aidan died on 4 January 1972.[2]

Sister Mary St Aidan's years at the helm were made even more challenging by the Second World War, which affected Australia – and Queensland in particular – far more directly than the First World War. The people of the city felt the Japanese threat acutely. Precautions to protect the civilian population from possible bombing included the construction of air raid shelters around the city, digging slit trenches in school grounds and at work places, and sandbagging buildings, including hospitals. At the Mater, several nurses were trained in air-raid patrol work. The windows at the Mater Children's Hospital were blacked out and the walls were sandbagged.[3] The main wharves of the Port of Brisbane at South Brisbane, a likely target in any air raid, were very close to the Mater.

War worries notwithstanding, important milestones in children's lives were not overlooked. Lola, a patient in the Mater Children's Hospital, wrote a charming Christmas 'thank you' letter to the *Courier-Mail* in 1941:

> All the children in the hospital enjoyed the toys we got and we send you our greatest gratitude. We wish you and all your friends a very happy New Year, and hope that you will be happy all the years of your life. The children all feel very much better now.[4]

Many Mater nurses and doctors joined the armed services, and the hospitals were very short of staff – and extremely busy – throughout the war. In 1942–43, 1,560 children were treated in the 90 beds crammed into the Mater Children's Hospital wards and, in 1943–44, the patient load increased to 1,687 patients treated for a total of 23,031 bed days.[5] PA Earnshaw and Harry Windsor shouldered very heavy loads and resident medical officers had very hectic terms.[6] Well-known Sisters of Mercy on the Mater Children's Hospital staff included Sister Mary Domitilla Kelly, who remained from the earliest days, Sister Mary Mechtilde Slattery, the renowned 'Auntie Moll', who arrived to take charge of the medical wards in 1941, and Sister Mary Lea Kelly, who took charge of the babies' ward in 1942.[7]

In 1944, Sister Mary St Pierre McCormack RSM was appointed matron.

MARY IRENE MCCORMACK was born in Western Australia in 1906, fourth in a family of nine children. The family moved to Queensland and she became a student nurse at the Mater in 1924 and entered the Sisters of Mercy. As Sister Mary St Pierre, she joined the Mater staff in 1929 and worked at the Mater Adult Hospital for two years before beginning many

continued overleaf

> years in the theatres at the Mater Children's Hospital. At exceptionally busy times, she also helped out in casualty. Sister Mary St Pierre remained as matron of the Mater Children's Hospital until she retired from nursing in 1972. She was then the only remaining Sister of Mercy from the group that opened the hospital in 1931. She had played key roles in establishing a formal ladies auxiliary committee to support the hospital, and knitted or crocheted numerous rugs and ponchos for raffles.[8] Sister Mary St Pierre died on 29 March 1977.[9] Her successor at the Mater Children's Hospital, Sister Mary Dorothea Sheehan RSM, remembered Sister Mary St Pierre as having 'a calmness and serenity which appeared to invade a room when she entered, bringing peace with her presence'.

Even though staff shortages remained, the hospital was abuzz with plans for the future. The advisory board was reconvened in 1944 after a three-year break. This hiatus, the chairman, JP Kelly, ruefully remarked, was necessary because so many doctors were absent on war service. The honorary medical staff had many ideas to improve paediatric care. A special clinic to treat juvenile diabetes was one of the first matters discussed by the advisory board.[10] There were compelling reasons for a diabetes clinic. Children whose diabetes was well managed needed fewer hospital admissions, reducing the pressure on both beds and the hospital's finances. The clinic would be an effective means of educating both parents and children in the correct management of the condition, a matter that greatly worried PA Earnshaw, who saw children with diabetes return repeatedly to the hospital, sometimes in a coma.[11] Children who returned home after long periods as in-patients relapsed unless the good work in balancing diet and insulin to the child's needs was maintained.

A diabetes clinic was possible, but the board rejected the suggestion that the Mater appoint a general medical superintendent who could assist the honoraries at particularly busy times. Mater finances could not stretch to cover a medical superintendent's salary and JP Kelly was aware that an old sensitivity might resurface: the appointment of a medical superintendent might leave the Sisters feeling that their role was reduced from managing the hospital to merely paying the bills.[12] In any case, the employment of doctors was subject to the approval of the Commonwealth government's Commission for Manpower, created in 1942 to direct the workforce to essential industries. Even the suggestion that a second resident medical officer be appointed to assist with anaesthetics had to be approved by the Commission; a Manpower directive moved a Mater orthopaedic registrar, Dr Michael Gallagher, to become temporary superintendent at Cairns Base Hospital.[13]

JP Kelly was preoccupied with the difficulties in attracting sufficient government financial and moral support. Hospital financing changed forever in Australia in 1945, when the Commonwealth government legislated to introduce its Hospital Benefits Scheme, which would pay a sufficiently high subsidy to introduce public hospital care free of charge. Until this scheme began in January 1946, public hospital patients in all states, including Queensland, were expected to contribute towards the cost of their treatment to the extent of their 'means', an expectation honoured far more in the breach than in the observance.[14]

In Kelly's opinion, the proposed Commonwealth subsidy – six shillings per day – represented no more than the loss per bed in government hospitals, already supported handsomely by the government, an advantage not available to the Mater even though privately owned public hospitals in the other states received substantial government grants.[15] To add insult to injury, the Queensland government tried to leave the Mater hospitals out of the new arrangement, a sleight of hand that distressed the Sisters and infuriated Kelly. He telegraphed the Prime Minister and took his case to the *Courier-Mail*.[16] The Commonwealth immediately ensured that the Mater was included.

The staffing situation gradually improved when peace was declared. The original core of the Mater Children's Hospital medical staff – PA Earnshaw, Harry Windsor, Alban Lynch, AV Meehan and John Lahz – remained and was joined by some new staff members. They included Dr PB English in ophthalmology and Dr BLW Clarke in radiology, both of whom also held appointments at the Mater Adult Hospital. Some of the doctors appointed in the immediate post-war era became long-standing members of the medical staff.

The number of new staff members with specialist qualifications also increased. Dr Dermot Clark Ryan, always known as Steve, studied paediatrics in England and Amsterdam and opened his paediatric practice in Coorparoo. He was encouraged to become a surgeon, but remained a physician, developing a particular interest in children with disabilities. In the 1950s, he began many years' involvement with the Xavier Home.[17] Dr Michael Gallagher completed his post-graduate qualifications in 1948.[18] Dr Anthony McSweeny completed his master's degree in orthopaedic surgery in 1949 and, in 1950, Dr David Jackson and Dr Neville Anderson gained their post-graduate diplomas in child health. Tony McSweeny and Michael Gallagher were appointed as assistants in orthopaedics and David Jackson as assistant physician.[19]

DAVID CLEMENTS JACKSON, MBBS, DCH, FRACP, FRACGP, was born at Kangaroo Point on 7 September 1912. He was educated at the Kangaroo Point State School and the Church of England Grammar School ('Churchie').[20] David Jackson graduated in medicine at the University of Melbourne in 1937 and began his life-long association with the Mater Children's Hospital. He left for England in 1939 and worked at Birmingham Children's Hospital until he began active duty in 1941 as Surgeon Lieutenant in the Royal Naval Volunteer Reserve on the destroyer HMS *Worcester*. On 12 February 1942, *Worcester* was badly damaged in battle and Jackson was knocked unconscious by an exploding shell.[21] Upon recovering, working in appalling conditions, he treated the wounded, many with multiple shrapnel wounds, some requiring amputation. Jackson was awarded the Distinguished Service Cross. While serving ashore, he found time to complete a Diploma of Child Health through the Royal College of Physicians. David Jackson returned to Australia in 1946 and devoted his life to paediatrics for the next 45 years. In Brisbane in 1949, he chaired the first meeting that resolved to establish a professional association of paediatricians. David Jackson was made a Member of the Order of Australia in 1984 for his service to medicine, particularly to people with disabilities; he had a particular interest in children with cerebral palsy. He was a prolific writer with a fascination for history. After he retired from full-time practice, David Jackson continued to cut a distinctive figure in his light-coloured suits, with his monocle always in place.[22]

David Jackson spent his early years at the Mater Children's Hospital in out-patients and, before long, suggested several improvements. He believed that the out-patient section was the hospital's front line in contact with the community and, therefore, very important to the hospital's reputation. Jackson suggested two levels of care, the first by general practitioners and the second by specialist consultants. He thought the flow of patients would be improved if a resident medical officer, or a clinical assistant, screened patients as they arrived and directed them either to a specialist or to a general practitioner. Resident medical officers should also deal with simple matters, such as issuing repeat prescriptions, but only consultants should order special examinations and X-rays. He thought that clinical assistants and resident medical officers – and, where possible, out-patient nurses – should attend the specialist consultations, which were very important arenas for medical teaching and essential in attracting promising young doctors.[23] Jackson also recommended improved education for general practitioners, so that they would refer patients to the specialist out-patient clinics; many general practitioners seemed unaware that specialist advice could be obtained this way.[24]

Jackson's ideas were courteously received. Screening patients had merit and his suggestion of improved advertising of out-patient services was welcomed.[25] John Lahz cautioned against instituting different levels of consultations in out-patients as a junior doctor might miss something and 'the consultant has to exercise the greatest care … not to injure himself or the hospital'.[26]

David Jackson prepared another report on desirable levels of service at the Mater Children's Hospital, suggesting that three senior resident medical officers, three registrars and nine junior resident medical officers would be required so that each doctor in training could spend four months working with a senior specialist.[27] This level of staffing was, however, in the realm of pipe dreams. The Sisters did, however, agree that appointing an almoner would improve liaison with patients in their own homes.[28]

The cause of improving Queensland's medical services had a powerful ally in Archbishop Duhig, who, at the opening of the Mater Children's Hospital in 1931, pleaded for government action to establish a medical school in Queensland.[29] The Sisters were equally enthusiastic and, even during the arguments with the honorary medical officers over the composition of the advisory board, said that they would be willing to modify the board's membership if the university requested a seat for one of its staff.[30]

The University of Queensland Medical School took its first students in 1936 and graduated its first doctors in 1941, including Tony McSweeny, appointed to the Mater Children's Hospital in 1946. During the war, honoraries at the children's hospital had emphasised the need to promote the Mater hospitals as teaching hospitals for the new medical school.[31] The Mater became a training school and the first students were seen in the wards in February 1950.[32]

Life in the wards was hectic. Almost as soon as the war was over, some of the old troubles of childhood filled the wards. Gastroenteritis was a persistent enemy. The 1946–47 epidemic was particularly severe; 65 adults and children died in 14 months. Many children were admitted to the Mater. Parents were urged to protect food from flies, and to avoid buying food that had been handled by previous customers in shops.[33] In 1951, an outbreak in the hot month of December, which brought 12 patients to the Mater Children's Hospital in one week, was blamed on milk that had been kept too long and had become contaminated. Ice chests, the Health Department warned, did not keep milk sufficiently cool; refrigeration was necessary.[34]

Poliomyelitis was never far away. In the 1945–46 summer, 400 cases were reported in Queensland and struck teenagers and young adults particularly severely. 'Iron lungs', as electrically driven tank respirators were known, had been installed at both Brisbane children's hospitals in the late 1930s with the support of the Nuffield Foundation. These machines were needed to care for children whose chest muscles were paralysed. Queensland was spared the worst of a very serious outbreak that affected Victoria and New South Wales in 1949, but the disease returned to Queensland with a vengeance in the 1950s.

The epidemic, which began in October 1950 and persisted through the winter of 1951, was the worst in Queensland's history. Compulsory notification recorded almost 1,200 people with the disease; Brisbane recorded its highest number of victims in the cooler months of 1951. The papers publicised the precautions that could be taken against infection and also recorded the stories of some of the children who came to the Mater Children's Hospital. Fay Thacker from Maryborough was admitted in February 1951 and it seemed that her prospects for recovery were poor. However, by early January 1952, Faye was able to walk with the support of calipers on her legs.[35] Mary Case was affected more severely. At the time her story appeared in the *Courier-Mail* in 1954, she was unable to walk and was hoping for books as gifts at Christmas, her second in hospital.[36]

Mercy flights bringing very ill children to the Mater Children's Hospital were newsworthy events in the 1950s. In 1950, a seriously ill baby who lived near Injune was flown from Roma to the Archerfield aerodrome and taken to the hospital. In 1954, a five-week-old baby, seriously ill with anaemia, was flown from Roma to Brisbane with a registered nurse administering oxygen during the flight.[37]

The Bush Children's Health Scheme (now BUSHkids), which began in 1935, assisted many children, aged from birth to 13 years, from outback Queensland to receive treatment in Brisbane. A little girl aged 18 months, one of a family of ten children, was brought from Blackall in the Central West to the Mater for surgery on her hip. It was hoped that she would be fully recovered after six weeks in splints and a plaster cast.[38]

Accidents continued to hospitalise many children. In 1954, a serious incident that killed one child and seriously injured his brother was directly related to Brisbane's experience as a major military base in the Second World War. The children were injured by shrapnel when an American mortar bomb exploded on vacant land at Inala, then a new housing development on Brisbane's south-western outskirts.[39] The surviving boy was treated at the Mater Children's Hospital for a shattered right hand and a punctured lung.

Child accident victims were only a portion of the patients that the hospital treated in its eventful first 20 years. The statistics were impressive: 20,000 children had been treated as in-patients in the hospitals' 90 beds; there had been 300,000 out-patient attendances and 200,000 casualties. The twentieth anniversary in 1951 was celebrated modestly with a campaign to raise £12,000 to air-condition the main operating theatre and heat the wards.[40] In 1953, unexpected praise came from a member of the British Medical Association's Queensland branch (now the Australian Medical Association), who said that the Brisbane and South Coast Hospitals Board should build hospitals that were comparable with the Royal Melbourne and Mater Children's hospitals.[41]

There were, however, bigger plans afoot on Mater Hill. In 1935, Mother Alban promoted the idea of a maternity hospital on Brisbane's growing south side. A hospital training students and resident medical officers in obstetrics addressed the 1943 amendments to the *Hospitals Act 1936*, which required all graduating doctors to spend their year as resident medical officers in public hospitals with obstetric beds.[42] In February 1936, plans were revealed. The maternity hospital for private, intermediate and public patients would work in conjunction with the Mater Children's Hospital. The architects, Prentice & Atkinson, were instructed to ensure that the new hospital would harmonise with the existing buildings on Mater Hill.[43]

The Queensland government began a concerted effort to improve antenatal care and conditions for childbirth in the 1920s. This was the first serious attempt to improve maternity care in the nation. The program included the establishment of antenatal clinics and the construction of specially equipped maternity sections in hospitals – large and small – all over Queensland. The crowning jewel was replacing the Lady Bowen Hospital on Wickham Terrace with a new Brisbane Women's Hospital at Herston on the campus already shared by the government's adult and children's hospitals. This large new hospital, opened in 1938, put considerable pressure on private maternity hospitals of varying standards dotting Brisbane's suburbs. By 1940, obstetric care in hospitals had almost completely replaced home births with a doctor or midwife in attendance, once preferred for the delivery of babies.[44]

No doubt the Mater did not want to be left out of the move towards centralised maternity care, but the lingering Depression and the advent of the Second World War delayed the project. The proposal was resuscitated vigorously in 1946.[45] Where once the Mater balls raised money for the Mater Children's Hospital, profits from these newsworthy annual events were transferred to the maternity hospital, estimated to cost three-quarters of a million pounds.[46] The Mater Mothers' Hospital on the opposite side of the campus from the ageing Mater Children's Hospital grew brick by brick, floor by floor, during the 1950s, consuming almost all the Sisters of Mercy's available resources; little could be done at either the children's hospital or the adult hospital.

Fortunately, the staff at the Mater Children's Hospital was well used to managing with slim resources. There was little relief in the 1950s. New generations of drugs – particularly antibiotics – were making enormous impact on paediatric care, but they were expensive. The Commonwealth free hospital scheme did not stretch to unlimited supplies of drugs. At the Mater Children's Hospital, junior members of staff were instructed to refer to the senior specialists if they wanted to prescribe expensive drugs, particularly sulfa drugs and penicillin.[47]

There was also pressure to reduce the length of time children spent in hospital. Referring children with disabilities to the Montrose or Xavier homes was one strategy, as was Dr AW St Ledger's successful advocacy for a special clinic to deal with patients with allergic conditions and diabetes. Some time-honoured practices came to an end in this era. In the hospital's early days, when diphtheria was a menace, the throat of every child treated at the hospital was swabbed to find out whether they carried the infection. At PA Earnshaw's suggestion this practice was discontinued, unless a child had not been immunised. The improved acceptance of immunisation against a range of serious illnesses – diphtheria, whooping cough and tetanus – had greatly reduced the risk to children's lives and also the likelihood of cross-infection in hospital.[48]

The nursing staff bore much of the brunt of managing with scarce equipment.

When Sister Marie Fitzgerald RSM joined the Mater Children's Hospital staff in 1948, the hospital had only one electric suction machine 'which we trundled upstairs or downstairs' to and from its home in the ear, nose and throat ward on the ground floor. Sister Mary Colette Anderson RSM, who began work at the children's hospital in 1950, was plunged into the work of making plaster of Paris bandages and dressings, rolling and sterilising catgut sutures and concocting the hospital's acriflavine wool, the oil-impregnated 'tulle gras' dressings, and vaseline gauze. Gloves and syringes were sterilised and re-used. In Sister Mary Colette's view, the warm friendliness in the hospital was great compensation for hard work.[49]

PA Earnshaw remained at the helm of paediatric practice, even though he offered to retire in 1951 when he was then in his late fifties, but the Sisters and his medical colleagues unanimously persuaded him to stay. There were still some specialties shared with the Mater Adult Hospital, but the number of specific appointments to the Mater Children's Hospital gradually increased in the 1950s. Dr AW St Ledger became the first honorary allergist, Dr Llewellyn Swiss Davies was appointed to the surgical staff, Dr EJ McGuinness was appointed as honorary ophthalmologist, assisted by Dr Yeates, and Dr Rae Robinson was the honorary anaesthetist. In 1952, Dr Winifred Suggit and Dr Stephen Suggit were appointed to the honorary ear, nose and throat staff.[50]

In 1953, Dr George Christensen's proposal for the establishment of a facio-maxillary surgery unit was discussed, but the hospital was not yet in the position to open a complex new field.[51]

In the midst of the hectic 1951–52 polio epidemic, John Lahz suggested improvements to orthopaedic services. Effective specialist care would, however, be dependent on the appointment of well-trained registrars who would screen all out-patients to ensure the appropriate priorities were followed. There were orthopaedic registrars on the Mater staff in the late 1940s, but they were shared between the adult and children's hospitals. There was some frustration at the shortage of beds in the Mater Children's Hospital when the work of the orthopaedic section was growing fast. Lahz believed that, if economies had to be made, 'staff trimming is more practicable than bed slimming'.[52]

John Lahz also believed that service in the casualty section could be improved. There were many instances of acute trauma, which flooded the casualty and orthopaedic sections. In 1956, the orthopaedic staff appealed for the appointment of an additional registrar.[53] The hospital's high reputation for orthopaedics, they believed, had greatly increased the number of patients presenting for treatment. The matron, Sister Mary St Pierre McCormack RSM, also believed that additions to the registrar staff would greatly help; she was particularly concerned about the growing load of general surgery.[54]

The 1950s drew to a close with the celebration of the centenary of the achievement of separate representative government in Queensland in 1959. At the Mater, there was a considerable focus on government. The publication of annual reports – in recess since 1935 – was revived with the particular purpose of reminding the government and the people of Queensland about the Mater:

> It is absurd to leave these hospitals with their long tradition of
> efficient public hospital service in constant danger of falling behind
> modern requirements, because of the refusal by public authorities
> to subsidise them at capital level.[55]

The government had provided only £70,000 towards the cost of the Mater Mothers' Hospital. All other improvements had drawn on the Sisters' own resources.

The children's hospital was once again overcrowded. In the 1958–59 year, the hospital had cared for 3,148 in-patients, two-thirds of the number at the larger Mater Adult Hospital. Although the Mater community was looking forward to the opening of the Mater Mothers' Hospital, there was no doubt that a maternity hospital on the campus would put extra pressure on the children's hospital.[56] Sister Mary Lea Kelly's babies' ward would be very busy.

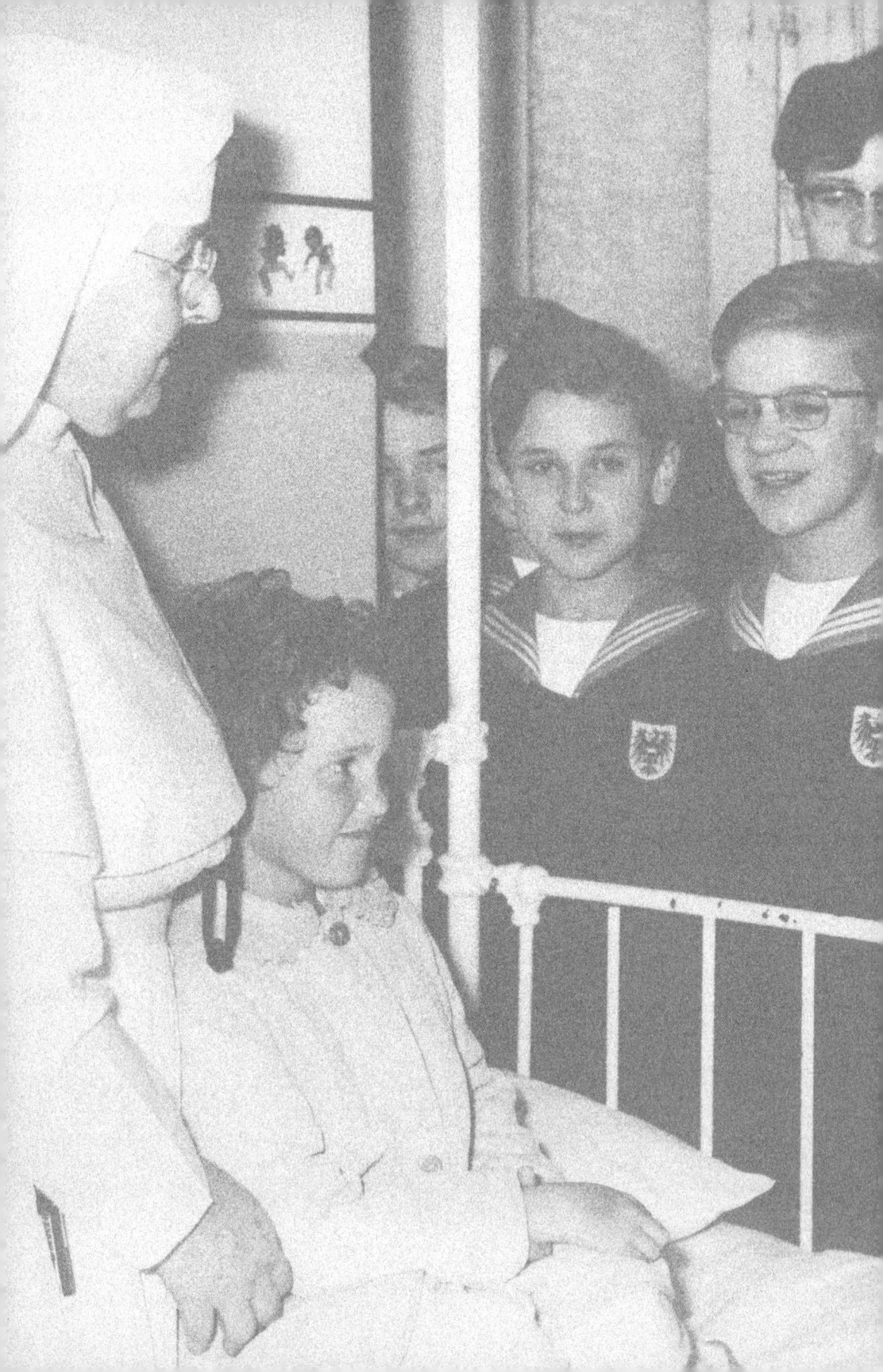

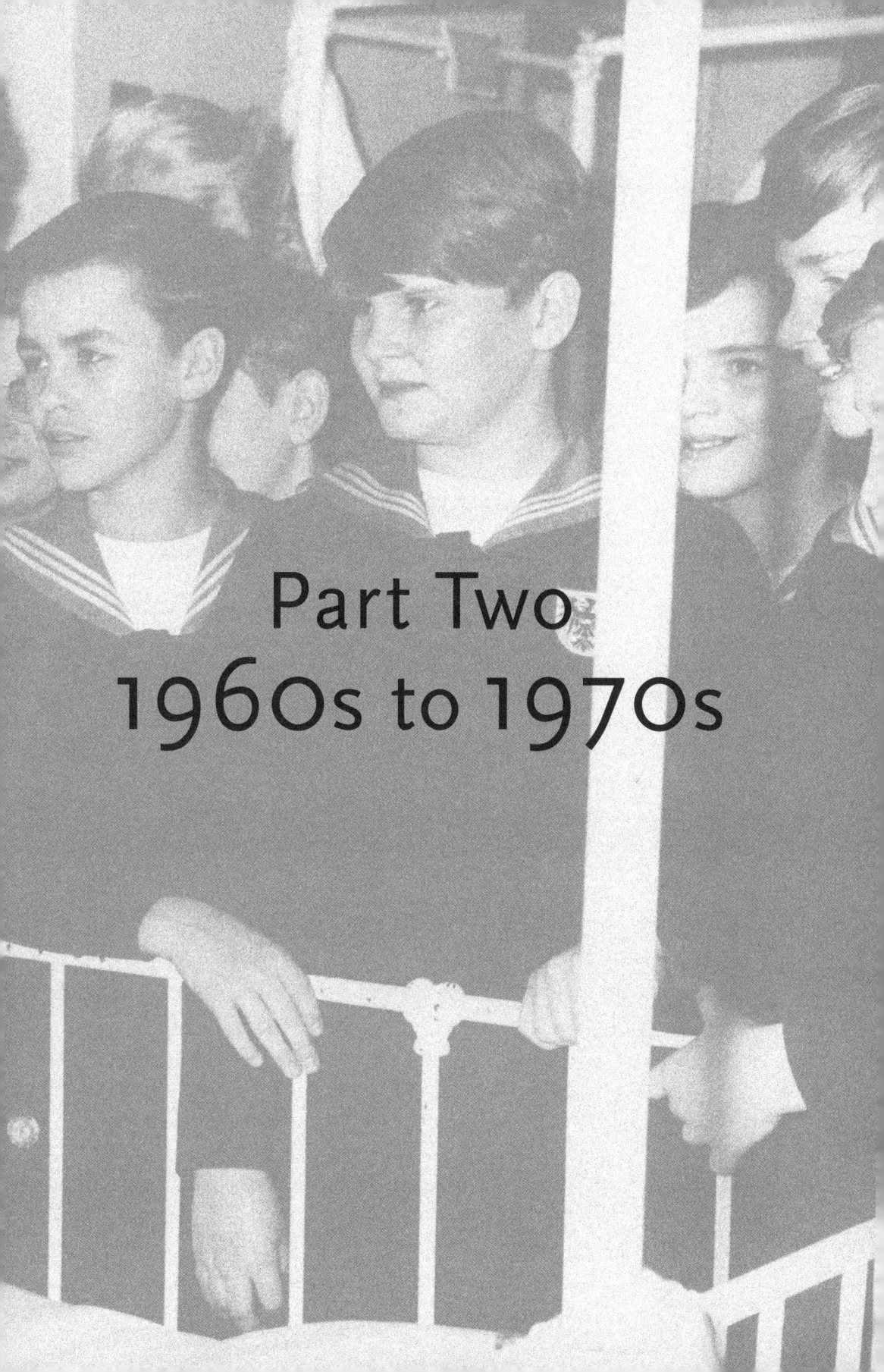

Part Two
1960s to 1970s

Chapter 4

Growth and Pressure

The modern hospital has the problem of providing highly complex and expensive equipment to keep pace with rapid advancement of medical research and patient care.

Sister Angela Mary Doyle RSM, 1968[1]

Growth and turmoil, protests and political upheavals punctuated the 1960s all over the world. The Mater Children's Hospital was not spared either trouble or turmoil, and was also subject to pressure generated by the great demographic feature of the era: the post-war 'baby boom'. More and more children attended the hospital; many lived in the new suburbs sprawling further and further to the south and west from Brisbane's central business district. Brisbane's growth in the post-war decades was, indeed, startling: from 453,660 at the 1951 census to 692,924 at the 1961 census and 891,100 at the 1971 census, a growth of more than 28 per cent in the 1960s alone.[2]

The rising birth rate ensured that the new Mater Mothers' Hospital was in great demand from the moment it opened its doors in February 1961.[3] The new maternity hospital brought the number of public hospital beds in the Mater complex to 615, making it the largest Australian hospital group controlled by a religious body.[4] Babies needing hospital care in their early months came to the Mater Children's Hospital. The 1960s were, therefore, testing years as the hospital coped with population pressures, while navigating changes in the steadily more complex post-war medical world.

The first year of the decade, 1961, was an exciting year. The Sisters of Mercy celebrated four very important milestones: the centenary of the arrival of the first Sisters in Queensland; the Golden Jubilee of the opening of the Mater Adult Hospital; the opening of the Mater Mothers' Hospital; and the thirtieth birthday of the Mater Children's Hospital.

Despite this development, an old injury continued to hurt: the government had contributed very little to the capital cost of the three hospitals and was often late in paying the maintenance subsidy on public beds. The chairman of the Mater Advisory Board, JP Kelly, was always ready to point out the inequity in hospital funding in Queensland.[5] The effect of the government's overlooking the Mater was more than a mere slight; it was a constant constraint on the ability to expand facilities and modernise services. The Mater Children's Hospital felt this disability acutely.

The years devoted to fundraising for the Mater Mothers' Hospital had created the situation where the Mater Adult and Children's hospitals were described as being at 'danger level' in 1964.[6] At the very least, the Mater Children's Hospital needed a new ward to accommodate 20 sick babies and an additional operating theatre. Kelly also believed that the government should subsidise the casualty department, the only such service on Brisbane's south side, providing one-third of emergency services to children in the entire city.

By the middle years of the decade, the Mater estimated that coping with the population in its catchment area would require 400 beds in the adult hospital, 200 beds in the children's hospital, 140 beds in the maternity hospital, 150 beds in the private hospital and 50 beds in the planned hospital for chronically ill patients discharged from the acute care adult hospital.[7] Development of this order would require considerable capital development and a large medical and nursing staff.

The matron of the Mater Children's Hospital, Sister Mary St Pierre McCormack RSM, had her own vision for the hospital's future. In 1961, she attended the first congress of the International Council of Nursing to be held in Australia and reported a significant change in the nursing of sick children, which she had seen demonstrated at Prince Henry Hospital in Sydney. Children there were taken to treatment areas and nursed in glassed-in private cubicles, rather than in large 'Nightingale' wards – like those at the Mater Children's Hospital – where treatment was administered at the bedside.[8]

Refinements had, however, to wait. In the early 1960s, simply keeping up with the demand for existing accommodation and services occupied all energies and all available finance. In 1963, for instance, 3,946 children were treated as in-patients, there were 25,184 attendances at the various out-patient clinics and 24,683 children were treated in the casualty department.[9] The problems the hospital faced in coping with its patient load were the subject of a great deal of thought and analysis in the 1960s.

The formal administrative structure was refined in the early 1960s to lay the foundations for modern hospital management. Two boards – both advisory to the Sisters of Mercy who retained all decision-making power – oversaw the day-to-day running of the hospital. The board of management dealt with the 'business' side and the medical advisory board dealt with clinical issues.[10] The Sister Administrator remained the main channel of communication between the Mater and the Superior General of the Sisters of Mercy.

An entirely new position created in 1959 brought the Mater more in line with state public hospitals. A Queensland graduate, Dr Brian Purssey, took up his duty as the first director of medical services for the Mater hospitals on 1 January 1959. A Fellow of the Royal College of Surgeons, London, Brian Purssey had considerable experience in teaching medical students at the Central Middlesex Hospital and the Middlesex Medical School. On returning to Queensland, Brian Purssey became assistant director of the Red Cross Blood Bank and a surgeon at Brisbane Hospital.[11] Missing the opportunity to practise surgery, he resigned from the Mater in 1962.

Brian Purssey was succeeded by Dr Eugene Desmond (Des) O'Callaghan, who had been a senior Mater resident medical officer in 1958.

Des O'Callaghan, known around the hospital as 'EDoc' from the way he initialled documents, began work at the beginning of a very testing decade. He regarded his time in the United Kingdom as invaluable in giving him an insight into modern hospital administration; his teaching experience convinced him that a hospital, 'if it is to advance, must inevitably become a great teaching medical school'.[12] The struggling Mater Children's Hospital became one of his biggest worries.

A separate Mater Children's Hospital sub-committee of the advisory board met regularly to discuss staffing, out-patient and casualty organisation, the place of post-graduate teaching and specialists' appointments to both the adult and children's hospitals.¹³ Some of these topics were controversial, revealing that points of view could differ between those who treated children only and those who treated both children and adults. The paediatrician Dr Geoffrey Bourke had several ideas.

> DES O'CALLAGHAN, MBBS, MRACP, MRCP, FRACMA, born in Bundaberg in 1931, graduated in medicine at the University of Queensland in 1955 and completed the clinical years of his undergraduate degree at the Mater. After one year as paediatric registrar at the Mater Children's Hospital in 1957, Des O'Callaghan became a registrar at the Mater Adult Hospital in 1958. He studied in London in 1959 and 1960 and gained his membership of the Royal College of Physicians, London. Returning to Brisbane, Des O'Callaghan became the senior teaching medical registrar in the University of Queensland's Department of Medicine and a member of the Royal Australasian College of Physicians. In his application, Des O'Callaghan said that he wanted the position as director of medical services to be his 'permanent career'. Des O'Callaghan died in office on 9 January 1988.

> GEOFFREY MERWIN BOURKE, MBBS, FRACP, D.ObstFRCOG, graduated in medicine with honours at the University of Sydney in 1952. He was a resident medical officer at Sydney Hospital in 1952 and 1953 and at the Royal Children's Hospital, Melbourne, in 1953 and 1954. After six months as a general practitioner in Queensland, Geoffrey Bourke was a paediatric registrar at the Crown Street Women's Hospital in Sydney. His application for a paediatric registrar's position at the Mater Children's Hospital was strongly supported by references from the Royal Children's Hospital in Melbourne and the endorsement of the senior paediatrician at the Mater, who described his qualifications as 'excellent'. In 1968, Dr Bourke twice worked as a member of civilian medical teams at Bien Hoa in Vietnam and led the Australian civilian team in Vietnam in 1971. Geoffrey Bourke retired some years before his death on 11 June 2013.¹⁴

Geoffrey Bourke was concerned that the hospital was standing still, rather than keeping abreast of the advances in paediatrics that followed the Second World War. He felt that the Mater Children's Hospital had not advanced in organisation and practice for almost a quarter of a century. In his paper on the Mater's further development, Geoffrey Bourke stated that he was communicating the views of many doctors who thought that the hospital needed to develop in three main areas: patient care, teaching and research.[15]

Concerns such as those expressed by Geoffrey Bourke came as no surprise to JP Kelly. He was well aware that ancillary services were in 'dire need of expansion' and was particularly concerned about the casualty department at the children's hospital, as well as pathology and diagnostic services generally. Kelly stated frankly that 'the efficiency of the hospital will be inhibited until these services are modernised and extended'.[16] Attendances at the casualty department at the Mater Children's Hospital had been increasing steadily to about 100 to 150 each day in the early 1960s; the need for more staff was becoming self-evident, as was the need for additional space to cope with the increase in neonatal and infant patients.[17] There was, however, a factor inhibiting both capital development and staff increases: the debt on the Mater Mothers' Hospital, which would not be repaid until the middle years of the 1960s.

Staff shortages prevented over-taxed specialists from taking advantage of available research grants.[18] The hospital's capacity for research was an important matter for John Rendle-Short, the University of Queensland's first Professor of Child Health. A Cambridge graduate, Professor Rendle-Short had experience of tropical medicine during service in India, Burma, Thailand and Malaya in the final stages of the Second World War and immediately afterwards. John Rendle-Short had decided to be a paediatrician during his clinical training years in Bristol and became a lecturer in child health at the University of Sheffield. In 1957, John Rendle-Short was awarded his doctorate for work on William Cadogan, an eighteenth-century founder of the discipline of paediatrics.[19]

On 8 May 1961, Professor Rendle-Short took up his chair and his consultancy to Brisbane's two children's hospitals with alacrity. He analysed the situation at the Mater Children's Hospital in 1962, and found that much more than shortage of medical staff and lack of research capacity needed to be remedied. He was asked his views on a suggestion that the children's hospital might need to share a building with adult services. Professor Rendle-Short was not overly concerned about a shared building, but regarded as mandatory the retention of the principle that staff and services for children should always be separate. A completely separate entrance for children and separate waiting rooms and procedure rooms were essential.

The existing hospital, the professor believed, was 'at present inadequate both for teaching purposes and for its case load'. There needed to be accommodation for infants, teaching rooms, a library, a milk kitchen, therapy departments, play rooms, a school room, a mothers' room and, ideally, mother and baby units. A shortage of space for a professorial unit was another issue. Both the hospital and the university hoped that the unit would be established by the mid-1960s. Somehow, the university department would need to be contiguous with the children's hospital, but separate from it, as the Australian Universities Commission funded university developments, not ordinary hospital facilities.

The university's requirements were challenging: teaching rooms adjacent to the wards on both surgical and medical floors. Ideally, teaching areas would be large enough to accommodate 12 students during a ward round, a child in a cot brought in for clinical review, a clinician, a blackboard, X-ray screens, a washbasin and storage. There would also need to be reading rooms, possibly separated from the teaching rooms by folding doors. A university staff member and a paediatric registrar would each need an office on the medical floor. University staff members were researchers as well as clinicians and, therefore, records in any teaching hospital had to be of the highest order as the 'contribution that sick children make to medical progress lies in their records'.[20]

Existing ward arrangements needed to be reviewed with a view to more efficient use of the available space, perhaps by subdividing wards. Professor Rendle-Short identified the need for an additional operating theatre and improved anaesthetic and recovery facilities. An eight-bed isolation ward was recommended, with a washbasin, an exterior window and air-conditioning in each glass-walled cubicle. Further, the ear, nose and throat ward and its operating theatre should be moved from the ground floor to make more space for out-patients.

It was inevitable, the professor thought, that out-patient numbers would rise as 'more and more investigation and treatment should be done at out-patient level'. Ideally, there should be two or three consulting-room suites in out-patients, each large enough for 12 students and an examination area for the child, a smaller registrar's room opening into the consulting room and a waiting room with space for three or four families. A play area common to all suites was desirable. The out-patient floor needed a treatment room, weighing and urine-testing rooms, two or three consulting suites, and a room for breast-feeding mothers.

There should also be an X-ray department in the children's hospital. The existing system of transporting very sick young patients outdoors and then to the adult X-ray department was unsatisfactory; too many children had to mix with adults in the combined department. A new X-ray area – perhaps in the existing out-patient waiting room – should be close to the casualty and out-patient areas and the lift; its staff should be specially trained in paediatric radiology. Two tables, an image intensifier, dark rooms, storage and an office for the radiologist would be required.

Extensions to the casualty section were underway when Professor Rendle-Short wrote his assessment, but he was disappointed that there was not to be an operating theatre for minor surgical procedures or provision for teaching students. The extension added rooms by dividing the original casualty area into two cubicles.[21] He also recommended an observation ward close to casualty for children who needed to be watched while recovering from such emergencies as asthma attacks or poisoning.

Better provision for parents was mentioned in every section of Professor Rendle-Short's report. Modern developments in paediatrics had emphasised the importance of the mother's presence with a child in hospital, a great departure from 'once a week' visiting hours in practice at the Mater Children's Hospital and many other children's hospitals. He recommended that at least one room be provided for a mother to stay in the hospital with her child. He favoured unrestricted parental daily visiting in all wards. It was also apparent to the professor that there needed to be opportunities for children to be out of bed and mobile more often than was the hospital's present practice. Play areas convenient to all wards were, therefore, necessary; access to a garden or an outdoor area was also highly desirable.

Fortunately, the hospital had already prepared plans for a nursery ward that would expand accommodation for babies from 10 to 24, which the professor considered to be adequate. There would, however, need to be space for four intensive-care cots to keep the environment stable for very ill infants. The professor's long list of desirable alterations extended to ancillary services, also highlighted by the Mater Children's Hospital staff. Modern physiotherapy, occupational therapy, speech therapy, social work and psychology had their own requirements.

Professor Rendle-Short was pleased that the Mater Children's Hospital was taking steps to establish a hospital school, necessary even for short-stay children, not only so that they could keep abreast of their peers, but also to provide essential relief from the tedium of hospital life. Although most teaching could be accomplished in the wards, a school room was necessary.

The concept of a hospital school was by no means new. The Sick Children's Provisional School number 1650 opened at Brisbane's Hospital for Sick Children on 11 August 1919, following the kindergarten classes that had been held at the hospital informally since 1906. This was Australia's first hospital school. Ensuring education for children who could not attend their local schools was particularly important for children with disabilities. The polio epidemics of the earlier twentieth century created great concern that children who might be in hospital for months – perhaps years – needed at least a primary standard of education if they were to have any chance of leading independent adult lives. Teaching in hospitals and for those disabled by polio began in Victoria and South Australia and spread to Sydney in 1930 and to Montrose Home in Brisbane in 1934.[22] A special 'paralysis' section of the Hospital for Sick Children's school opened in O'Connell Ward in 1938.[23] For some years, Dr David Jackson, a senior paediatrician at the Mater Children's Hospital, had helped to improve educational opportunities for children with cerebral palsy and, in 1951, a school opened at their New Farm treatment centre.[24]

An extension of the Brisbane Children's Hospital school to include children at the Mater was approved by the Education Department in 1962, but only for a one-term trial. The department's demands for the trial included furniture: a teacher's table, chair, cupboards and small tables and chairs for up to five pupils.[25] Classes began at the Mater Children's Hospital in 1963 in a screened-off portion of the medical ward's verandah; children confined to bed used portable desks.[26]

The trial was a success, largely due to the efforts of the first teacher, Ailsa Chadwick. The staff appreciated the school regime, which ensured that the children were occupied – and quiet. At the weekends, 'bedlam' could prevail when boys got up to pranks, such as swinging from the top railings of the four-poster beds. The introduction of radios in every ward in the 1960s delighted the children – and the nurses, as they could listen to The Beatles. School life in hospital followed many of the traditions of any other school, including Christmas parties.[27]

Professor Rendle-Short's concern for the psychological and emotional wellbeing of children in hospital was not limited to education and visiting hours. In the early 1960s, the upper age limit at the Mater Children's Hospital was 12 years. Physically and emotionally immature children were admitted to adult wards and often confronted by unsuitable sights and smells. Some adult patients could be unpleasant to children and, conversely, noisy, convalescent teenagers could upset sick adults. Even more seriously, this practice disrupted the follow-up of those childhood diseases, which could have all-of-life consequences. In Adelaide, children were admitted to children's hospitals until they were almost 15, in Melbourne almost 17 and in Perth and Sydney until they were 14. An adolescent unit at the Mater Children's Hospital was, therefore, necessary.[28]

Professor Rendle-Short concluded his 1962 analysis with advice: it was of the utmost importance that further building was not undertaken at the Mater Children's Hospital until it could be certain that it would conform to the required standards. Sister Mary St Gabriel Corbett RSM, Sister Administrator at the Mater, immediately referred the professorial 'prescription' for the children's hospital to the Congregation's headquarters with a note: 'Mother, these are the circulars from Professor Rendle-Short ... it looks like another new Hospital!!'[29]

Despite the note of alarm in the Sister Administrator's memorandum – and the financial impossibility of creating an entirely new children's hospital – most of Professor Rendle-Short's recommendations were implemented in one way or another. In 1962, parental visiting hours were extended to 10.00am to 6.00pm every day except Sunday, when visiting was restricted to the afternoons. Grandparents, aunts and uncles could visit, but children under 14 were still forbidden to visit the wards. Nevertheless, relaxing the visiting hours paid dividends. Sister Marie Fitzgerald RSM observed, 'gone now are the days when toddlers clung to their mothers for six months or longer after hospitalisation, fearful to let them out of sight'.[30]

In April 1963, a small room under the stairs near the operating theatres was transformed into a developing room for X-rays filmed by a portable

X-ray machine. This was not quite the elaborate department Professor Rendle-Short had suggested, but at least the children no longer needed to be taken to the adult department. In 1965, extensions to the nursery ward and operating theatres were at last approved. Funding was released by the elimination of the debt on the Mater Mothers' Hospital, but the children's hospital was only one item on the list of urgent needs across the campus.[31]

Constructing a professorial unit at the Mater Children's Hospital should have been straightforward, as far as finance was concerned. This would be part of the University of Queensland and, therefore, financed by the Australian Universities Commission (AUC). In 1962, the AUC's allocation to the Mater to support the teaching of 81 medical students in five different courses – some 20 per cent of the total number of students in their clinical years – was bitterly disappointing.[32] The Mater's grant was only £3,000, which seemed miserly compared with more than £600,000 for the three hospitals on the government's Herston campus (Brisbane General Hospital, Brisbane Children's Hospital and Brisbane Women's Hospital) and £31,600 to the Princess Alexandra Hospital.[33] The Mater Advisory Board also believed that reliance on visiting 'honorary' medical staff, rather than employing a large number of staff specialists, had harmed its cause. This was, as JP Kelly put it, a 'grievous blow'.[34] The situation gradually improved and, in the mid-1960s, the University of Queensland was funded to construct teaching facilities and academic offices at the Mater Children's Hospital.[35]

These much-needed extensions were not accomplished without considerable noise and dust, uncomfortable for patients and staff. The children were fascinated by the huge crane that arrived to remove the roof from the kitchen so that the professorial unit could be constructed as a second floor. No-one mourned the departure of the old coal stove that had been in use since 1931.[36] On 18 May 1965, the Mater was notified that Cabinet had agreed to increase the rate of capital subsidy to 50 per cent of the cost of new beds and to subsidise the purchase of new life-saving equipment.[37] This change of governmental heart may have been purely expedient: the population was growing fast and new beds were urgently needed. The larger babies' ward, made necessary by the opening of the Mater Mothers' Hospital, was designed to accommodate all babies under 12 months of age, reducing the need to admit babies to general wards at busy times. Even better, there could be an additional operating theatre to supplement the original single theatre with its small annexe that sometimes had to be pressed into service as a second theatre.[38] The staff was not overlooked in the flurry of extensions and renovations in the 1960s: lunch rooms were renovated and new quarters for trained nurses, overlooking Clarence Street, were completed in 1962, without the benefit of government subsidy.[39]

Even when the extensions were complete, the Mater Children's Hospital still strained to accommodate patients from its ever-expanding catchment. Coping with the demand meant a higher turnover of patients. Even in an era that emphasised shorter hospital stays for children and treatment as out-patients whenever possible, discharging children in order to admit new patients was an unwelcome pressure. The improvements, however, implemented Professor Rendle-Short's recommendation that children should be treated in privacy. However, the aim of introducing separate accommodation for teenagers and accommodation for the mothers of sick babies had not yet been realised. Separate intensive care and infectious diseases sections were also still on the wish list; the need to refer some patients with gastroenteritis to the Royal Children's Hospital irritated both hospitals.[40]

The patients kept coming. Growth in the mid-1960s was spectacular. In 1931, there had been 1,266 admissions, 7,375 out-patients and 1,153 treatments in the casualty section. In the 1965–66 year, there were 4,092 admissions, 28,410 out-patient attendances and 44,885 casualty treatments. In 1966–67 – only one year later – there had been a 25 per cent increase to 5,029 in-patients and a 25 per cent increase in attendances in the casualty section; the number of out-patients, however, remained stable.[41] As David Jackson remarked, 'it is a matter of some wonder that these staggering increases in patient load have been accommodated and efficiently treated with so little structural alteration to one small building'.[42]

The advent of a government subsidy for capital works in the mid-1960s made an enormous difference, but did not eliminate the need for fundraising for the equipment that helped to make advances in treatment possible. The Mater Children's Hospital allocation from the Lord Mayor's command performance in 1966 produced a much-needed ventilator. The Mater Children's Ladies Auxiliary, led for many years by Mrs Beth Dittmer, produced intensive care cots, playpens, radiators, cardiac monitors, hip frames and a resuscitation trolley.[43] Instruments for the children's percussion band, recommended by their teacher, was an important auxiliary project that addressed recreational and educational needs rather than strictly necessary medical equipment. The Mater Younger Set also kept the children's hospital in mind and donated a machine that blew a stream of moist air over a croupy child, eliminating the need for dangerous boiling kettles.

The auxiliary raised its funds through raffles and at morning teas, gala dinners, Melbourne Cup parties, cake stalls and the annual Mater Debutante Ball. As well as its impressive array of gifts in the 1960s, the auxiliary had an ambitious project in mind: a Zeiss operating microscope for delicate surgery, which would cost £1,400. The hard work that produced these gifts had an additional benefit: the public relations dividend generated by extensive publicity of auxiliary parties and events helped to keep the Mater Children's Hospital in the public eye. Larger fundraising efforts were also necessary. The door-to-door appeal in 1965 helped to generate the Mater's share of funding for the new nursery and operating theatre extensions.[44]

Even this was not enough. In 1969, an exhaustive review of the Mater's prospects of raising the money it needed for urgent capital works produced some chastening findings. The Mater Children's Hospital was found to be most in need of attention, but a new adult hospital was the Sisters of Mercy's highest priority, a position difficult to understand as the Princess Alexandra Hospital had opened as the second adult hospital on Brisbane's south side. There was only one south-side paediatric hospital – the Mater Children's Hospital – where pressures had increased following the opening of the Mater Mothers' Hospital.

Some doctors said that the Mater Children's Hospital was 'so disgraceful it should be closed down immediately' and many others believed that the Mater would have to spend at least $20,000,000 by 1980 to create first-class adult and children's hospitals.[45] Ironically, many people in the wider community thought that the Mater was affluent because the standard of the new Mater Mothers' Hospital was so high. Photographs of the old sections of the adult and children's hospitals might have shocked the public. If the real situation at the children's was publicised, the 1969 review contended, the project to extend it would have great public relations potential.

Difficult and overcrowded conditions in out-patient, casualty and many other sections of the hospital were not the only challenges facing the nursing and medical staff at the Mater Children's Hospital in the 1960s. These were years of transition in patient care.

Chapter 5

Transition

Your help in seeing that every necessary attention – and more – was given each child eased one's responsibilities and gave a sense of security.

PA Earnshaw to Sister Mary Mechtilde Slattery RSM, 1961

The matron of the Mater Children's Hospital, Sister Mary St Pierre McCormack RSM, and Sisters of Mercy in each ward or department led a growing corps of nursing staff. There were inevitable changes. Sister Mary Audrey Lucy RSM, one of the most experienced nursing sisters in the casualty department and the operating theatres, left the children's hospital to become the first matron of the Mater Mothers' Hospital. Sister Mary John Patch RSM, who completed nurse training before entering the Sisters of Mercy, was both an operating theatre nurse and a ward sister at the children's hospital before following Sister Mary Audrey as matron of the Mater Mothers' Hospital in 1964. The children's hospital lost another of the Sisters of Mercy's rising stars in 1963, when Sister Angela Mary Doyle RSM transferred to the Mater Adult Hospital. She had found her two years at the children's hospital the hardest of her nursing career and later wrote: 'I doubt that anyone can watch sick children without feeling pain, especially pain for the parents'.[1] Sister Angela Mary became Sister Administrator of the whole campus in 1966.

Sister Mary Lea Kelly RSM, who had been in charge of the babies' ward since 1942, witnessed many changes in the treatment of very ill babies, as well as the transformation of her ward in the 1960s extensions. Sister Mary Lea had every reason to have particular sympathy with tiny babies.[2]

> MARY THERESA KELLY was born prematurely in 1916, and was said to be too small to sleep in an ordinary bassinet. She completed her general nurse and midwifery training before entering the Sisters of Mercy in 1935. As Sister Mary Lea, she joined the staff at the Mater Children's Hospital in 1942 and remained there for a remarkable 32 years. One of her young patients once referred to her as 'boss Sister', a nickname which stuck, although she was also referred to as 'the nursery lady'. A poem composed to celebrate the Silver Jubilee of her profession captured both the circumstances of her birth and her insistence on high standards:
>
> > 'When Ma brought her home to Clifton,
> > All the church bells rang and rang',
>
> and, in a later verse,
>
> > 'For in straight lines must always be,
> > The legs of every cot,
> > To sit on a bed a major crime'.
>
> Sister Mary Lea died on 1 April 1992.[3]

Sister Mary Lea's standards were so exacting that one of the 1960s nurse trainees, Patricia Mexted (nee Mahoney), found that, when she was transferred to the babies' ward from the adult hospital, she had to 'learn all over again'.[4]

The Mater's longest-serving paediatrician, PA Earnshaw, recognised the skill of the Sisters of Mercy by, for instance, thanking Sister Mary Mechtilde RSM, charge sister of the medical ward, for her 'splendid support and loyal assistance', acknowledging that her help 'made the care and treatment of the patients much smoother and so much more effective'. This, he said was a 'debt I cannot repay'.[5]

The number of nurses working at the Mater Children's Hospital grew from 57 in 1956 to 70 in 1966. Additional trained lay staff were appointed to senior ward positions as the 1960s progressed.[6] In 1965, Sister Pamela Cashen RN and two Sisters of Mercy, Mary Winifrede Patterson RSM and Mary Dorothea Sheehan RSM, managed the surgical wards; Sister Anne Begg RN and Sister Mary Mechtilde Slattery RSM were in charge of the medical wards; Sister Mary Lea Kelly RSM and Sister Mary Wagner RN reigned over the nursery; Sister Marie Fitzgerald RSM, Sister Mary Colette Anderson RSM and Sister Margaret Conanan RN looked after the operating theatres; and Sister Olga Dewhurst RN and Sister Jennifer Munro RN cared for the busy ear, nose and throat ward. A large cast of full-time and part-time qualified sisters managed the out-patient and casualty departments.[7]

The trained staff did not rest on their laurels. Several Sisters of Mercy, including Sister Mary Dorothea Sheehan RSM, Sister Michaeleen Mary Ahern RSM and Sister Jill (Mary Raymond) Stringer RSM, completed their certificates in child welfare. Sister Mary St Pierre McCormack RSM and Sister Imelda Mary Shannon RSM attended a meeting in July 1965 to form an association for the welfare of autistic children. The trained staff frequently attended lectures at the University of Queensland Department of Child Health on topics such as 'oesophageal atresia – two-stage operation', 'neonatal subdural collection' and 'Klippel-Feil Syndrome with other congenital abnormalities'. Sister Regis Mary Dunne RSM was one of the lecturers in 1965 when she spoke on genetics, an area in which her expertise was widely recognised.[8]

Nurses, whether qualified or still in their training years, faced considerable change, both in their work in the wards and in their education. Establishing preliminary training schools for nurses reflected the first major change in the Queensland nurse training curriculum since 1928.[9] The academic content of the course remained low – only 148 hours over four years – but, for the first time, trainee nurses spent time in the classroom for a short time before being assigned to the wards. Sister Josephine (Imelda Mary) Shannon RSM was the first of the Sisters of Mercy at the Mater to complete her qualifications as a tutor sister, followed by Sister Eileen (Mary Gerarda) Pollard RSM, who became responsible for 300 nursing students spread across the Mater hospitals.[10]

The preliminary training school was based at a property acquired in 1958, Raymond Court in Raymond Terrace, close to the Mater Mothers' Hospital where, in 1965, an old garage became a lecture theatre – the 'McAuley Study'. Quite apart from managing changes to the nurse training curriculum, the increased number of nurses made necessary by growth across the campus had to be accommodated.[11] St Mary's Nurses Home was benevolently ruled by Sister Alphonsus Mary Kennedy RSM, known as Alfie, who 'always appeared when you hoped she wouldn't'.[12] Many student nurses felt that the companionship of St Mary's Nurses Home eased the tough four years of the training regime. Accommodation pressures were relieved when a new four-storey building for the trained staff was opened in 1962 and, in 1966, when fourth-year students were allowed to live outside the hospital for the first time.[13] Conditions for Mater nurses were considerably boosted when five weeks' annual leave for student nurses commenced in 1963; their recreational opportunities improved when a squash court and swimming pool were opened in September 1966.[14]

Shortage of medical staff was a persistent issue at the Mater Children's Hospital. In 1964, there were only one paediatric registrar, Geoffrey Bourke; one senior resident medical officer in casualty; two second-year resident medical officers; and three first-year residents.[15] The 'doctor scarcity' affected most Western countries in the 1960s. Indeed, the decade began with one of the senior resident medical officer positions at the Mater Children's Hospital unfilled and no ear, nose and throat registrars at either the adult or children's hospitals.[16] There was also a significant loss from the staff: the longest-serving paediatrician at the Mater Children's Hospital, PA Earnshaw, retired from the active staff in 1961. He was badly missed.

Confusion and embarrassment often came the way of resident medical officers: at the Mater Children's Hospital in 1963, a senior orthopaedic surgeon asked a new doctor to arrange a 'below the knee' splint for a child. The resident heard this as a 'Baloney' splint and had great trouble procuring it, much to Sister Mary St Pierre's great amusement.[17]

The operating theatres at the Mater Children's Hospital were never still. Demands on the surgeons and the operating theatres were intense. On any given day, there were about 30 patients in the general surgical wards and another 10 or 11 tonsillectomy patients in the ear, nose and throat ward.[18] In February 1969, Sister Mary St Pierre wrote that she had 'spent most of the time writing 'I am sorry' letters, telling mothers that their children's ear, nose and throat bookings had been deferred.[19]

Issues of demarcation arose with the development of modern paediatric surgery. Should, for instance, a paediatric surgeon or a urologist operate on a child with a kidney or urinary tract problem? Should there be specialist paediatric ear, nose and throat surgeons? The issue was raised at meetings of the Mater Advisory Board. Three visiting surgeons who served Brisbane's two children's hospitals, Drs Des McGuckin, Llew Swiss Davies and Len

Marriott, unlikely to press the claims of one hospital over the other, staunchly advocated the full-time appointment of a paediatric surgeon without 'anatomical boundaries' being assigned to the surgeon's responsibilities.[20] Professor Rendle-Short and Dr David Jackson supported them, believing that children should always be cared for by those specially trained in paediatrics.[21]

There was some concern that the Mater's anaesthetics system was falling behind 1960s standards. Without citing evidence or examples, a group of registrars wrote alarmingly of 'the untoward large number of tragedies, near tragedies and an occasional last-minute aversion of tragedy associated with surgery and anaesthetics in this hospital group'.[22] They were concerned at the lack of a full-time director of anaesthetics, the practice of allowing 'junior and inexperienced resident medical officers' to administer anaesthetics, and 'cost factors', which might be restricting the 'large selection of anaesthetic agents and drugs [and the] ... wide range of equipment and a choice of technique', all of which, in the registrars' view, were necessary in modern anaesthesia.[23]

At that stage, there were 11 honorary anaesthetists – five with higher degrees in anaesthesia – on the Mater staff, but none attended emergency operations and the anaesthetists rarely had time to teach junior staff. The situation improved when Dr CF Conway was appointed as director of anaesthetics for the Mater group. His patients benefited in 1963 when the non-flammable anaesthetic agent Fluothane was introduced, with a much more pleasant odour than the ether it replaced.[24]

The trend to specialisation in medical practice became more and more evident as the 1960s progressed, creating some tensions at the Mater Children's Hospital, where cost was an issue, particularly in developing specialties within paediatrics. Financial issues inhibited the employment of full-time specialists in a hospital still reliant on the honorary system.[25] The recommendation that all babies – whether admitted for surgery or not – be assigned to the care of the receiving physician was not popular.[26] Brisbane's first neurosurgeon, Dr Geoff Toakley, argued against assigning surgical patients in the nursery to the overall care of a physician. He maintained that he should be responsible for his patients and free to choose any physician who might be needed to see them.[27]

In 1964, a proposal to abandon the traditional practice of offering specialists conjoint appointments at the Mater Adult and Children's hospitals raised considerable protest. The ear, nose and throat specialist, Dr Stephen Suggit, for instance, thought that:

> ... the interest for the specialist in a purely children's appointment is limited ... the tendency now is against special hospitals of all sorts. In the interests of economy special units are being incorporated into general hospitals wherever possible.[28]

Stephen Suggit wanted to integrate his work at the children's hospital with work at the adult hospital and found that his practice was made more difficult as the department was 'scattered in bits and pieces'.[29] Dr EF McGuinness was 'totally against' a divorced staff at the two hospitals as there was no adult–child division in the ear, nose and throat specialty and, therefore, a separate staff would deny the full practice of the specialty.

Others saw the issue of separate or conjoint specialties as going to the heart of Mater philosophy. Dr James Hynes said simply: 'I do not like our hospital being divided like this'. Dr Toakley wrote: 'one should realise that the Children's Hospital is not a children's hospital in the Mater grounds but part and parcel of the Mater hospitals as a group'. In addition, 'a specialty does not end at age 12 and then start again at 12 years and one month'. There was also a practical consideration. It was proving very difficult to find a neurosurgeon to be appointed to the Mater Children's Hospital. The urologists had a similar view about the difficulty in attracting specialists in the paediatric dimension of their specialty.[30]

In 1964, the University of Queensland eased the situation by deciding to appoint a Reader in paediatric surgery, who would take charge of surgical teaching at the Mater Children's Hospital.[31] This step may have been just in time to ease student complaints. One group did not believe that teaching by long ward rounds was satisfactory and, in addition, there were insufficient opportunities to observe paediatric surgeons at work.[32] The administration commented that the standard of teaching was inevitably dropping with increasing numbers of students without much addition to the number of teachers. All registrars were, therefore, instructed to regard teaching as part of their duties. There was also a changing of the guard: in 1966, Dr Llew Swiss Davies, one of the longest-standing visiting surgeons at the children's hospital, retired, believing that he should make way for a younger surgeon.[33]

Whether specialist paediatric surgeon or not, whether trained nurse or the newest student, the staff at the Mater Children's Hospital dealt with a wide range of childhood conditions, problems and tragedies. In the mid-1960s, for instance, there were usually an average of about 30 patients in the general surgical and orthopaedic wards, 11 who had had their tonsils removed; another 8 with other ear, nose and throat conditions; 4 patients treated by the neurologists and neurosurgeons; 2 with suspected heart conditions; 34 children in the general medical wards; and at least 14 babies in the nursery.[34] In 1964–65, as in-patients, boys at 2,414 outnumbered girls at 1,748.

The casualty section was so busy that the Director of Medical Services for the Mater group, Des O'Callaghan, recognised that the children's hospital needed its own casualty registrar supported by two junior resident medical officers, rather than rely on the surgical registrars. Between 1963 and 1965, there were 41,002 attendances at casualty and more than 29,000 out-patient attendances.[35] Many of the patients brought to the casualty department needed care for the ordinary woes of childhood, rather than emergency treatment. In the 1960s, fewer general practitioners saw patients at nights and weekends and these were the times the strain in the casualty department was greatest, as nurses often discovered. In May 1967, Sister Mary St Pierre wrote about disturbed preparations for the Mater Ball: there were 'many beautiful heads of hair in evidence … The Debs look lovely and so excited. Four children decided to break their arms, much to the disgust of the Medics and Nursing Personnel who wished to make an early start to the Ball'.[36]

There were, however, many emergencies. In 1963, a child needed eight operations after swallowing corrosive caustic soda; children ingesting chemicals and medications left within their reach were emergencies with sometimes fatal consequences. Burns, often as a result of playing with matches, were also responsible for lengthy hospital stays. A new mesh bed acquired in 1965 eased the pain for some young burns patients.[37] Cars had become more numerous and faster and more and more children were injured in road accidents. In the affluent 1960s, swimming pools began to appear more frequently in backyards and more public swimming pools attracted crowds in Brisbane's hot and humid summer. Child drownings – and near-drownings – were recorded more frequently.[38] As well as common falls at home and spills from bicycles, there were incidents of more unusual childhood accidents: swallowing a one-cent piece shortly after decimal currency was introduced in Australia in 1966 and the serious consequence of a hand in a mincing machine, which resulted in the amputation of three fingers.

Life-saving surgery on newborn babies also became more commonplace. Sister Mary St Pierre noted several such procedures in her journal, including procedures to correct oesophageal malformations. Correcting oesophageal obstructions and fistulas was exacting, lengthy surgery. A baby born with several gastrointestinal malformations underwent many hours of surgery on the day she was born. The baby died after weeks of struggle. Surgery on a baby boy with oesophageal atresia, weighing only four pounds, was one of the surgeons' successes. He was nursed in an intensive care cot for a month, transferred to an ordinary cot and discharged six weeks after his surgery.[39]

Some patients came from far afield. In 1967, a child was brought from Port Moresby for treatment of his head injury. He recovered well, assisted by a favourite treat: onion sandwiches 'which are tearfully prepared by Sister Mary Winifrede'.[40] In 1967, baby Annette was flown from Darwin when she was three days old for surgery for oesophageal atresia. She made many return flights to and from Darwin and became a 'much travelled little lady, quite happy in the air'.[41] A baby from Stanthorpe with oesophageal atresia had a long operation when he was only a few hours old and went home 'fit and fat' two months later. The surgical team and nursing staff were greatly relieved in 1968, when a six-year-old boy was able to do without his oesophageal tube that had been in position for three years following ingestion of caustic soda. Sister Mary St Pierre observed that he 'would like to be drinking and eating all the time just to prove to himself that the tube is not still there'.[42]

There were also special treats. Special arrangements were made to take a child with brittle bones, who had sustained many fractures in his short life and many admissions to hospital, to see a soccer match between an English team and Queensland in 1967. In July 1967, the Vienna Boys' Choir sang for the children; while they were there, Dr Len Marriott removed the sutures from one chorister who had had his appendix removed six days earlier.[43]

Injuries to the brain, whether caused by illness or accident, were always worrying. In 1969, a child who had been unconscious for three months gave the staff a great thrill when she began to wake, smile and nod her head. Some childhood illnesses could also affect the brain; cases of encephalitis following chicken pox were recorded.[44] In 1965, Sister Mary St Pierre was very concerned by three cases of osteomyelitis – a condition thought to have been defeated by penicillin – which seemed resistant to antibiotics.

One of the Mater Children's Hospital's early patients, Peggy Flenady, returned to the hospital as a visitor from the United States in 1966, recalling the many times she spent in the hospital in the three years following a very bad fall. She left the hospital when she was six years old – in a full-length brace and crutches – and spent considerable time at the Montrose Home for children with disabilities. She returned to the hospital when she was 15 for Dr Meehan to perform further surgery on her injuries. At last, she was free of her brace.[45] Peggy is likely to have qualified for the doll presented by an anonymous donor to the girl who spent the longest time in hospital in any year. The doll had appeared annually since the hospital's foundation and continued to be presented in the late 1960s.[46]

Although fewer children needed to remain in hospital as long as Peggy Flenady, the Mater Children's Hospital was still the most rapidly expanding part of the Mater campus in the late 1960s. Patients came from all over Queensland and northern New South Wales. Infectious conditions – most commonly influenza and gastroenteritis – frequently spread to the staff, causing considerable strain in the wards at busy times.

In September 1969, the newspapers reported grave concern over the shortage of beds available in Brisbane's two children's hospitals. The total number of beds – 319 – was inadequate.[47] At peak times, the situation could become more than frantic. In August 1969, for instance, the Brisbane Exhibition seemed to account for 'huge crowds' – including entire families – at the Mater Children's Hospital out-patient and casualty departments. Sister Angela Mary Doyle RSM and Dr Des O'Callaghan revealed the situation in casualty on the ABC television program *Today Tonight*, setting the tone for many debates and discussions in the 1970s.[48]

Chapter 6

Phoenix Rising

No longer must the children's hospital be the Cinderella of the Queensland health system.
Professor John Rendle-Short, November 1970

In the early 1970s, the Mater Children's Hospital – and children's hospitals all over Australia – were dealing with the pressures of rapid developments in paediatrics against the background of ever-growing child populations. The 1970s were difficult years to balance these pressures. A severe economic recession in Australia in the middle years of the decade added to the challenge all hospitals faced in modernising their services to match rising public expectations. A potentially disastrous fire at the Mater Children's Hospital in 1971 could have hampered modernisation but, ironically, became the signal for the construction of the long-awaited second wing.

In 1970, within ten years of his first comprehensive 'prescription' for the Mater Children's Hospital, Professor Rendle-Short communicated even more radical ideas for the future of children's hospitals in Brisbane.[1] Brisbane, he said, would need 400 children's beds within ten years. His ideas for achieving this goal were startling: advocacy for one self-contained large hospital with good facilities, rather than two separate hospitals – the Mater Children's and the Royal Children's – on opposite sides of the Brisbane River.

This vision for the hospital included preventive health services, an important focus for the professor with his characteristic emphasis on child health, rather than illness. Services that could be included were, for example, the Maternal and Child Welfare Service, the School Health Service, the government's Child Protection Unit and, perhaps, a children's dental hospital. Such a comprehensive hospital would, he thought, be convenient for parents, referring doctors, research and university teaching.

On the other hand, two children's hospitals of equal calibre, the professor thought, delayed the implementation of a full range of paediatric services, impeded university teaching as students had to travel from one to the other, and confused referring doctors in other parts of Queensland, if they did not know which service was available at which hospital. Neither hospital, he thought, could be large enough to have comprehensive facilities of sufficiently high standard. Although it might be possible to divide the hospitals according to various services – psychiatry, neurology and neurosurgery could, for instance, be available at one but not the other – Professor Rendle-Short doubted that this would be feasible.

Many visiting specialists already served both hospitals, easing the way for an amalgamation of the two children's hospitals administratively, while maintaining a physical separation. Full-time staff could also rotate from one hospital to the other, encouraging a free interchange of expertise. An amalgamated hospital should also encourage the development of paediatric nurse training, an innovation Queensland badly needed, as it was the only Australian state without it.

Professor Rendle-Short introduced an enticing thought: the Mater could build the major children's hospital in Queensland and the majority of university teaching could be done there. At the very least, he suggested, the Mater should create a large, efficient out-patient department with a 'day' ward to accommodate patients who did not need to stay overnight. It should also be equipped with comprehensive ancillary services, canteens, car parks and, perhaps, a few motel-type rooms where mothers could stay with their children. The professor's emphasis on improving out-patient facilities did not surprise the Sister Administrator, Sister Angela Mary Doyle RSM. She was also appalled at the crowded conditions in the existing out-patient department and said, 'I could go through the floor with shame'.[2]

The efficiency of a complex hospital on the professor's model would depend on well-coordinated services, a large secretarial staff and a first-class ancillary staff in all the therapies, radiology and pathology. Although the professor dismissed his plan as 'random thoughts', rather than 'informed or definite opinions', future events revealed the prescience of his suggestions.

Professor Rendle-Short saw some advantage in the disappointment that only one half of the planned hospital could be completed when the hospital was originally built: the second half 'would be outmoded and impractical if built to the same design as the 1931 wing'. The new nursery and operating theatre – completed in the 1960s – were not sufficient to address the 'dramatic changes in the management of sick children' in the previous decade. The profile of child illness was changing significantly. Illnesses such as osteomyelitis, poliomyelitis, and meningitis were far less common than they had been in the immediate post-war years.

A hospital with acute and subacute wards, rather than the conventional division into medical and surgical wards, was more appropriate in the 1970s. The Mater had already implemented this acute–subacute system in the new nursery. Such a change would also facilitate modern treatment for older children. The turnover of patients was more rapid; surgical patients were leaving hospital much earlier than had once been the case. A specialised surgical ward could be nearly empty, for example, at the same time as a medical ward was bulging at the seams during an epidemic.

The Mater Children's Hospital casualty department was also in the spotlight. Professor Rendle-Short recommended an entirely new combined casualty and out-patient block, perhaps replacing the old timber 'Queenslander' house adjacent to the hospital that accommodated the adult out-patient department and pharmacy. The slow floor-by-floor construction of the Mater Mothers' Hospital had, he thought, provided a suitable model: one floor of the new building could be constructed with additional floors added when funds became available. This building would also be suitable for an intensive care ward. Professor Rendle-Short ended his suggestions with a ringing plea on behalf of Queensland children: 'No longer must the children's hospital be the Cinderella of the Queensland health system' and continued:

> Whatever action the Mater administration takes with regard to increasing children's services at the present time is of far reaching importance and could well determine the whole course of paediatrics in the State of Queensland for the next hundred years or so.[3]

New ideas in paediatrics were discussed many times at the Mater in the 1970s. Dr Alan Dugdale, a former senior lecturer in the University of Queensland Department of Child Health who became inaugural professor of paediatrics at the University of Malaysia in 1967, addressed a meeting at the Mater in November 1970.[4] It was imperative, Dr Dugdale said, that children's hospitals become more like general medical centres, extending their reach into the community, rather than restricting their services to in-patient care. There was a very good reason for this approach: 'Repeatedly the hospital treats a child for sickness and returns the child to the sub-standard environment that caused the sickness'. Community orientation would, however, require increased services in social work, care at home and extensive out-patient facilities. Employing semi-retired general practitioners in out-patient clinics, as was the practice in New Zealand, was a suggestion in harmony with community outreach.

The visiting medical staff was also aware of the challenges confronting the hospital. In a letter to the Sisters, the president of the Mater Children's Hospital Honorary Medical Staff Association, Dr Steve Clark Ryan, set out his views. Reflecting on the development of paediatrics as a distinct specialty since the Second World War, he thought the community was placing increasing value on child health. Nevertheless, there was a problem in Queensland: government money was spent where votes could be attracted and, for that reason, the lion's share of resources was allocated to adult hospitals and repatriation services for members of the armed services. In Clark Ryan's opinion, resource starvation had allowed the Royal Children's Hospital to become outdated and the Mater Children's Hospital to languish. The new – rapidly overwhelmed – casualty block completed in the early 1960s had been the only major extension to the hospital since 1931.[5]

Dr John Eckert, appointed paediatric supervisor in 1971, saw the Mater Children's Hospital's needs in the context of both the rising standards of medical care in the community and the growing population on Brisbane's south side. The situation in the overcrowded casualty and out-patient departments worried him: 'Out-patients ... wait in crowded corridors, to be interviewed and examined in noisy cubicles, often with two doctors working side by side sharing the same table'.[6] The cramped X-ray and physiotherapy departments did not match modern standards. There was, he thought, a need for more public beds for orthopaedic and surgical patients and more beds for 'intermediate' patients – children whose parents paid a fee for treatment by their chosen specialist. The planned increase in ear, nose and throat surgery would require a separate ward. The current waiting time for ear, nose and throat treatment – nine to 12 months – was unacceptable. Eckert also advocated a separate intensive care area, an anaesthetic recovery area and a larger section where children with gastroenteritis could be nursed in isolation.

Dr Eckert also identified emerging needs, which became more obvious and more urgent as the 1970s progressed – wards for adolescents, in-patient facilities for children with psychiatric disorders, wards for 'day' patients who needed only limited time in hospital to recuperate after simple procedures, occupational therapy rooms with a play area and, in Brisbane's hot, humid climate, air-conditioning throughout. A modern records department was urgently needed to track patient care efficiently and to provide necessary data for research.

Dr Ray Tiernan, a visiting paediatrician, reported that the government statistician expected Brisbane's child population to double between 1970 and 1990.[7] Although the trend towards day and out-patient treatment would reduce the need for in-patient beds, the two children's hospitals would, nevertheless, be inadequate. The government, as far as he could see, had no plans to rectify the situation. As well as a much larger out-patient department, Dr Tiernan thought a specialised day hospital would be necessary. On the other hand, if sophisticated children's wards were included in major district hospitals, the number of patients seeking routine treatment at the specialised children's hospitals might decline. There was another anomaly that Dr Tiernan thought could be corrected: all treatment for children with heart conditions occurred at The Prince Charles Hospital at Chermside on Brisbane's northern edge, but some cardiac and thoracic procedures could be undertaken at the Mater Children's Hospital. He also hoped for a large research department to stimulate evidence-based practice, energise clinicians and attract top-quality staff not to mention better funding from external sources.

The Mater's long-serving paediatrician, David Jackson, and a more recent addition, Neville Anderson, appointed in the 1960s, were frustrated that the $9,000,000 building program earmarked for the Mater Adult Hospital would do nothing for the children's hospital, where the most rapidly increasing demand existed.[8] They maintained that if the Mater Children's Hospital or the Mater Mothers' Hospital closed, the result would be chaos. This might not be the case if the Mater Adult Hospital no longer existed as it 'merely duplicated', on a smaller scale, services available at the nearby Princess Alexandra Hospital, but the Mater Children's Hospital provided a service that was 'unique and manifestly in real demand'. They also believed that a large children's out-patient area was necessary and wanted it to be the first stage of a 'new and comprehensive children's hospital' adjacent to – and possibly connected with – the Mater Mothers' Hospital. This would, they said, emphasise that the 'role of the Sisters of Mercy in the community would increasingly be in the care of mothers and children'.

The nursing staff also took the opportunity to make their own suggestions. The matron, Sister Mary St Pierre McCormack RSM, believing that children should be treated out of sight of other children, was concerned about privacy in crowded areas. As well as treatment rooms, she also wanted playrooms and was concerned about a practical issue: the existing incinerator was 'not hygienic and soot blew over children and their beds'. The matron also suggested an amenities block for staff who didn't live at the hospital, a recognition of the change from the traditional requirement that nursing staff live at the hospital. A cafeteria, she thought, had also become necessary – parents and families spent more time at the hospital with the introduction of much more generous visiting hours.[9] Sister Marie Fitzgerald RSM suggested a childminding centre for the well children of visiting parents.[10]

On 31 January 1971, Sister Mary St Pierre McCormack completed her many years in charge of the Mater Children's Hospital. Sister Mary Dorothea Sheehan RSM succeeded her as nursing superintendent, as the former role of matron became known.

Although her appointment as nursing superintendent coincided with the beginning of a period of rapid development in medical specialisation and technology, Sister Mary Dorothea maintained the tradition of humane, expert nursing. She was rarely desk-bound and continued to take a pastoral and nursing interest in the children. She believed that 'humanity will always be the most important part of nursing because nursing is human caring'. 'Sister Dot', as Sister Mary Dorothea was invariably known, kept toys for visiting children in her office, where a notice on the wall read: 'happiness is not perfect until it is shared'.

The nursing standards maintained and developed during Sister Mary Dorothea's regime were recognised more widely. The anaesthetist Professor Tess Brophy later wrote:

I look back with great affection on my time at the Mater Children's Hospital and the development of paediatric anaesthesia in Queensland. I have said many times that the nursing at the Mater Children's Hospital was the best I have ever seen.[11]

> YVONNE MARY SHEEHAN was born at Warwick on the Darling Downs and completed her nurse training at the Mater in 1940, after entering the Sisters of Mercy in 1938 and taking the religious name Mary Dorothea. Sister Mary Dorothea regarded her time working at St Vincent's Orphanage as very important training for her years at the Mater Children's Hospital, where many children had social problems of various kinds. 'Sister Dot', as she was affectionately known, joined the children's hospital staff in 1961 and worked in almost all departments. She studied nursing administration at the College of Nursing in 1970 and initiated post-graduate paediatric nurse training at the Mater. The Australian College of Children & Young People's Nurses named a scholarship in her honour. In 1985, she became the first nurse to receive an award from the Paediatric Society of Queensland for her 'meritorious contribution towards the betterment of the health and welfare of children'. Sister Mary Dorothea became a Member of the Order of the British Empire in 1987 and received an Advance Australia award in 1988. She retired in 1986 and died on 9 July 1999.[12]

The Sisters' leadership, Professor Brophy said, developed that standard. Sister Mary Colette Anderson RSM was clinical supervisor and deputy matron.

> EILEEN ANDERSON was born in Roma in South West Queensland in 1923. Both her parents died when Eileen was very young and she was cared for by the Sisters at St Vincent's Home for Children (formerly known as St Vincent's Orphanage) in Nudgee. Eileen Anderson commenced her nurse training at the Mater in 1945 and entered the Sisters of Mercy in 1948. As Sister Mary Colette, she returned to the Mater in 1950 and began
>
> *continued overleaf*

> 36 years of tireless work at the Mater Children's Hospital. Her sense of humour was legendary and she communicated effortlessly with the children. Sister Mary Colette was almost as well known for her beautiful embroidery and crochet and the fruit cakes and jams she produced for fundraising events. Following her official 'retirement' in 1986, Sister Mary Colette worked in pastoral care for eight years; she frequently stayed all night with the parents of a very ill or dying child. Sister Mary Colette Anderson died on 10 August 2006.[13]

Sister Mary Dorothea and Sister Mary Colette had several ideas for the development of the hospital: a special plaster room for children with fractures and moving the ear, nose and throat theatre to create space for a larger out-patient area. 'Sister Dot' also recommended moving children from the casualty area without taking them past waiting children and their parents and finding a private space for parents when a child died.[14]

The Sister Administrator, Sister Angela Mary Doyle RSM, was aware of the serious shortcomings at the Mater Children's Hospital, but these were only some of the challenges confronting her. She reported in 1971 that 'the point is now reached where nearly every section of the hospital has to be ... renovated, extended or even completely replaced' – at the formidable cost of $15,000,000. Sister Angela Mary did not let her catalogue of deficiencies rest; she had a plan, to be accomplished in stages over ten years, prepared by the Sisters' architect, Harry Chapman.[15]

The plan drew on the ideas put forward by the Mater Children's Hospital staff and Professor Rendle-Short. Stage 1 involved relocating the adult out-patient department and the pharmacy from the old Queenslander house on the southern side of Mater Children's Hospital and replacing it with a three-storey extension to the children's hospital, creating a new casualty department with an improved ambulance entry, a new X-ray department and an additional 20 beds. This, however, would be a purely interim measure until a completely new Mater Children's Hospital could be constructed on the other side of the campus, close to the Mater Mothers' Hospital.[16] Future planning also explored the possibility of incorporating the Mater Children's Hospital into the adult hospital. This, Sister Angela believed, was becoming a trend in paediatrics. In the Mater's case, such a combined facility would bring a children's hospital physically closer to the obstetric hospital.[17]

Some promise of financial assistance from government came only after years of tense negotiations. The Sisters' priority was major modernisation of the Mater Adult Hospital, struggling in a building that had been little changed for decades. In 1968, Cabinet had approved a subsidy of $2,453,333 towards the $9,000,000 needed to redevelop the adult hospital.[18] There was no provision for the children's hospital and the Mater's overdraft was growing.[19] The only hope for rejuvenation of the Mater Children's Hospital lay in greater government generosity.

In 1971, Sister Angela Mary pounced on the Health Minister's announcement that the government intended to spend $100,000,000 on public hospitals. What provision, she wanted to know, had the government made for the Mater? Sister Angela Mary was blunt: 'The Mater can no longer go on as a "private" hospital providing a free public hospital service. This issue is as vital and fundamental as that'.[20] She reminded the Health Minister, Douglas Tooth, that the Mater hospitals had been built by 'charity' and that private citizens, some with international reputations, reacted with:

… dismay and incredulity that we were attempting to raise from
public charity the amount of approximately $9,000,000 for a minimum
capital development necessary to cope with the pressing demands by
the public.[21]

To illustrate, Sister Angela Mary pointed out that the Mater Children's Hospital dealt with 30 per cent more trauma patients than the Royal Children's Hospital, and asked a pertinent question: 'Is a $15,000,000 outlay too much to consider in the light of 60 long unsubsidised years?'

The most immediate needs were increased capacity in diagnostic services, modernised adult in-patient accommodation and an enlarged Mater Children's Hospital. The plan for coordinated services between the adult and children's hospitals would cost $14,000,000 over ten years. The government should, therefore, abandon its policy of providing a subsidy only for new beds: the Mater's proposal was not expansion, but provision of 'good facilities to care for patients properly'.

On the very day Sister Angela Mary wrote her plea to the Health Minister – 12 May 1971 – fire, the horror of all hospitals, broke out at the

Mater Children's Hospital at midday. The fire erupted in the ceiling of the University of Queensland section above the kitchen, only ten metres from the babies' nursery. Black smoke billowed, the police closed all surrounding streets to allow the fire brigade easy access and 119 children were evacuated. The evacuation – accomplished in ten minutes – was no mean feat: some patients were very ill, many patients could not walk, and others had to be carried with nurses holding their drip bottles aloft. The evacuation was accomplished without a single injury or one case of smoke inhalation.

It might have been so much worse: some children were on oxygen, which could have exploded near sparks or flames. There were instances of real heroism.[22] Sister Mary Lea Kelly RSM went back into her nursery ward and, in the dense smoke, put her hands into every cot to make sure that no baby had been overlooked. In the operating theatre, Dr Des McGuckin was operating on a tiny baby with oesophageal atresia, with Dr Tess Brophy administering the anaesthetic. The theatre was plunged into darkness when the power failed but, fortunately, the lights came on again when the emergency generator sprang into life.[23] The operation continued successfully against the background of wailing sirens. The baby recovered in the nursery at the Mater Mothers' Hospital.

Children who were not well enough to go home were transferred to the Royal Children's Hospital, to a ward at the Mater Private Hospital or to the television room at the nurses' quarters. Fortunately, the damage was confined to the university section and most of the hospital was re-opened the next day.[24] The death of Stan Anderson, the Mater's superintendent of works, from a heart attack on the day after the fire was the most tragic result of the fire. As Sister Angela Mary said, 'a building can be replaced; Mr Anderson cannot'.[25]

The fire was extensively covered in newspapers throughout Australia. Press coverage stimulated many offers of help ranging from engineering companies offering to replace damaged equipment and food companies offering provisions.[26] Significantly, media coverage generated much greater public awareness of the hospital, its work and the challenges it faced. On the very day of the fire, for instance, Brisbane's *Telegraph* newspaper cited arresting statistics: more than 65,000 casualty attendances each year and 32,000 out-patients examined and treated in the clinics. Not to be outdone, the *Courier-Mail* informed the public that the three previous annual reports had highlighted the pressure on the Mater Children's Hospital, information that had apparently fallen on deaf government ears.

The government relented. In July 1971, the Health Minister issued the glad news that the government now recognised 'the Mater Public Hospital as filling an important role in the free Public Hospital system of Queensland and in its association with Queensland University in the teaching of medical students'.[27] In future, capital subsidies would not simply relate to the provision of additional public beds, but would take into account the whole range of accommodation and services associated with the conduct of a public hospital and out-patient service.

The need to expand and develop diagnostic services recognised the expansion in the range and accuracy of pathology tests and radiological investigations since the Second World War. The government subsidy was increased to $2 for each $3 of approved expenditure. It was not, however, an open cheque: development had to be staged and was only for services that were 'integral and contributory' in the development and provision of hospital services.[28]

Increased government beneficence introduced a term that frequently brought tremors to the hospital world in ensuing decades: rationalisation. There was to be no duplication of services. Sister Angela Mary reassured the minister that 'It was not our intention ... to duplicate any unusual or highly expensive specialties, especially in the adult section'. She explained further, 'we see ourselves as playing an important part in obstetrics, possibly gynaecology, certainly paediatrics, and that we have a limited but definite role in adult public hospital medicine'. The minister was 'particularly pleased' to hear this and said 'that it would greatly strengthen his case when he presented it to Cabinet'.

The frank exchange of views between the government and the Mater continued. The Mater Children's Hospital had considerable difficulty in accommodating children with infectious diseases. They were no longer transferred to the Royal Children's Hospital because, as Sister Angela Mary told the minister, 'They were unhappy about taking any patients that they felt belonged to us'. She also told him about needing a special piece of equipment to remove a foreign body from a ten-month-old baby – an instrument the government had neglected to supply – and which the Royal Children's Hospital had refused to lend. The equipment was eventually borrowed from a private doctor. 'Mr Tooth remarked that these are the things that never come to his ears. We have, subsequently, made a further appeal for this essential equipment'.[29]

Cracks of light began to lighten the funding gloom. Government funding – $2,500,000 – was approved for new adults' and children's out-patient departments; further funding was possible for a second building to accommodate diagnostic radiology, pathology, operating theatres, a central sterilising department, an intensive care unit and a pharmacy.[30]

A lurid description in the *Courier-Mail* demonstrated that the Mater Children's Hospital needed urgent relief. A single day, 20 October 1971, was described as a 'sublime and ridiculous day'. More than 350 people had been packed into the 'poky' out-patient department for orthopaedic; ear, nose and throat; skin; and general medical clinics. The narrow corridors, as well as the waiting room, were jammed; an overflow of patients waited outside the hospital. In one room, measuring seven by fourteen feet, a doctor worked surrounded by 13 people – members of staff and patients. Five doctors were working non-stop in casualty. The situation was so bad that, if there was no emergency patient at the casualty area, four children were treated in the emergency room. They – and their doctors – had to move very quickly if a very ill child arrived for emergency treatment. It was not uncommon for ward beds to overflow into corridors and doctors' desks summarily moved to make room for beds. The casualty section was one-quarter the necessary size and the out-patient department was half the necessary size, with consequent risk of cross-infection.[31]

The physiotherapy department, where physiotherapists were treating four girls with spina bifida when the journalist visited, was described as 'bedroom size'. One of the physiotherapists commented that 'an Indian Army tent would be an improvement'. An intensive care unit and a burns unit were also mentioned as urgent requirements. Sister Angela Mary was direct in her view: 'I am past the point of shame. Something has to be done'. As the population on the south side of Brisbane was expected to 'explode' from 282,641 in 1961 to 530,130 in 1981, it was clear that the Mater Children's Hospital would never be able to cope, particularly as about one-third of the population would be under 15 years of age.[32]

Forced to respond, the minister replied that accommodation in the wards was adequate, but out-patient and casualty departments were overstretched at both Brisbane children's hospitals.[33] The Royal Children's Hospital was also struggling. Its superintendent, Dr DC Fison, reported that his out-patient department was so congested that doctors couldn't hear children's heartbeats. Soundproofing and a day hospital were urgently needed at the Royal Children's Hospital, where the hospital buildings inconveniently flowed down the hill, connected by a series of flights of stairs.

The needs of Brisbane's two children's hospitals were, however, greater than the government's capacity to finance additions and renovations. Telethons, usually featuring Sister Mary Dorothea – a natural 'performer' – continued to be successful, but more was needed. It was the perfect time for a door-to-door appeal. In October 1971, the *Courier-Mail* and the *Telegraph* announced a new Children's Hospitals Appeal to absorb the *Courier-Mail* Toy Fund, which had provided cheering gifts to children in hospital since 1910.[34] Thus began the Mater's long association with the managing director of Queensland Newspapers, Reg (later Sir Reginald) Leonard, and the *Courier-Mail's* appeal, which benefited both children's hospitals.

The *Courier-Mail* recognised that no state government could ever produce the amount of money that the children's hospitals needed and that this 'has become a matter for every citizen's conscience and help'. The new appeal aimed to provide equipment and funding for research; the causes and treatment of cystic fibrosis were mentioned particularly. The *Courier-Mail* started the ball rolling with a $5,000 donation and encouraged Brisbane people to take advantage of tax deductibility for all donations over $2. The *Courier's* sister newspapers, the *Sunday Mail* and the *Telegraph*, country and suburban newspapers and two radio stations – 4BK and 4AK – joined in.[35]

The Children's Hospitals Appeal soon bore fruit. Within a few months, the Mater Children's Hospital had acquired two 'IVAC' intravenous drip control systems to regulate the flow of intravenous feeding for premature and very small babies,[36] and was eagerly awaiting the arrival of an operating microscope and the first paediatric neurosurgery operating table in Queensland, products of its first allocation of $20,244.[37] The appeal kept on giving: special intensive care recovery cots for children injured in road accidents, an 'Oxydom' tent to ease breathing after operations and in serious illnesses, a respirator to revive children after drowning accidents, nebulisers to support children with asthma, a cardiac oscilloscope, a cryosurgical unit and portacots to transport very ill, tiny babies.[38]

Despite these acquisitions, the Mater Children's Hospital continued to struggle. In December 1971, the green light flashed for the second three-storey wing to complete the original 1931 scheme.[39] Tenders were called in May 1973. The prospect was exciting: the new, much larger, casualty department, with its own six-bed observation ward, was designed so that a child could be admitted out of sight of other children and be taken directly either to the operating theatre or a ward.[40] The much larger ground floor was allocated to the admissions office, out-patients – with a much larger waiting area – the pharmacy and physiotherapy.

There were to be 22 beds in the nursery, 28 in the original surgical ward, 32 in the medical ward and 45 in the new building. There would be two beds in the area near the operating theatre for children with burns. There would also be four intensive care beds near the lift, piped oxygen, suction and air-conditioning in the new wing. There would also be ten beds for fee-paying patients, a mixed medical and surgical ward with 15 beds, a six-bed casualty observation ward, an isolation unit, a playroom and a childminding room for 'well' children. A room for distressed relatives was furnished by the Mt Gravatt Rotary Club.[41]

Flooring – apart from carpet tiles in the main entrance and some waiting rooms – would be practical vinyl tiles. The needs of the staff were also included in the plan with provision for additional toilet facilities. No detail was overlooked; there were plans for the design of the internal signs, the colours of laminex benchtops, light fittings and furnishings right down to the wastepaper baskets.[42] The plan to build a new children's hospital near the Mater Mothers' Hospital was deferred – for almost 30 years.

Groundwork for the new building was underway by September 1973, but the project struck trouble. There were many casualties in the serious recession blighting the Australian economy in the mid-1970s, including the construction company, KD Morris & Sons, engaged on the Mater project. The firm went into liquidation in October 1974. Work stopped, and it appeared that it would be a very long time before the new wing would be completed.[43]

Fortunately, Underwood Constructions took over and, in August 1975, the new wing was completed.[44] The Health Minister, Dr Llew Edwards, opened the new wing on 9 March 1976, marking the completion of a plan first conceived almost 50 years earlier.

A 'flyover' link between the Mater Children's and Adult hospitals, funded partly by the Children's Hospitals Appeal, was completed with much less stress and drama. Work on the flyover began in February 1973. The flyover, named for Sir Reginald Leonard, was designed to address fire brigade requirements for additional fire escapes from both the adult and children's hospitals and to accommodate important medical facilities: the electroencephalograph and electrocardiograph machines and an important new addition, Sister Regis Mary Dunne's cytogenetics department.[45] Cytogenetics offered the prospect of diagnosing whether or not abnormalities were hereditary. The cytogenetics department was a taste of the rich range of future possibilities.

Chapter 7

Future Visions

Nursing cannot be regarded simply as an art, simply concerned with the physical care of the patient, for nursing is also a science in a scientific age.

Sister Eileen (Mary Gerarda) Pollard RSM, 1971

The long-awaited completion of the second wing of the Mater Children's Hospital transformed its physical fabric. Changes in the hospital's paediatric services in the 1970s were not as visible, but were transformative.

Sisters of Mercy, in their pristine white habits, were no longer as dominant a presence in the wards. In a world of burgeoning career opportunities for women and the developing women's movement, many young women who might once have entered religious orders found worthwhile paths in the secular world. In the aftermath of a decree of the Second Vatican Council, which instructed them to be equipped to interact with the contemporary world, many women in religious orders also looked for other opportunities.[1]

The evolution to the employment of greater numbers of lay nurses had a significant impact on the Mater's finances: religious Sisters received small stipends; secular nurses were paid salaries at award rates. At the same time, the nurse training system changed considerably. Pressure also grew for improvement in the training of paediatric registrars and senior resident medical officers.

As always, the hospital's effectiveness depended on the skill and dedication of the staff. Nurses were in great demand at the Mater Children's Hospital, indeed at all hospitals on the Mater campus. In 1973, when Sister Rosalie Lewis RN – a future director of nursing at the Mater Children's Hospital – was interviewed for a part-time job at the Mater Private Hospital, Sister Mary St Gabriel Corbett RSM concluded the interview with a request: 'Sister, can you start tonight?'[2]

Obtaining and retaining sufficient numbers of trained staff and nurse trainees was a constant pressure. Nursing was still an essentially female profession but, when university courses became more accessible in the 1960s and 1970s, women pursued a wider range of careers than the traditional office work, teaching and nursing. Opportunities for further education also expanded in nursing. In 1971, Sister Marie Fitzgerald RSM was awarded an Australian Nursing Federation scholarship to study ward management at the Royal College of Nursing, Australia (RCNA) (now Australian College of Nursing) in Melbourne.[3] She was one of several members of the Mater Children's Hospital staff to undertake advanced courses, which helped them to keep abreast of developments in patient care, curriculum and fields such as occupational health and safety.[4]

Newly qualified nurses in the middle and later years of the 1970s had been trained differently from their predecessors. A revised nurse training curriculum was introduced in 1970, reducing training time from four years to three, a change that had a considerable impact in hospitals. Fourth-year nurses – almost as qualified as fully trained nurses, but less expensive to employ – had been very important in maintaining staffing levels economically.

This was not the only change. The new curriculum was designed to enable nursing to reflect developments in medicine. The introduction of patient assignment and team nursing to replace task-oriented nursing brought many changes at ward level. No longer were tasks such as bedpans and bathing allocated to the most junior nurses. In the new system, nurses in teams were responsible for the total care of the patients assigned to them. There was concern at all the Mater hospitals and, probably, in all Queensland hospitals, that increased clinical supervision and bedside teaching was necessary, as well as considerable support and education for existing trained staff adapting to the new system.[5]

The final group in the four-year course completed their training in June 1972, but there was a shortage of senior experienced nurses. Qualified nurses who had left the profession – often for marriage and motherhood –

were a valuable, badly needed resource. Courses to bring them up to date with modern nursing were held regularly at the Mater hospitals.

Nursing became steadily more sophisticated. Research was increasingly emphasised, particularly work-study projects that explored ways of offering optimal care at the bedside; administrative tasks were to be left to the charge sister in each ward.[6] As the Senior Nurse Educator Sister Eileen Pollard RSM put it: 'Nursing cannot be regarded simply as an art, simply concerned with the physical care of the patient, for nursing is also a science in a scientific age'.[7] Nurses in two new categories appeared in the wards. 'Hospital assistants', as they were known, performed non-nursing duties; a special course trained nursing aides to perform some nursing duties.[8]

Increasing specialisation in paediatrics put additional pressure on general nurse training. Even in the late 1970s, the paediatric content in the general nursing course was disappointing. Although many principles of nursing applied equally to patients from birth to old age, children were very different patients. Paediatrics was a different, highly complex medical and nursing discipline. Some childhood conditions were not encountered in adults and the effect of hospitalisation was very different for child patients and their families. Clinicians needed particular awareness of the social and psychological factors that affected sick children. Patient-assignment nursing encouraged a closer working relationship with the allied health professions.

A course in paediatric nursing was essential.[9] Before such a course for qualified nurses could be introduced, experts on the government's Paediatric Advisory Committee engaged in considerable debate on the nature of paediatric nursing. Some believed that a new specialist course would turn nurses into social workers; others thought that procedures for carrying out a doctor's orders were only part of a nurse's responsibilities and that nursing should be directed towards helping people to cope with health problems.[10]

With the enhanced emphasis on preventive medicine in paediatrics, the role of the paediatric nurse was, Sister Marie Fitzgerald RSM thought, 'extending from the life-saving role to the supportive, educative role'.[11] Reflecting the trend to shorter hospital stays, the Paediatric Advisory Committee wanted a paediatric nursing course to instruct nurses in assisting parents to nurse children at home. There was also considerable discussion on including developmental paediatrics and the characteristics of the well child in the course.

In approving a post-basic course, Queensland's Nurses Registration Board looked at a whole range of states from wellness to illness and *vice versa*, endorsing current thinking that nurses should be able to cope with every state – a considerable change from previous ideas, which concentrated on illness.[12] Clarifying the scope of paediatric nursing was a factor in delaying the introduction of a post-basic paediatric nursing course. A range of meanings was discussed: caring for the child in hospital, or in the community as well as in hospital, keeping the child healthy, as well as attending to the sick child.[13] Even though nursing was defined as differing from medicine in its focus on caring for the patient and the family, these ideas mirrored developments in paediatric medicine generally. Aspects of the nursing 'process', covering topics such as health and illness, developmental and lifestyle phases, stress, coping strategies and adaptation to unfamiliar situations, were also part of the overall evolution of paediatrics.

Medicine was also moving towards managing patients in their whole social contexts and increasingly emphasising strategies to keep people well. No longer was the focus purely on illness and organs. New subspecialties in paediatrics had the potential to save the lives of many children who would have died in earlier decades when highly developed expertise was unavailable. Children's hospitals would need to accommodate two different cohorts: short-stay patients, for whom day hospital facilities were appropriate; and children with complex or chronic conditions, who needed lengthy hospital stays.

Assessing needs and opportunities for paediatric services on a broader scale was on the minds of policy makers in the Queensland government. The Paediatric Advisory Committee, established by the Health Minister, Dr Llew Edwards, in 1975, investigated patterns of illness among Queensland children and whether or not public health education would improve child health. Augmenting the training of doctors and members of the allied health professions was also in the committee's remit.[14]

The committee, including Dr Geoffrey Bourke as the Mater Children's Hospital representative, considered many suggestions.[15] The meeting in September 1976, for instance, reprised the concept of a single Brisbane children's hospital, which Professor Rendle-Short had promoted years earlier. In 1976, however, the committee foresaw a single hospital physically divided into two campuses and fed by peripheral paediatric units, each with 30 beds, at Redcliffe, Ipswich, Southport and Mt Gravatt. This would yield a total of 440 paediatric beds in South East Queensland. This integrated children's hospital would have its own board and a medical superintendent; all medical, nursing, paramedical and administrative staff would be completely interchangeable between the two campuses. In this model, The Prince Charles Hospital at Chermside would retain the paediatric cardiothoracic unit.[16] Although these ideas bore no fruit in the 1970s, they regularly reappeared in succeeding decades.

The inclusion of a unit of the University of Queensland Department of Child Health at the Mater Children's Hospital opened avenues for increased discussion on the way the hospital could best progress. The limited opportunities for post-graduate paediatric medical education was a major problem. The Royal Australasian College of Physicians did not believe that the Mater Children's Hospital offered registrars the necessary training to achieve full College membership.[17] More subspecialties were necessary.

Alan Dugdale, who had returned to Brisbane in 1972 as senior lecturer at the Mater unit of the Department of Child Health, echoed the view that two highly specialised children's hospitals in Brisbane, each offering all specialties, was impractical. The development of an effective children's hospital could, Dr Dugdale said, depend on improving specialties and services that would become inducements to attracting top-quality staff. A practical approach to the increasing sophistication in paediatric specialties might require an allocation of specialties between Brisbane's two children's hospitals to avoid expensive duplication. The Mater could, for instance, develop a children's renal unit in liaison with the renowned adult renal service at the nearby Princess Alexandra Hospital. Similarly, there were opportunities for a specialist respiratory unit. Any suggestion that the Mater Children's Hospital could be an annexe of the Royal Children's Hospital was unlikely to win many hearts at the Mater.

Alan Dugdale set out the options as he saw them: the Mater Children's Hospital could cease to specialise in paediatrics, but this would leave Brisbane's south side without a children's hospital; the Mater Children's Hospital could be a convalescent or 'long-stay' hospital, but there might not be sufficient need; it could be entirely a private children's hospital – and the potential existed – if the new casualty department was converted into consulting rooms. There was, he thought, great possibility in another option – a community-oriented teaching hospital.

Most Australian teaching hospitals concentrated on in-patient medicine and almost ignored preventive medicine and home care. The concentration on training to meet College requirements for specialist registration had left no space for training general practitioners, who were actually responsible for most paediatric care. The community-oriented model focused on the out-patient and casualty departments. To be successful, this model needed senior full-time paediatricians so that registrars would be sufficiently trained to satisfy the College of General Practitioners. As had Professor Rendle-Short a few years earlier, Dr Dugdale advocated the inclusion of infant welfare clinics and the School Health Service and other allied health organisations. This scheme would be unique in Australia, but there were suitable overseas models in London, and in Canada at McMaster University in Hamilton, Ontario.[18]

Doctors at the Mater Children's Hospital had similar ideas. They believed that the hospital's strengths lay in its casualty and out-patient departments, which offered a wide range of excellent experience, particularly in managing trauma, respiratory disease and gastrointestinal illnesses. There was an opportunity to offer general practitioners intensive training in these areas and, perhaps, at least one year of intensive training for paediatric registrars.[19]

In 1977, just over a year after the second wing of the Mater Children's Hospital had opened, the Mater Advisory Board appointed its own committee, chaired by the orthopaedic surgeon, Dr Tony McSweeny. It was to examine all aspects of the Mater Children's Hospital and to make recommendations for patient care, the facilities appropriate to its present and future needs, the standards and systems necessary for full accreditation of its paediatric training program, teaching programs for medical students and nurses, and ways to attract the most highly qualified staff.[20] The committee also set itself an ambitious goal: to achieve 'the greatest benefit to every individual child and to the family of that child'.[21] The committee members were the neurosurgeon Dr Leigh Atkinson; the paediatrician Dr Geoffrey Bourke; the superintendent of the children's hospital, Dr Barrie Heyworth; the director of post-graduate studies, Dr Peter O'Regan; Dr Alan Dugdale; the nursing superintendent, Sister Mary Dorothea Sheehan RSM; and the assistant to the sister administrator, Sister Geraldine Doyle RSM. The committee held weekly meetings for 16 weeks and received 42 submissions.

The committee's recommendations fell under four main headings: facilities, personnel, teaching and development. The list of facilities was long and very detailed, but contained few surprises. Flexibility was the keynote. Although some wards would retain the traditional medical–surgical division, the creation of see-through cubicles was recommended for children recovering from severe burns or neurosurgery. All wards – particularly the 27-bed orthopaedic ward – should be regarded as available to accommodate patient overflows from other wards at busy times. The committee suggested that beds for intermediate patients – those who paid a fee to choose their own specialist – could be distributed throughout the various medical and surgical wards.

The flexibility policy extended to the six-bed casualty department; day patients could occupy those beds when they were not required for emergencies. The trend towards not keeping patients in hospital overnight whenever possible was, the committee noted, creating problems in maintaining the essential patient statistics, which were the basis of the government's payments for maintaining patients in hospital. The 'bed count' was traditionally performed at midnight, but modern trends to 'day-only' admissions had rendered this methodology obsolete, to the hospital's disadvantage. On the other hand, the committee thought that the trend to day treatment could allow the hospital to reduce its bed capacity from 139 to 120. The nursery, however, should be maintained at a minimum of 24 beds.

The facilities section of the report also included a recommendation that an adolescent ward be created, perhaps in the old Ward 5 of the adult hospital, which was close to the flyover connecting the adult and children's hospitals. The Paediatric Advisory Committee had also pinpointed the dilemma that all children's hospitals faced: at what age did a child cease to be a child and should, therefore, be admitted to an adult hospital? The early years of adolescence were generally conceded to be far too early, yet admitting 14-year-olds to wards with very young children was almost as inappropriate.[22]

Compared with the new building, the original 1931 wing was tired and old-fashioned. Some parents had refused to enter the old section because it appeared so decrepit. A decade later, Director of Nursing Rosalie Lewis escorted a visitor touring the hospital who thought that a neat Nightingale ward – empty while the children were at school – was a museum.[23] The McSweeny-led committee received plenty of suggestions: improving electrical safety, adding a canteen, replacing the beds with modern mobile ones, turning the patios adjacent to the wards into play areas, repainting, re-carpeting and enlivening the decor with pictures of the childhood of Christ and examples of Australian flora and fauna on walls and ceilings. Families were not overlooked: the committee suggested that one of the Mater-owned houses in Clarence Street could become motel-type accommodation for country families.

The committee recommended extensive additions to the staff. A director of intensive care, perhaps combining this position with that of director of anaesthetics, was required, as were a plastic surgeon, a nephrologist and a cardiologist. Many more allied health professionals were also needed. In those days of developing multidisciplinary approaches, psychologists, audiologists, family therapists, social workers and play therapists – increasingly employed in children's hospitals overseas – were particularly mentioned. Instances of child abuse were increasingly reported in the 1970s and the committee thought that there should be a social worker on call, who could visit families in their own homes.

The committee also considered the touchy issue of rationalisation of paediatric services between Brisbane's two children's hospitals and saw advantages in sharing staff with the Princess Alexandra Hospital in neurosurgery and nephrology. Similarly, there would be advantages in closer collaboration with the Royal Children's Hospital on social, educational and clinical levels. The committee also referred to the notion of an Institute of Child Health, an idea that had been floated many times. However, the committee believed that 'the die is already cast for the continuance of two teaching children's hospitals in the City of Brisbane, each complete in its own right', a position the Health Minister had affirmed when he opened the new nursery in 1976.[24]

Affirmations of a future for the Mater Children's Hospital did not conflict with the development of the relationship between the hospital and the community and the strengthening of relationships with organisations caring for children with disabilities, as 'proliferations ... into many fields are essential if the hospital is to remain the central children's paediatric service for the south side of the Brisbane River'.[25] The committee's report was not, it believed, the end of assessing the hospital's future plans and recommended that a planning committee for the Mater Children's Hospital be a standing committee of the Board.

The recommendations of the 1977 committee on the need to expand the hospital's specialist staff came in a period when the staff was already rapidly growing. In 1971, Dr John Eckert, described as the 'paediatric supervisor', was the only paediatrician on the full-time staff. Geoffrey Bourke and Steve Clark Ryan were the senior honorary physicians with Malcolm Nasser and Kerry Sullivan as assistant physicians.[26] Kerry Sullivan, a graduate in medicine from the University of Queensland and a member of the Royal College of Physicians, London, succeeded John Eckert as paediatric clinical supervisor, a position renamed medical superintendent in 1976. Kerry Sullivan resigned in 1977 to enter private practice.[27]

In 1970, the honorary surgical staff included Dr Fred Leditschke of the Department of Child Health, Dr Des McGuckin, Dr Len Marriott and Dr Morgan Windsor, the honorary thoracic surgeon to both the adult and children's hospitals. At that time, there were seven formal subspecialties at the children's hospital: orthopaedics; ear, nose and throat; urology; ophthalmology; neurology; dermatology; and psychiatry. By 1977, the full-time staff had been augmented by the appointment of six paediatric registrars: PJ Egan, PJ Fletcher, KE Churchward, PPT Khoo, DC Hall and David Orme Wood, who became the first Mater paediatric registrar to achieve full membership of the Royal Australasian College of Physicians as a paediatrician. Anaesthetics and dentistry had been added to the 1970 list of hospital departments.[28] There was a major change in the orthopaedic department: Dr John Lahz, who had been part of the hospital since the beginning, retired in 1974.

The appointment of a Professor of Child Health at the Mater unit of the Department of Child Health marked an important stage in the hospital's development.[29] In 1977, when the decision to base a chair in Child Health at the Mater was made, the staff of the department at the Mater comprised Dr Alan Dugdale, the first full-time member of the academic staff; Dr John Thearle, appointed in 1973; Dr John Vance, appointed in 1976, and the psychologist Dr Heather Mohay, appointed in 1976. All were consultants to the hospital in their specialist fields: Alan Dugdale in nutrition and growth, John Thearle in neonatology, John Vance in community paediatrics and Heather Mohay in assisting children with hearing impairments.

An arduous selection process resulted in the appointment of the immunologist Yee-Hing Thong as Professor of Child Health at the Mater. He was a graduate of the University of Malaysia, and had studied in the United Kingdom and the United States.[30] Professor Thong advocated a research foundation similar to those at the Melbourne and Sydney children's hospitals.[31] He was frequently frustrated that a lack of resources impeded research at the Mater Children's Hospital, describing his laboratory as small and badly equipped. His research was constantly interrupted because he was the only immunologist at the hospital and was constantly called upon for clinical work.

In the late 1970s, the Mater Children's Hospital was envisaging the development of additional subspecialties: respiratory medicine, gastroenterology, plastic surgery, paediatric psychiatry and, possibly, endocrinology.[32] Dr Barrie Heyworth was appointed medical superintendent in August 1977. He was a graduate in medicine from the University of Manchester and a member of Royal College of Physicians, London. He had also obtained post-graduate diplomas in obstetrics, paediatrics and tropical medicine, and had worked in Gambia and Rwanda.[33] The Mater Children's Hospital achieved an important goal in the year of Barrie Heyworth's appointment: full accreditation of its training program in paediatrics. By 1980, the number of registrars had grown to ten.[34]

The registrars had plenty of work. Patient numbers grew rapidly in the late 1970s. In-patients – both public and intermediate – doubled between 1975 and 1979 to 11,631 and 1,050 respectively. Numbers presenting at casualty increased by 30 per cent in one year to 63,000, a similar increase to the number of out-patient attendances.[35] The pattern of presentations to the casualty section was examined in the 1970s. There were 62,000 casualties in 1972; the 1972 weekly average of 1,192 cases was generally maintained during the 1970s.[36]

It was a big load. Notices in three languages warned people coming to casualty that emergencies only would be seen at weekends. Even so, waiting times could be long.[37] A study of the casualty section in 1975 noted that there needed to be more training for resident medical officers in emergency work. The study revealed that many parents bringing children to casualty for comparatively minor conditions were reassured by a large institution with its facilities and resources, even though the cost of the trip to the Mater could exceed a local general practitioner's fee.[38]

About 10 per cent of all children arriving at casualty came from the suburb of Inala on Brisbane's south-western fringe. In 1971, Sister Assumpta Mary RSM, a former teacher at St Mark's Catholic Primary School at Inala, noted that parents in Inala faced particular difficulties when their children were ill or needed medicine. There were many single mothers and parents in poverty in this lower socio-economic area. In the days before general practitioner fees attracted a government rebate, they had little option but to travel many kilometres to the Mater by public transport. Sister Assumpta Mary suggested that this arduous trek deterred many mothers from seeking help early. Consequently, their children were frequently too sick to be treated as out-patients and were admitted to hospital. She suggested that the Mater Children's Hospital establish a mobile unit in Inala or, preferably, a day clinic or small hospital.[39]

In 1971, the government had acquired land in Inala for a community health centre, a proposal that interested the Sisters of Mercy.[40] The Inala initiative would directly link their acute health services to the care of the poor in their own community and to a variety of welfare projects funded by the Commonwealth in Inala.[41] There was an element of self-interest: involvement with Inala could ensure that patients would continue to be directed to the Mater, even if another general hospital was opened on Brisbane's south side.[42]

Children in country areas – and their parents – also faced great difficulties when serious illness or accidents came their way. There were many frightening stories of aircraft dashing to Brisbane from regional and rural Queensland with dangerously ill children needing urgent surgery, as well as sad stories of children spending long periods away from home.[43] The baby boy who was in the operating theatre when the fire at the hospital started in 1971 came from Rockhampton. Later that year, his mother said that she couldn't afford to come to Brisbane to visit him as she had several other children. A kind donor made it possible for the whole family to visit.[44] The kindness of a stranger also played a large part in bringing a baby from Thailand to Brisbane for throat surgery.[45]

In the late 1970s, the Paediatric Advisory Committee sought to bring expert care closer to country people with a scheme for paediatricians to visit regional centres. Mater paediatricians offered to visit Warwick, Stanthorpe and Goondiwindi, and hoped to include Inglewood and Texas in the country scheme. The University of Queensland staff was prepared to join the scheme and agreed to hold educational sessions for country general practitioners. The Director-General of Health thought that a benefit of a post-basic course in paediatric nursing could have the side effect of making nurse practitioners available in country areas.[46]

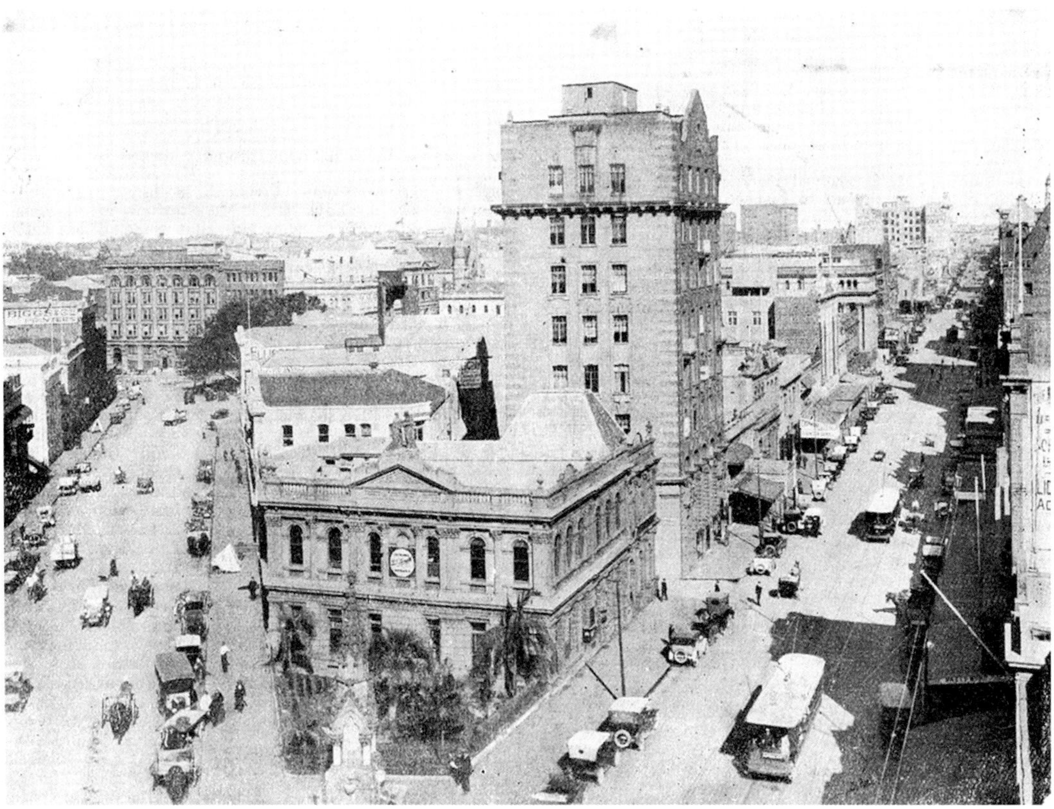

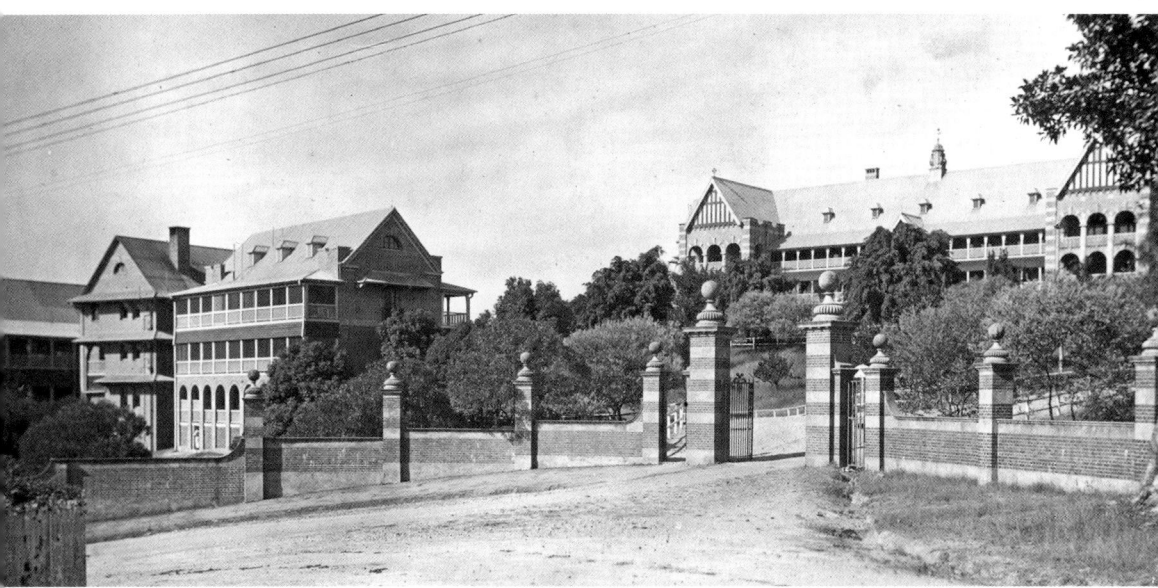

Brisbane in 1925, looking south from the corner of Eagle and Queen streets.
State Library of Queensland

The Mater campus in the 1920s, showing St Mary's Nurses Home in the foreground and the Mater Private Hospital at the top of the hill.

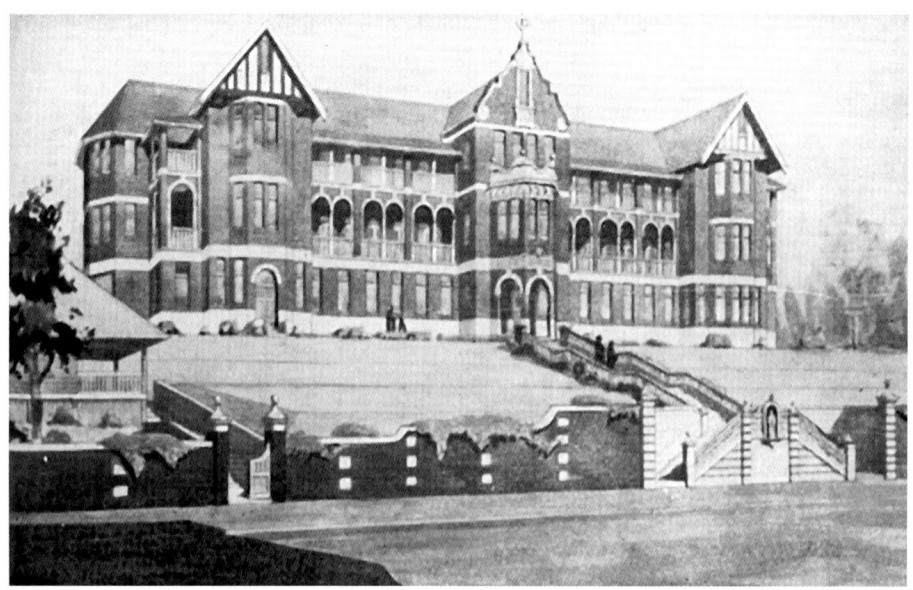

The original design for the Mater Children's Hospital.

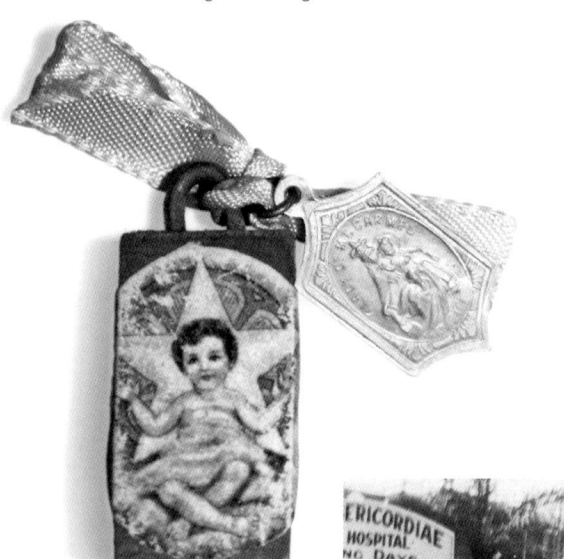

The miniature brick, decorated with a picture of a child, given to donors to the Mater Children's Hospital in the 1920s and 1930s.

BELOW: Mater nurses with the banner used to publicise a fundraising appeal in 1926.

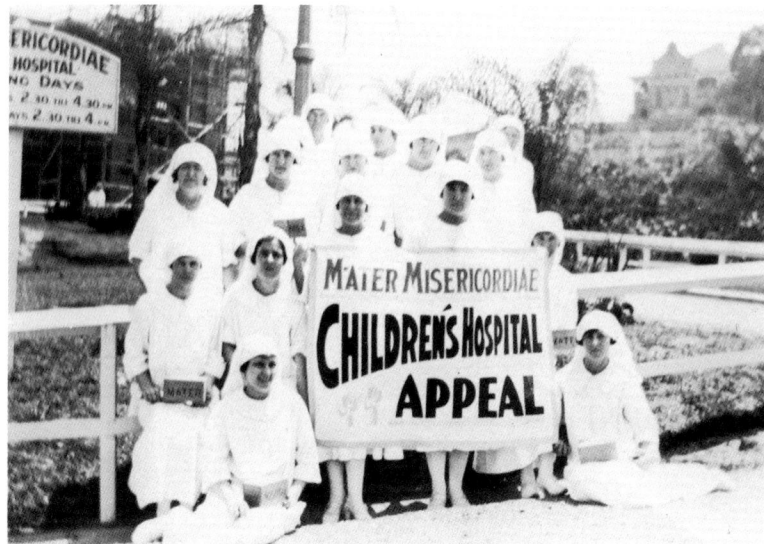

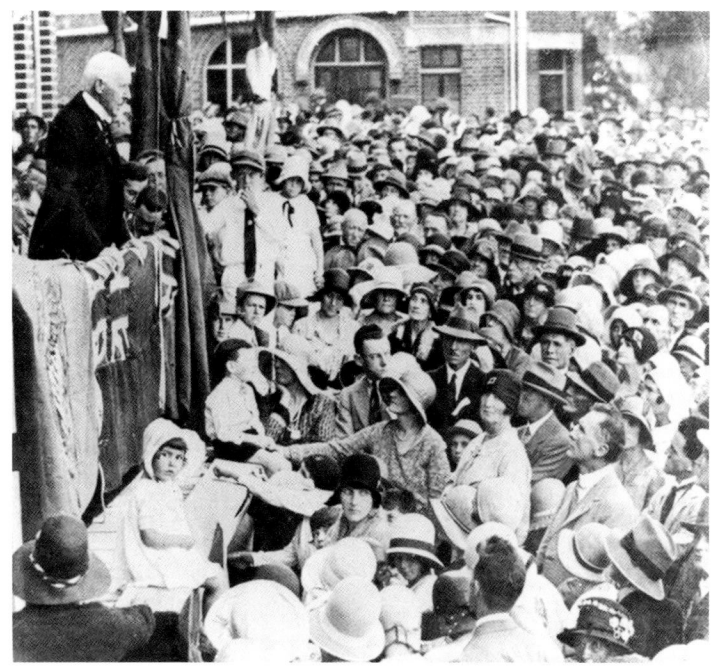

Crowds gathered in the hospital grounds to celebrate the opening of the Mater Children's Hospital in 1931.

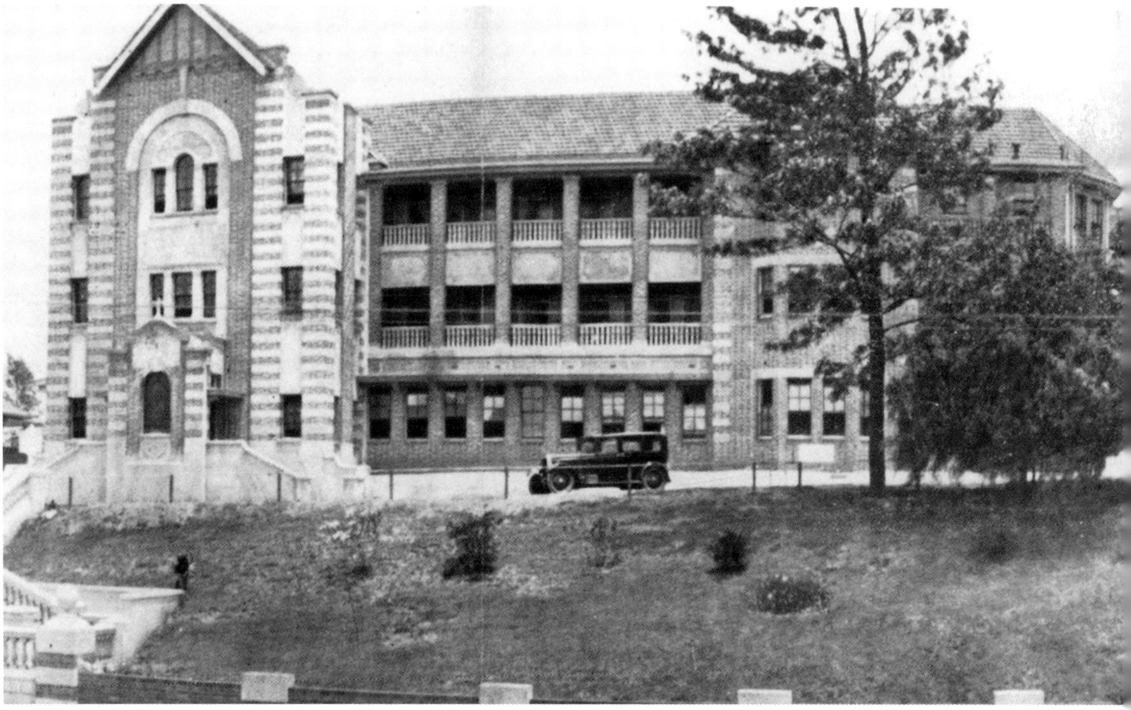

The Mater Children's Hospital was different from the original plan, but the distinctive stairs to Annerley Road can be glimpsed at far left.

FOLLOWING PAGES: A tidy Nightingale ward at the Mater Children's Hospital in the 1930s, with cots neatly arranged along the walls.

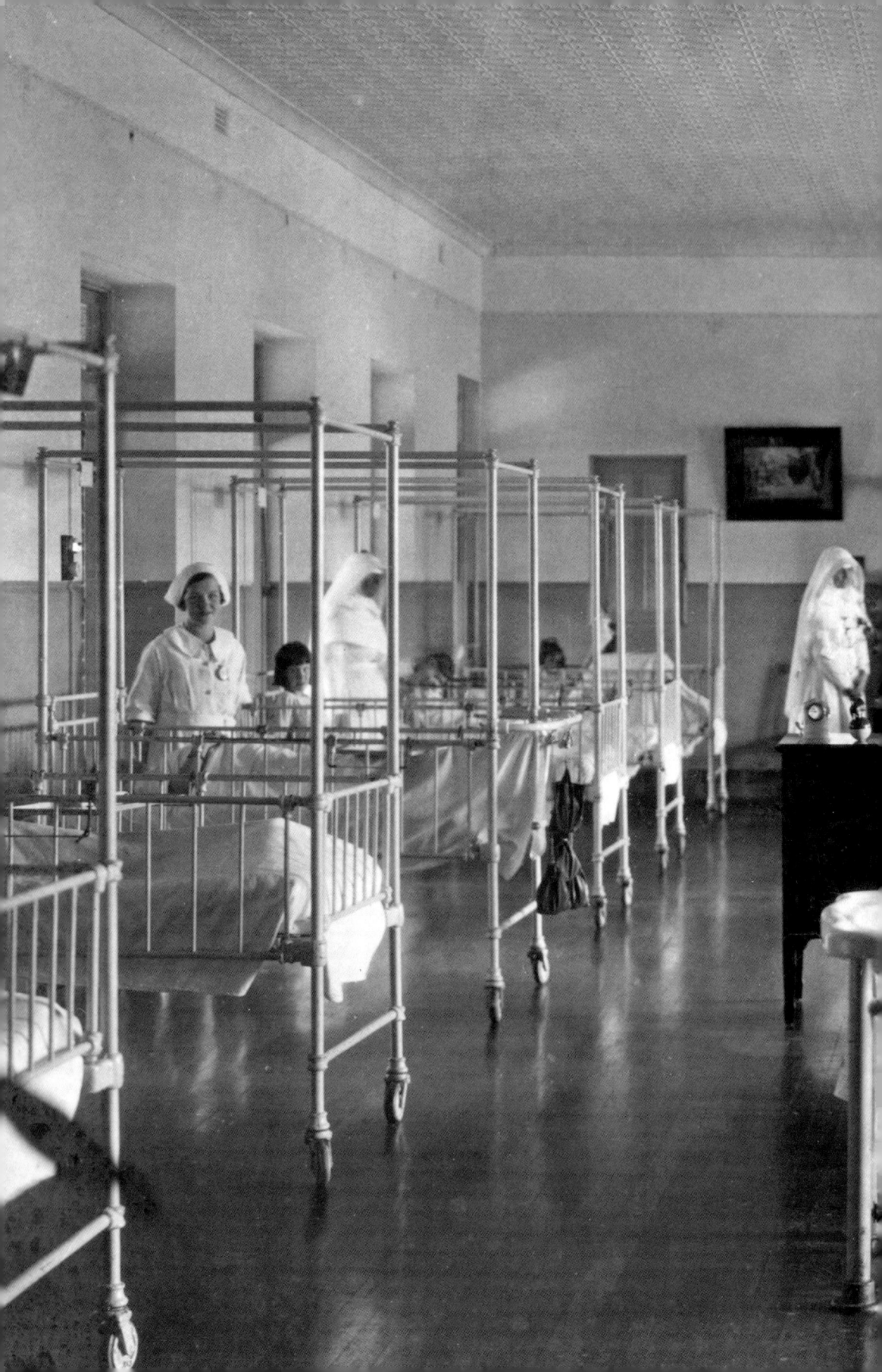

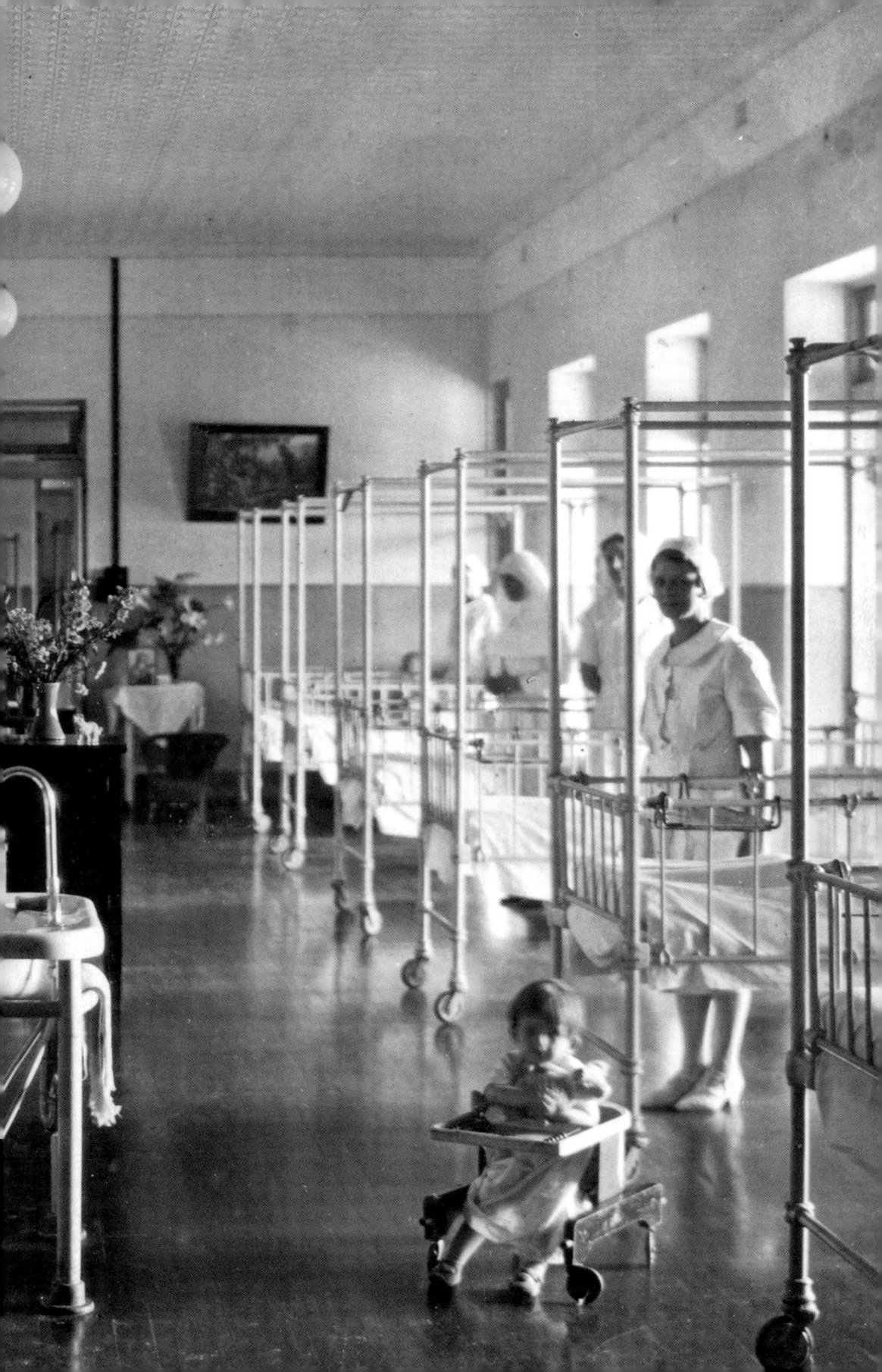

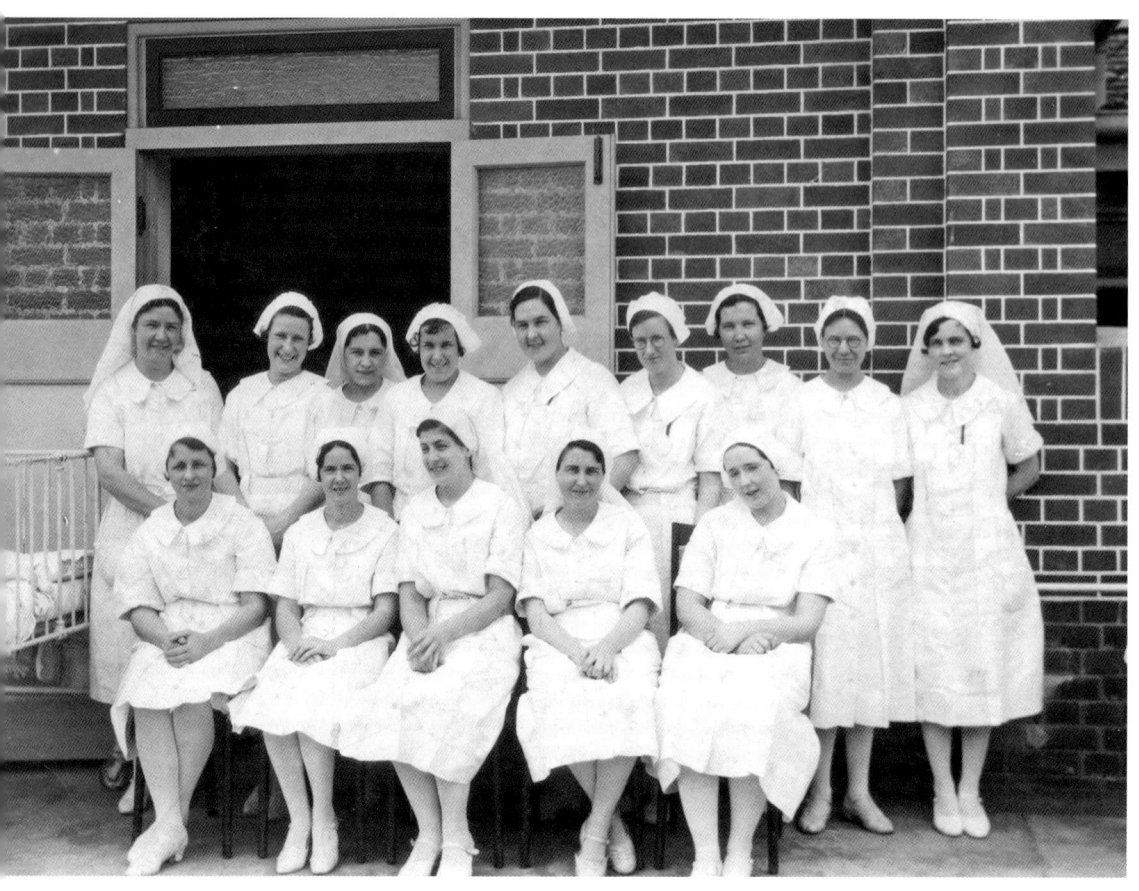

Mater Children's Hospital nurses photographed on the sun balcony at the rear of the hospital in the early 1930s.

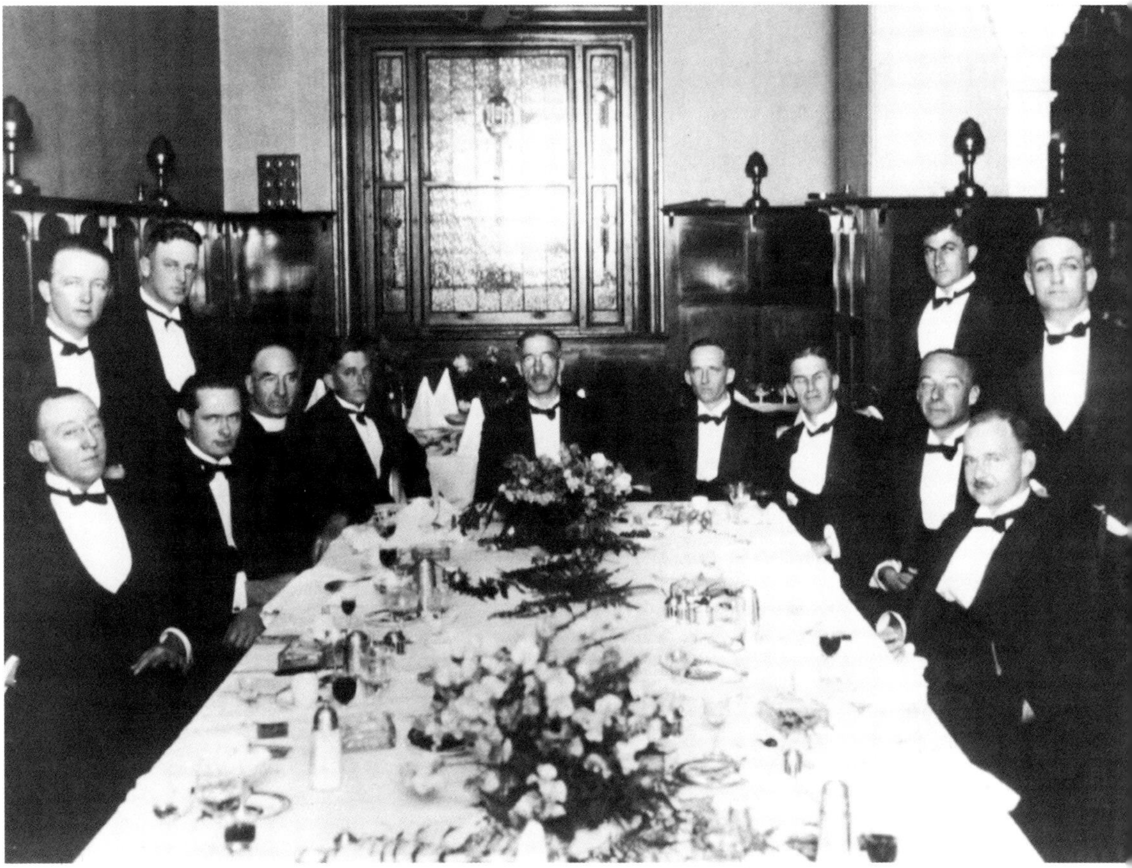

Mater specialists dining together in 1931. Seated, from left to right: WD Ryan, AJ Lynch, Father John Fagen, G Taylor, HJ Windsor, PA Earnshaw, H Mathewson, AV Meehan, E Earnshaw; standing, from left to right: John Lahz, AW St Ledger, BLW Clarke, A Murphy.

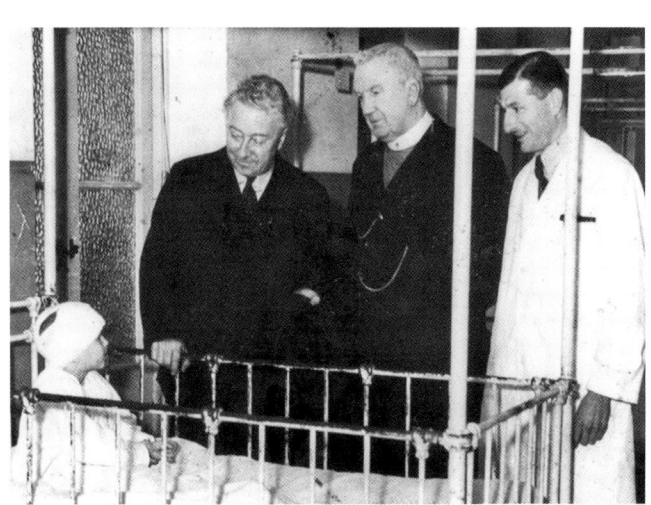

The Prime Minister, Joseph Lyons, visited the hospital in 1936 and is seen here chatting to a small child with Archbishop Duhig (centre) and Dr G Pasquerelli (right).

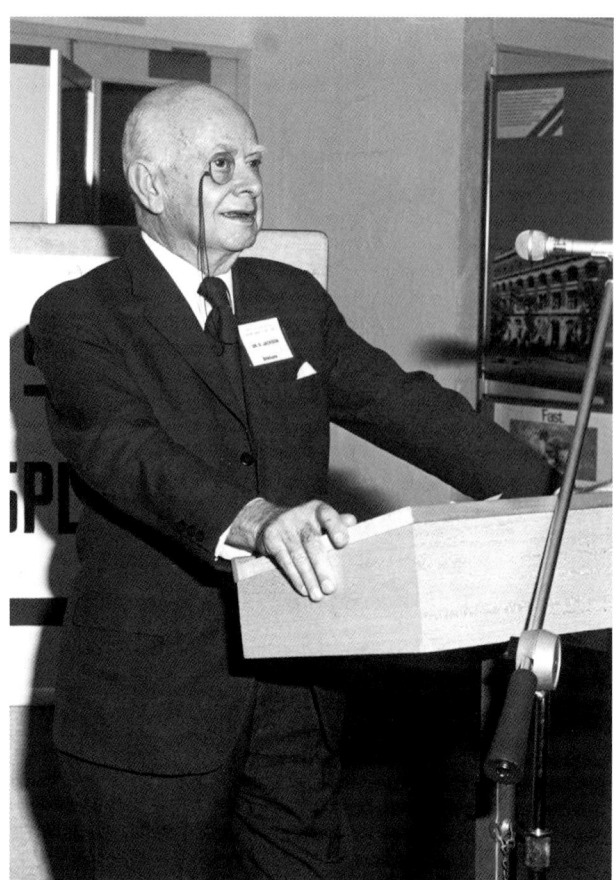

Dr David Jackson, complete with the monocle familiar to generations of children, opening an historical display in 1981.

BELOW: Crowds waiting in the out-patients' department, where there were not enough chairs for everyone in the busy years after the Second World War.

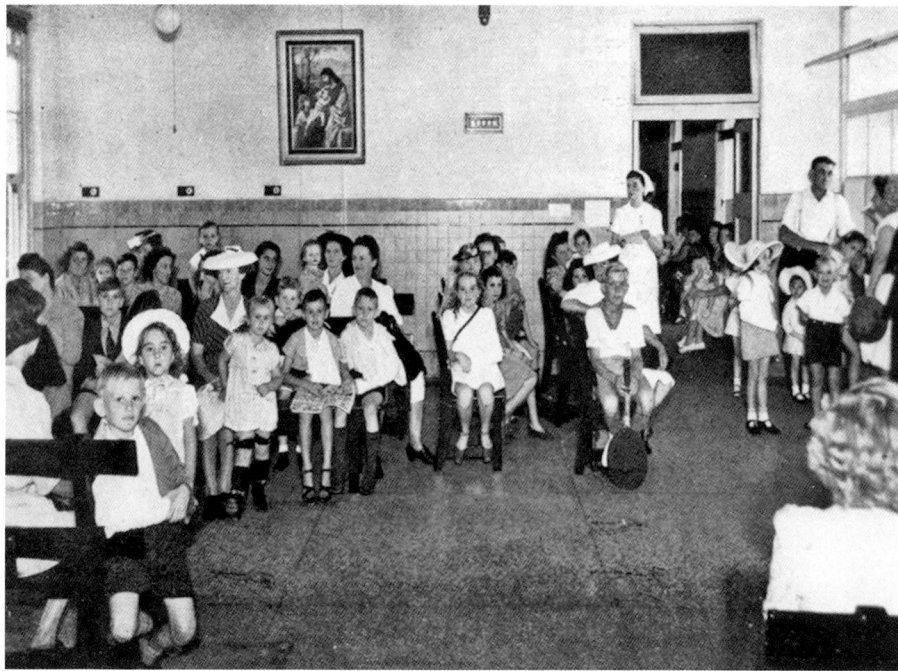

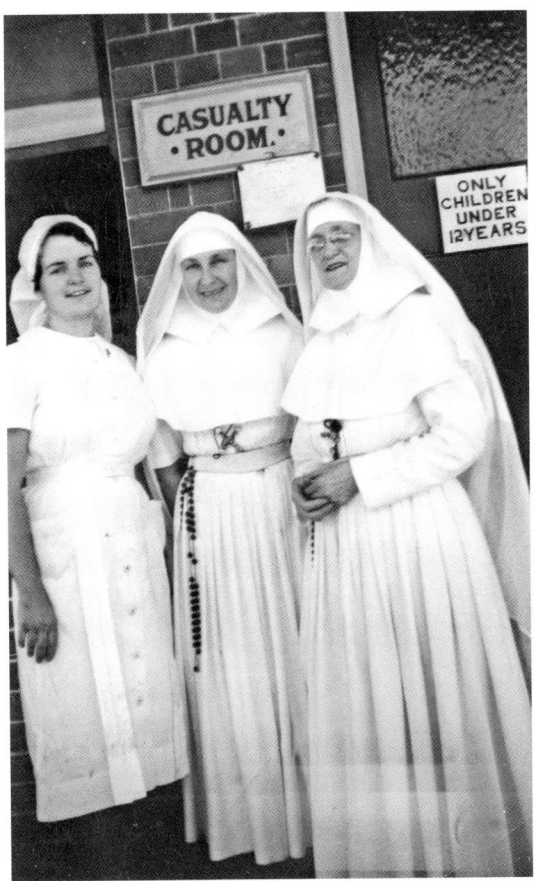

Nurse Jan Carey with Sister Mary Winifrede Patterson and Sister Mary St Bernard McNamara near the door to the casualty room.

BELOW: Dr John Lahz and a young patient photographed in 1950, with Sister Gertrude Mary Lyons and Sister Mary John Patch in theatre garb.

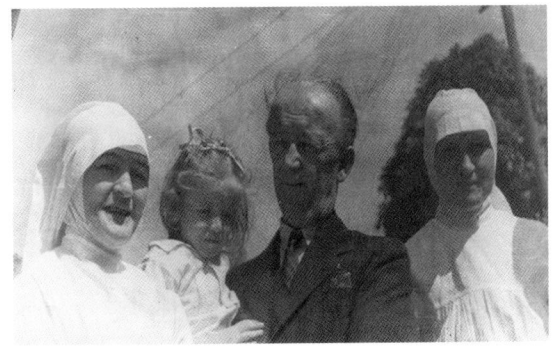

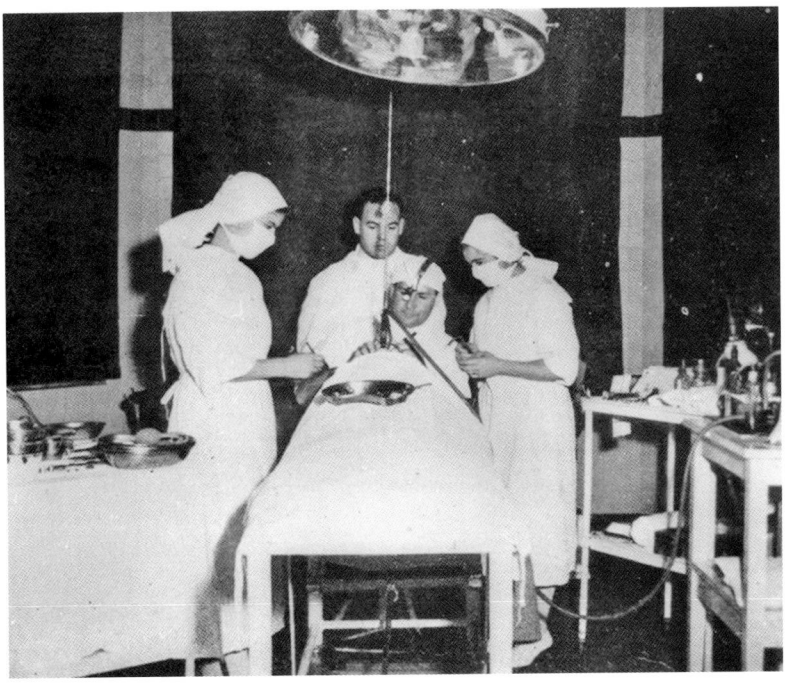

A tonsillectomy underway in the Mater Children's Hospital's operating theatre in 1947. Neither the anaesthetist nor the surgeon appears to be wearing a mask.

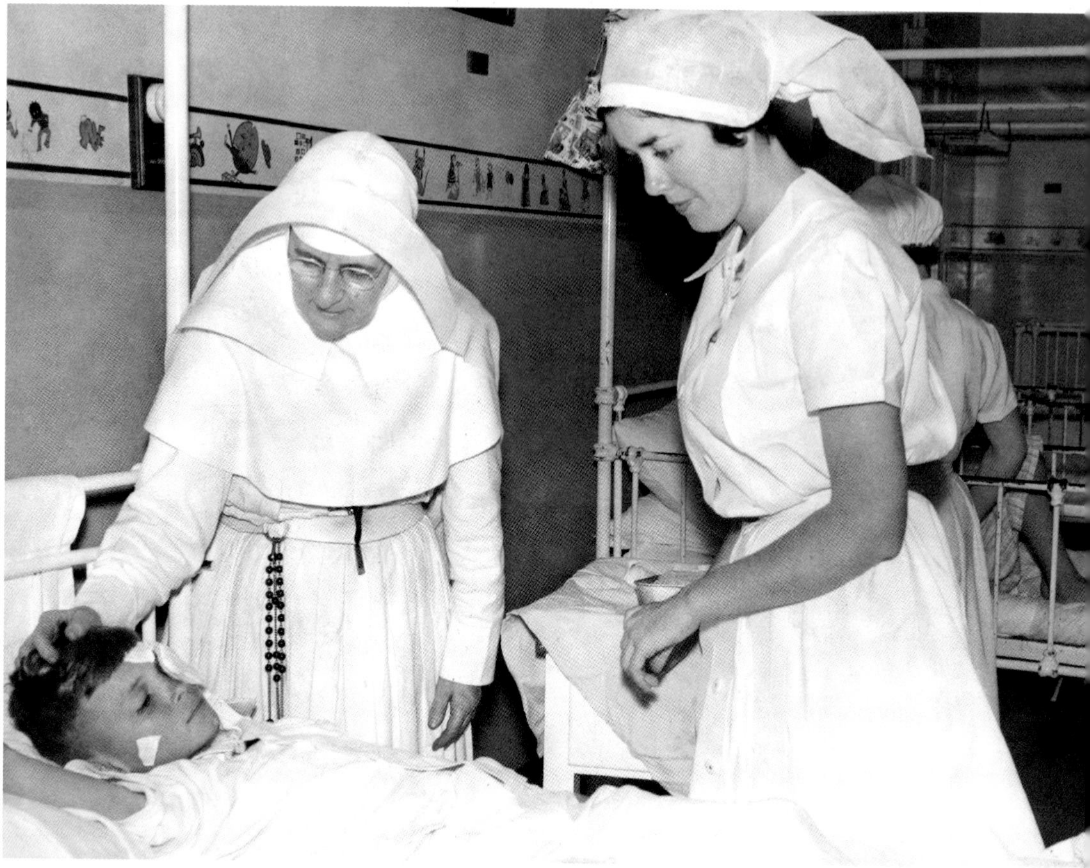

Sister Mary St Pierre McCormack and Nurse Karleen O'Reilly – a future director of nursing at the Mater Adult Hospital – with a patient in 1962.

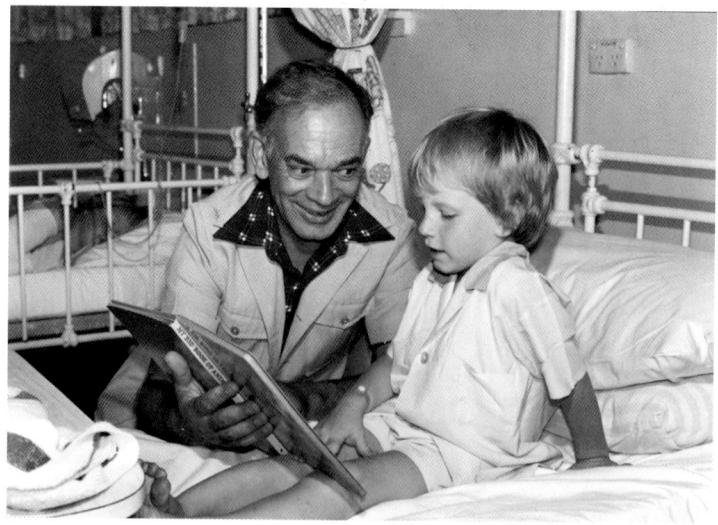

Dr Geoffrey Bourke and a patient enjoying a story in 1981.

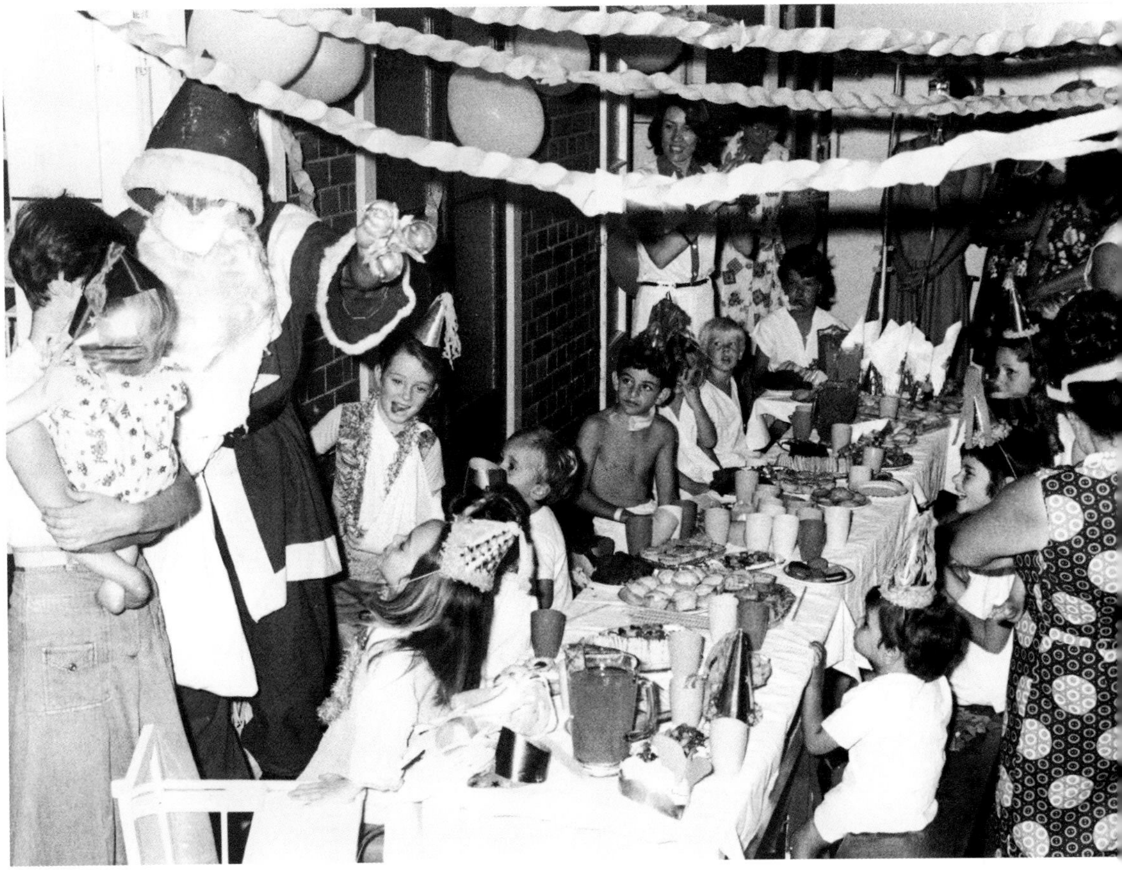

Although space was very tight, school end-of-year parties, like this one in 1964, were held at Christmas.

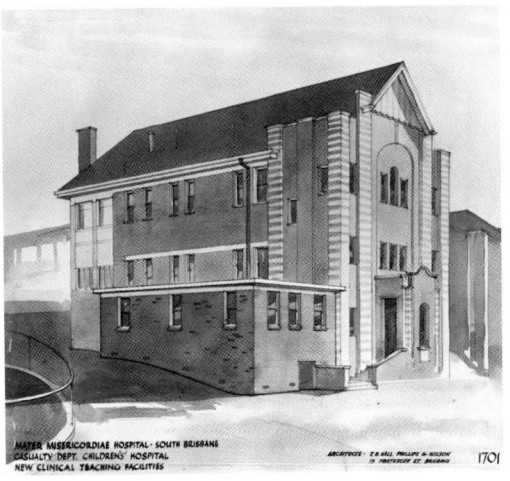

The 1966 architect's plan for the operating theatre and nursery extension.

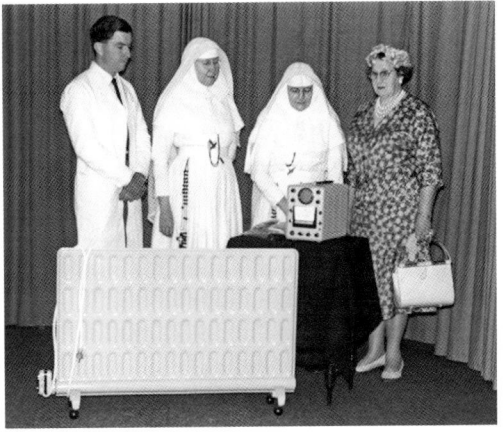

The auxiliary presented many gifts to the Mater Children's Hospital. In the mid-1960s, the auxiliary president, Mrs Beth Dittmer (right), presented a heater to Mater Children's Sisters, with (left to right) the medical superintendent, Dr Des O'Callaghan, Sister Mary St Gabriel Corbett and Sister Mary St Pierre McCormack looking on.

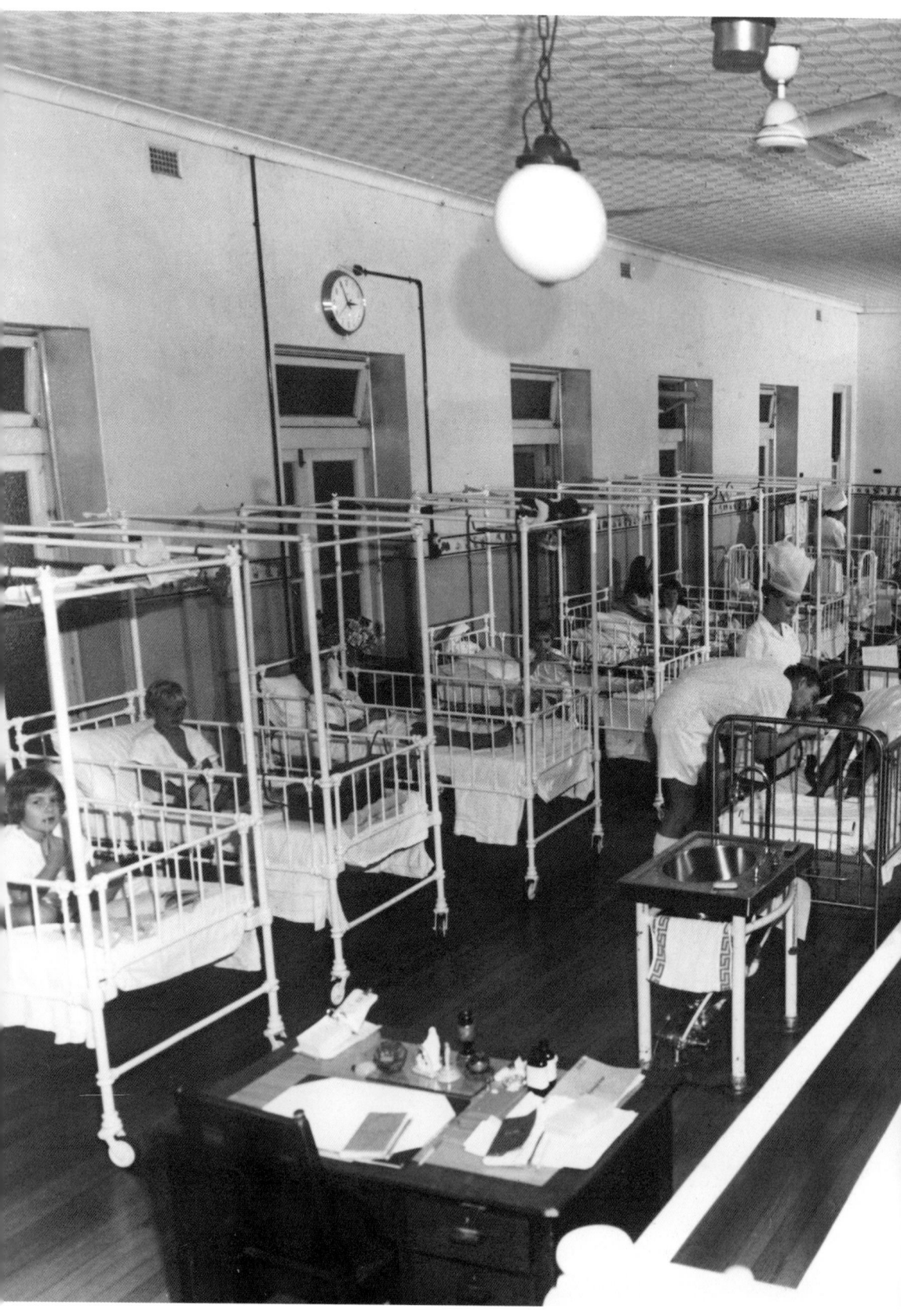

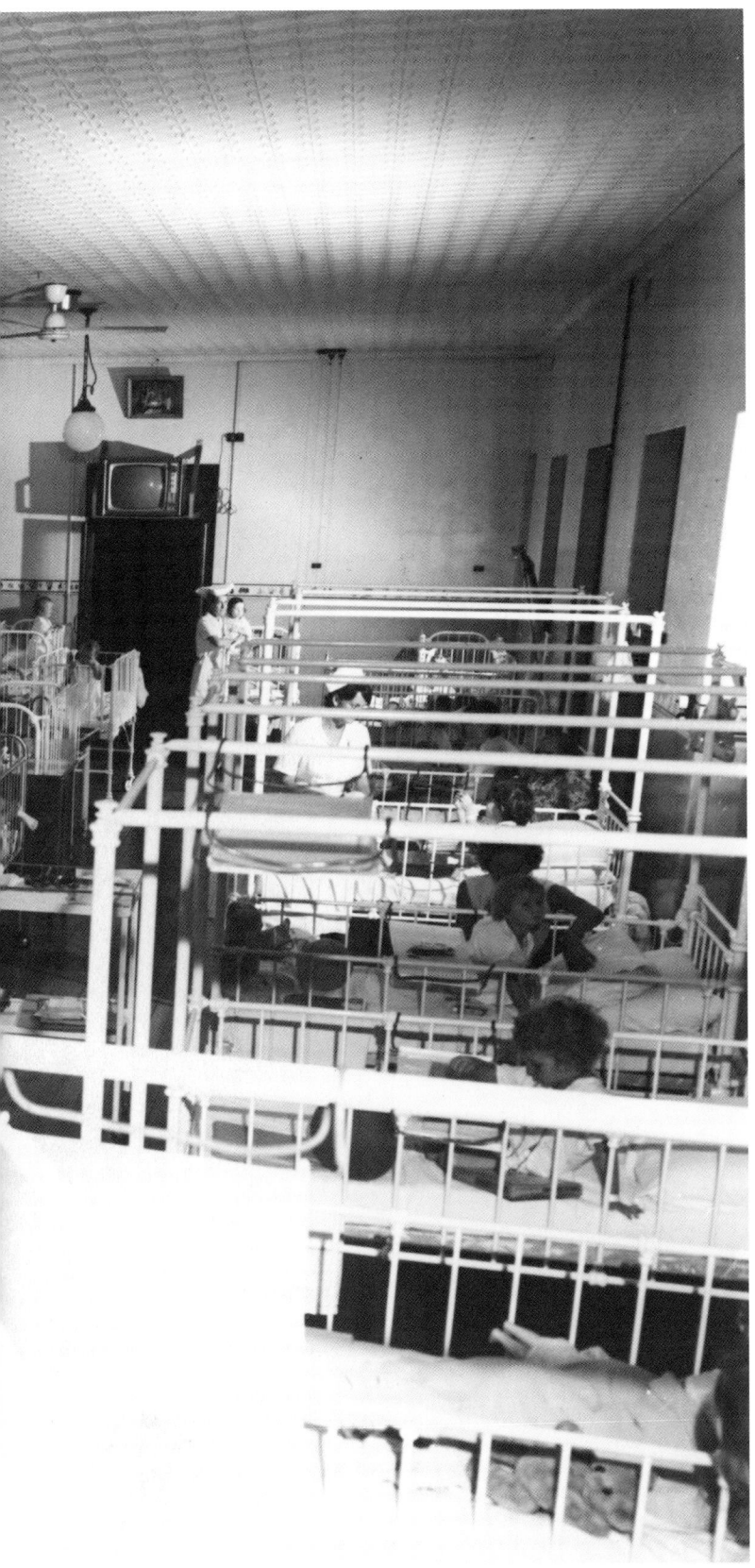

A crowded, regimented ward at the Mater Children's Hospital in the 1960s.

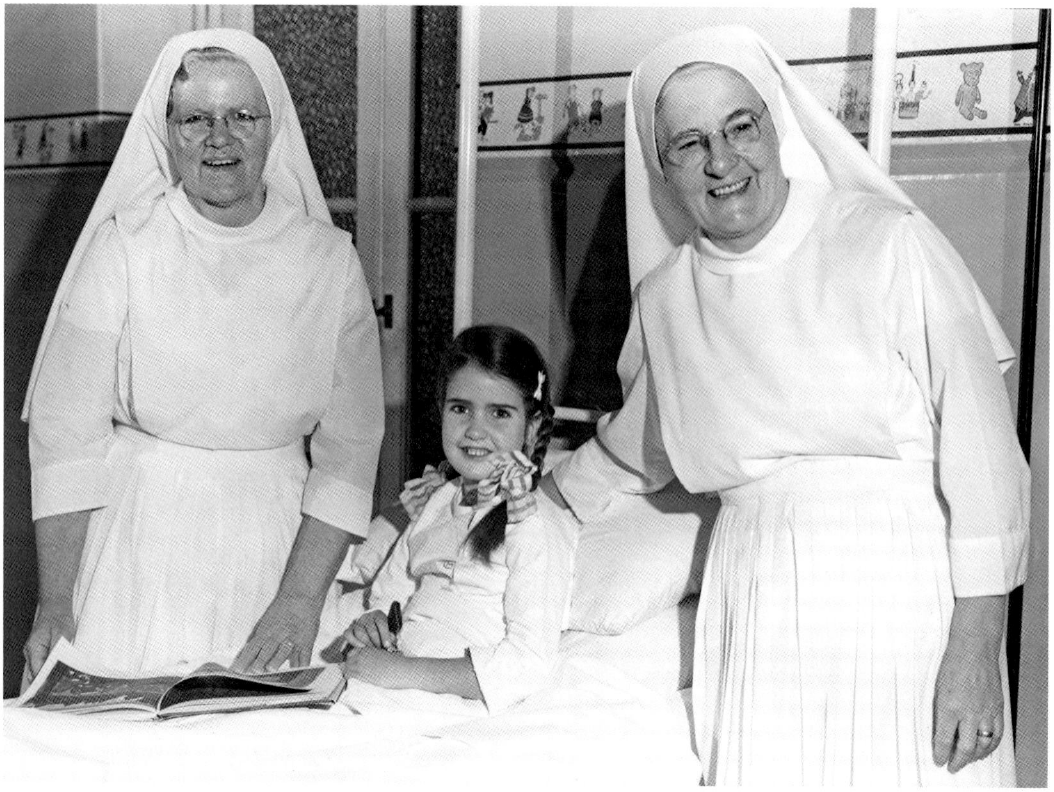

Sister Mary Lea Kelly (left) and Sister Mary St Pierre McCormack (right) with one of their young charges in 1970.

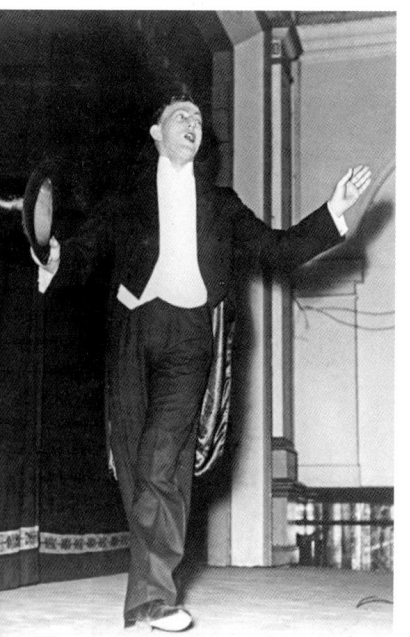

LEFT: His work was serious and demanding, but Dr Geoffrey Toakley enjoyed a lighter moment when he sang in the 1949 Mater concert.

A tiny patient 'retrieved' from an outlying community in 1968.

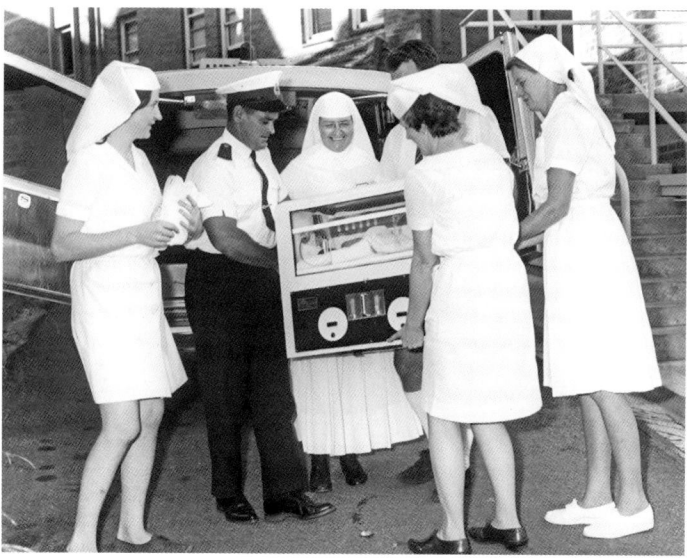

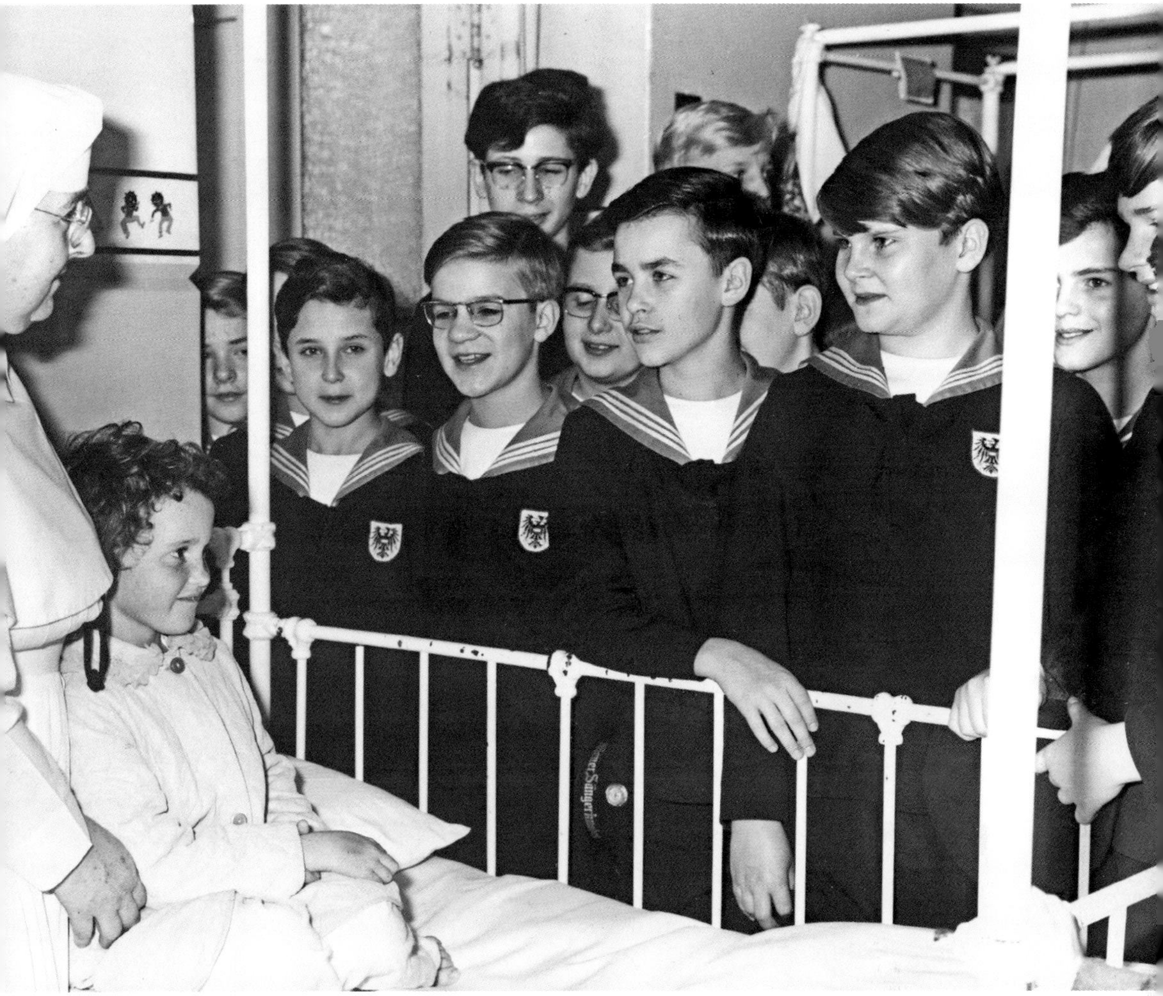

A young patient and Sister Mary Mechtilde Slattery enjoy the Vienna Boys' Choir's visit in 1967.

RIGHT: Fit and well, Peggy Flenady enjoys a return visit to the Mater Children's Hospital in 1966, meeting Sister Mary Dympna Hoare, who had nursed her many years earlier.

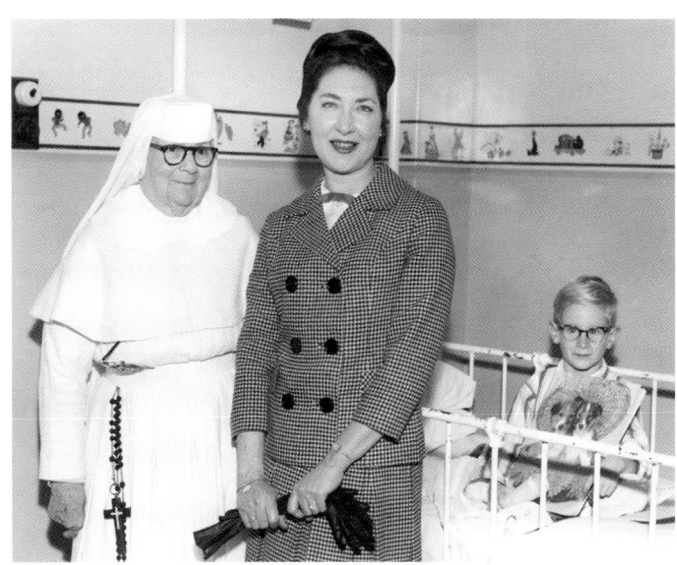

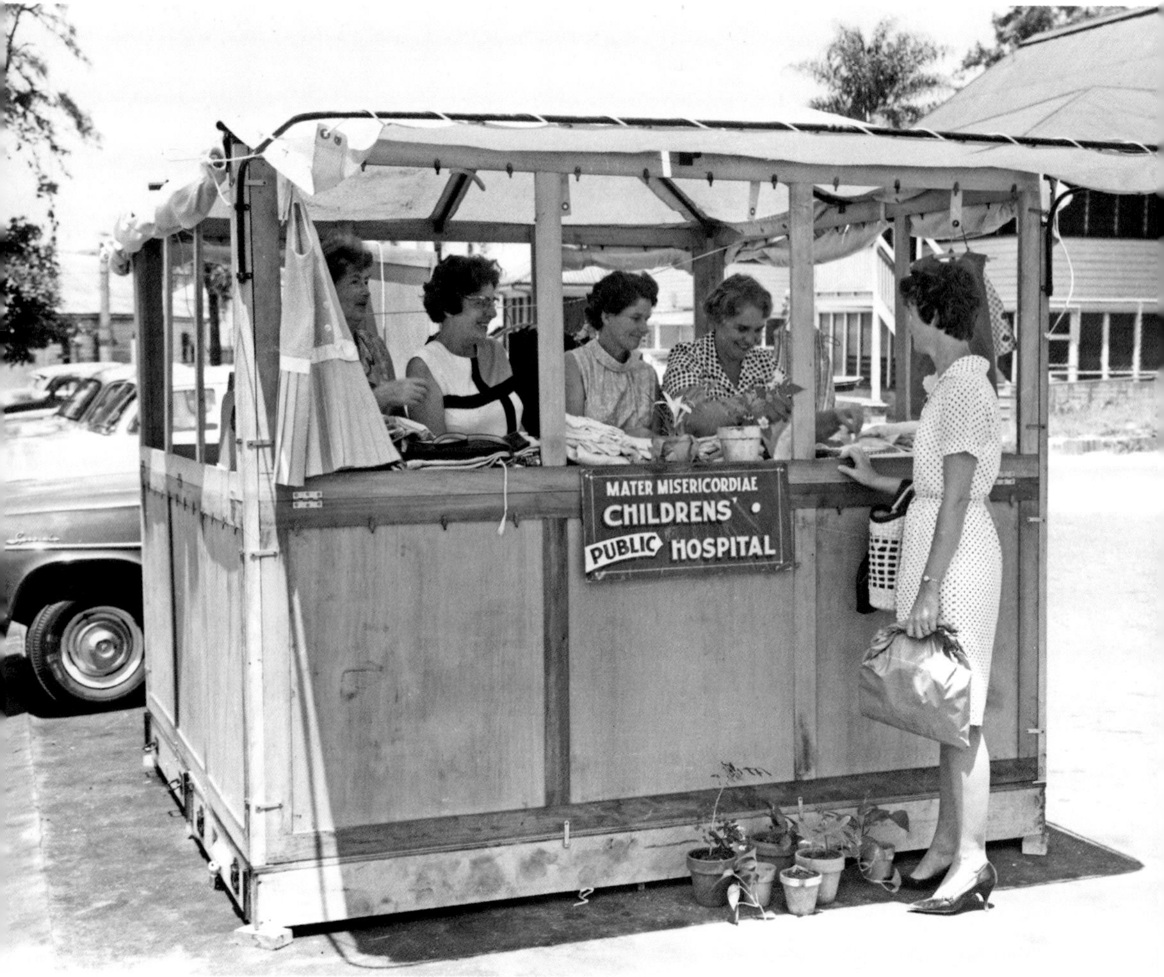

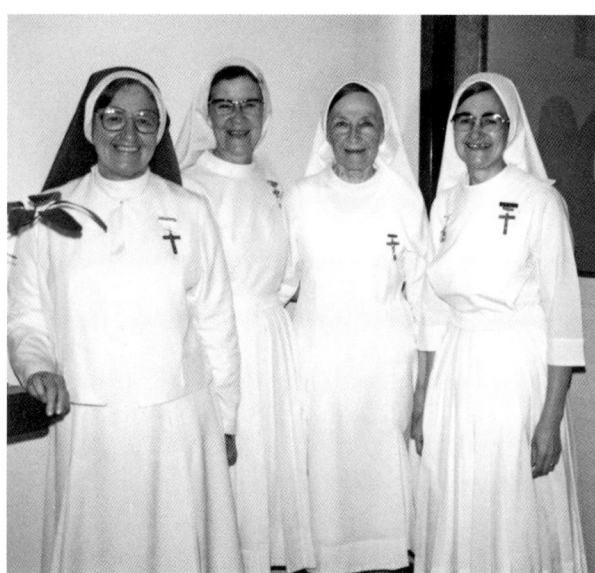

The jaunty Mater Children's Hospital Auxiliary 'caravan', 1967, where goods flowed out and funds flowed in.

LEFT: Long-serving Sisters of Mercy at the Mater Children's Hospital photographed in 1976. From left to right: Sister Mary Dorothea Sheehan, Sister Marie Fitzgerald, Sister Mary Winifrede Patterson, Sister Mary Colette Anderson.

Many of the suggestions emanating from the various enquiries and examinations of the hospital's services bore fruit. The program for general practitioners was up and running successfully and initiatives to conserve children's health were developing. Dr Michael O'Callaghan, appointed staff paediatrician in 1979, was one of Australia's first specialists in developmental paediatrics. As well as a development assessment and therapy program, he assisted Dr David Tudehope in his growth and development clinic at the Mater Mothers' Hospital.[47] These new initiatives – and ideas circulating in wider circles – reflected developments in paediatrics. Taking full advantage of new ideas would require considerable change at the Mater Children's Hospital.

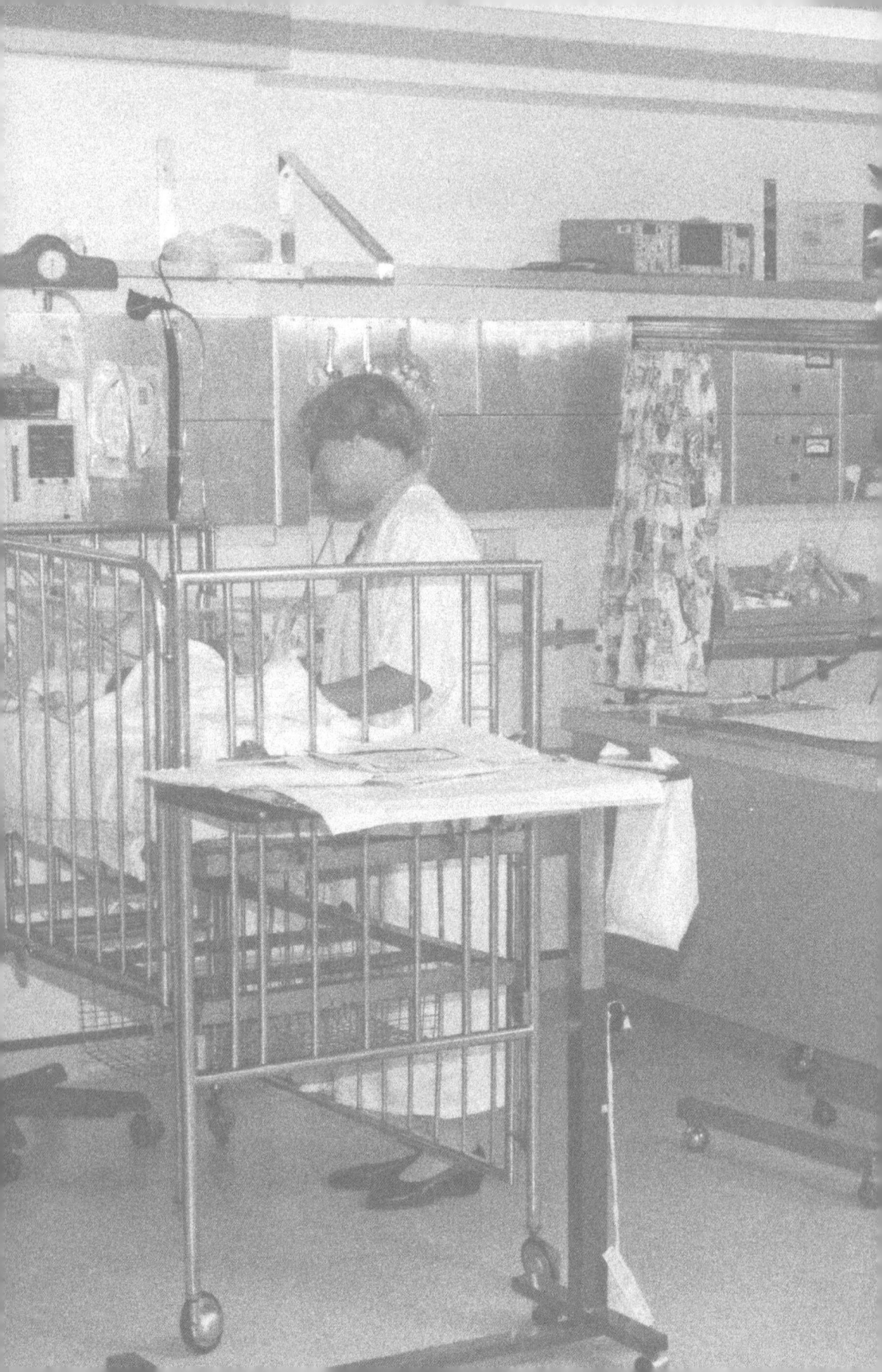

Part Three
1980s to 1990s

Chapter 8

Celebration and Construction

I thank God that He has given us such caring and committed people.

Sister Mary Dorothea Sheehan RSM, 1981

The 1980s began at the Mater Children's Hospital with preparations for the grand celebration of a major milestone: the Golden Jubilee of the hospital's opening in 1931. The year of celebration set the tone for a generally optimistic decade. New buildings eased the most acute congestion and new specialist clinics extended the hospital's services.

A multitude of events was planned to celebrate the Golden Jubilee; no interest was overlooked. There were visits from famous Australian cricketers, fashion parades, children's parties, champagne suppers, gala dinners, a visit from the Health Minister, morning teas, a Golden Jubilee Ball, a special orchestral concert in the hospital's honour and a reunion of past nurses.[1] The reunion featured two former Mater Children's Hospital nurses, Anne-Marie Malouf and Mary Butler, whose mother, Margaret Kelly, was a trainee in the 1930s.[2] There was also a special thrill: the hospital's float in the parade for Brisbane's 1981 Warana (blue skies) Festival was judged the best community service float.[3]

There were some very special events: the presentation of the first Mater Children's Hospital Humanitarian Award to Reg Leonard, managing director of Queensland Newspapers and the *éminence grise* of the *Courier-Mail* Children's Hospitals Appeal, a special Mass to commemorate the official opening of the hospital on 6 July 1931 and, in October, a visit from Mother Teresa of Calcutta.[4]

The Golden Jubilee also had its serious side. On 28 February 1981, a seminar on nursing, attended by 200 delegates, showcased a variety of innovations in paediatric care, particularly the multidisciplinary clinics and the hospital's initiatives in community care.[5]

A procession of experts in paediatrics visited the hospital in 1981. They included Dr Joseph Simone, paediatric oncologist and, later, director of St Jude Children's Research Hospital in Memphis, Tennessee; Dr Roderic Phibbs, director of neonatology at the University of California, San Francisco; Dr Cyril Chantler, professor of paediatric nephrology from Guy's Hospital in London; Professor Lyn Taussig, paediatric pulmonologist from the Arizona Health Sciences Centre at the University of Arizona; Dr Pat Bale, paediatric histopathologist from the Royal Alexandra Hospital for Children, in Camperdown, Sydney; and Dr Clifford Hosking, immunologist, from the Royal Children's Hospital in Melbourne.[6]

The Golden Jubilee Scientific Week was the highlight of the serious medical side of the celebrations. Geoffrey Bourke chaired the organising committee, which attracted an impressive array of speakers. The seminar program was opened by the Governor-General, Sir Zelman Cowen, on 30 August. The speakers included Professor C Berry, professor of pathology at the University of London; Dr N Carroll, orthopaedic surgeon, from the Hospital for Sick Children in Toronto; JES Scott, paediatric surgeon, from Newcastle upon Tyne, and Dr J Deeble, head of the Health Research Project at the Australian National University in Canberra.[7]

The Golden Jubilee was a perfect opportunity to promote the hospital. The Scientific Week was extensively covered in the newspapers, with reports on topics such as the need for special wards for adolescents and techniques for helping children to cope with impending death: their own and that of other children.[8] In April, Frank Warrick and a crew from Channel 7 spent all morning in the wards interviewing parents and filming children in preparation for a fundraising telethon for Brisbane's two children's hospitals.[9]

There was plenty of opportunity to spend money. There were three major constructions at the Mater Children's Hospital in the 1980s: a new school, a new out-patient department and an extension that combined the University of Queensland's Department of Child Health with a new nursery for 25 patients. The old nursery was too small, with insufficient space for large pieces of modern equipment; doctors sometimes had to carry out examinations and treatments – often on their knees – in the middle of the ward. There was no room for chairs beside some of the cots and no privacy for parents, even in extreme stress or if talking to a doctor. There were certainly no facilities for mothers to stay overnight with their babies.[10] The plans were scrutinised to ensure that the new ward would be efficient. One of the 'one-cot' rooms was changed to a bathroom with two deep sinks, a vast improvement on the practice of using a bathtub on the floor.

The new nursery was a revelation. There were cubicles separated by glass partitions, a four-bed intensive care unit, space for parents on fold-up beds and a parent lounge near the entrance to the ward. A small interview room helped to solve the privacy problem.[11] Staff comfort was improved with a shower added to their changing room.

The new McAuley wing was opened in March 1982. Constructed above the much larger babies' ward, the Department of Child Health was complete with laboratories, offices, seminar spaces and a lecture theatre. Two of the rooms were named in honour of early Mater Children's Hospital paediatricians PA Earnshaw and David Jackson.[12] The old nursery was renovated for psychiatric in-patients. The space was sufficiently large for beds, a dining room and a therapy support space.

These changes had not eliminated the wish list: an additional operating theatre, conference and seminar rooms, a modern medical records department, an area for developmental paediatrics and additional space for ancillary medicine disciplines.[13] About $50,000 raised from three art unions gave at least some confidence that these hopes might be realised.[14] The beleaguered operating theatres were the next to be relieved. In 1983, the old kitchen was transformed into change rooms for operating theatre staff, a lounge and storage space, but more was needed.[15] At last, in 1987, work on the surgical area created a suite of three A-class theatres, supplemented by a smaller theatre. New intensive care facilities, funded by the proceeds of a Channel 7 telethon, were opened in November 1987.[16]

An entirely new school came next. For almost 20 years, the Mater school had worked in makeshift accommodation on the second floor verandah of the 1931 wing. Some children worked at desks in the 'schoolroom' and other pupils on desks specially designed for use in bed. The one and only classroom had been divided into sections for preschool, primary school and secondary school children, who were taught by three teachers and three teachers' aides.

In the 1970s, the schoolroom was also used as the nurses' tutorial room.[17] Covering a patio gave an additional area for a play centre, where Helen McAllister entertained 35 children each weekday.[18]

The school had expanded to include young people at the Mater Mothers' and Mater Adult hospitals, the Princess Alexandra Hospital's spinal unit and at Ipswich Hospital. The educational program included music lessons on donated instruments and art therapy during the Christmas holidays. In 1977, the Mater school became independent of the school at the Royal Children's Hospital.[19]

The original plan in the late 1970s was to include the school in the extension developed for the new nursery and Department of Child Health at the rear of the hospital. The Sisters, however, wanted the new school to be larger. A more appropriate solution was found: a property the Mater owned in Clarence Street, adjacent to the hospital. The land was leased to the Education Department at a peppercorn rental: ten cents, payable upon demand.

This was an era of custom-built special schools, part of a wider discussion on integrating children with special needs into the general education system.[20] The Royal Children's Hospital school was rebuilt in 1976. The new four-storey Mater school, with its separate, brightly coloured classrooms for all year levels, a living skills area for cooking and manual arts, a library, computers and a grassed play area, opened on 24 May 1983.[21]

Carmen Smith, principal when the new school opened, wrote extensively about the importance of hospital schools. Children in hospital, she said, often had poor self-concept and saw themselves as different from their peers and, often, not as capable. School also helped the children's recovery because they were less worried about 'missing out'. Education, in Carmen Smith's view, was essential to caring for the whole child:

> As children can be more handicapped by their own feelings about themselves than by their actual physical conditions, it is important for medical and nursing staff, therapists and teachers to work together in helping each child to understand and accept their condition and to focus on their abilities rather than their disabilities.[22]

Carmen Smith had succeeded Rae Dommett in 1982 and was one of a series of remarkable principals at the Mater school.[23] In 1985, when Vicki Sykes became principal, there were more than 80 pupils and a total of

15 teachers, whose classrooms reflected the increasing diversity of Brisbane's population. Many of the children did not come from English-speaking backgrounds; the Mater's catchment area contained many locations favoured by settlers from overseas. Several children were refugees, and some had been victims of torture.

In 1987, Vicki Sykes developed the school's reach to include a home-visiting service, which included the school's pupils from the Princess Alexandra Hospital. The service was necessary because many children – particularly those with spinal and orthopaedic conditions – spent a long time at home after their stay in hospital before recovering sufficiently to return to school. Eight children were using the service shortly after it began in January 1987. Children were visited in districts as widely dispersed as Bellbowrie, Seventeen Mile Rocks and Ipswich in the western part of the Mater's large catchment, Woodridge and Loganholme in the south, and Wynnum and Redland Bay in the east – travelling more than 1,000 kilometres in a week was not uncommon for the visiting teachers. Parents, doctors and nurses all applauded the visiting service, but all were nervous that it could be vulnerable to any government funding cutbacks.[24]

Educational opportunities addressed one aspect of the social and emotional needs of children in hospital. Better facilities for their families addressed another. Assessments of the hospital in the 1960s and 1970s had stressed the need to improve facilities for visiting families. Accommodation for the families of sick children was particularly important as the Mater's huge catchment area included western Queensland and northern New South Wales. Self-contained apartments enabling families to stay close to their children in hospital was an important step.[25]

The apartment block in Clarence Street, opened on 3 September 1979, was named in honour of Reg Leonard, in recognition of his contribution to improving facilities at both children's hospitals. Families came from as far away as Papua New Guinea, Norfolk Island and the Northern Territory. Some parents had never previously visited Brisbane. It wasn't long before need exceeded supply and an extension was opened in 1982.[26]

Improvements to clinical services came next. Almost as soon as the hospital opened in 1931, its out-patient clinics were overwhelmed. The movement towards treating as many children as possible as out-patients, rather than admitting them as in-patients, put even more pressure on the out-patient area. The appointment of John McNee as director of ambulatory paediatrics in 1978 signified the new emphasis on reducing hospital stays and supporting general practitioners in managing the treatment of children at home.

> JOHN LEIGH MCNEE, MBBS, was a paediatric registrar at the Mater Children's Hospital between January and December 1973 and between July and December in 1974. On his appointment as director of ambulatory paediatrics, John McNee introduced a vigorous teaching program for general practitioners. He was also determined to improve the casualty section and the out-patient department. John McNee was appointed acting superintendent of the Mater Children's Hospital in August 1983 and was confirmed in that position in February 1985. He was a foundation Fellow of the new Australasian College of Emergency Medicine, a member of the Child Accident Prevention Foundation and a member of the Australian Sports Medicine Foundation. John McNee was known for both his capacity to develop a vision for the hospital and his practicality in implementing this vision. He had a well-developed sense of inclusiveness and a commitment to team building. His wit and sense of fun were legendary. John McNee resigned from the hospital in March 1988 to pursue his interest in sports medicine. John McNee died suddenly on 3 February 1999.[27]

The announcement in 1985 that an entirely new building would be constructed for out-patients was music to John McNee's ears. He had reported serious deficiencies: the plastic surgery clinic operated in the casualty section, and had to move if emergencies arose; the gastroenterology and neurosurgery clinics were located in the ear, nose and throat section of the adult hospital; the oncology clinic was in the Reg Leonard link; the craniofacial clinic could be held only on Saturday mornings. There was no separate children's audiology department, yet 75 per cent of the Mater's audiology patients were children.[28]

In addition to shortage of space for out-patients and emergencies, John McNee's assessment of the hospital's needs highlighted a critical shortage of space to meet the demands of the 1980s. There were no suitable facilities for the increasingly important social work department, or for speech therapy, psychiatry, clinical psychology, staff counselling, dietetics and play-workers, or for specialised services, such as respiratory medicine, gastroenterology, oncology, endocrinology or developmental medicine. Paediatric radiology, intensive care and day surgery were also housed in makeshift areas. There was no appropriate staff room for visiting specialists and no conference facilities.[29]

A demographic study based on the 1981 census demonstrated that this situation could not continue. There were 844,321 people in the Mater Children's Hospital catchment in 1981, compared with 627,746 in 1980. Even if this had been a population boom year, substantial growth could still be expected, leading to a population of 1,750,000 people in the year 2000.[30] As if these predictions were not enough, the number of out-patients had doubled from 36,502 in 1976–77 to 72,756 in 1986.[31]

A site on the corner of Clarence Street and Annerley Road, separated from the main children's hospital building only by an internal driveway, was suitable for a new building, but there was a worrying delay.[32] In May 1984, the Health Minister broke the bad news that, due to the government's 'financial difficulties', there could be no funding. Things changed and, in March 1985, the government announced a $3,100,000 grant for the building. With $600,000 from fundraising through the Mater Children's Hospital Art Union and $400,000 from the Children's Hospital Appeal – one of the final funding projects before the appeal was disbanded in 1987 – the government grant would be sufficient for the shell of the building, but there would be no spare money for outfitting.[33] Construction began in 1986, but the upper floors remained a shell for several years.

The building was officially opened on 28 September 1987. The Mater Children's Hospital was Queensland's first hospital to house all ambulatory services and clinics in a single block. Ear, nose and throat and eye out-patients were installed on the ground level with general out-patients and physiotherapy on the level above. Eventually, occupational therapy, speech therapy, audiology, dietetics, social work, child protection and the parent aide unit, psychology and psychiatry moved to the new building.

In 1985, when these new developments were underway, John McNee outlined his ideas for the hospital. Children's hospitals all over the world had become much less formal and full of bright colour. The days of treating children as miniature adults had well and truly gone. The Mater Children's

Hospital was, John McNee said, a family community because children's hospitals did not treat children alone, they treated whole families. This approach was in tune with the tenor of the times: the previous year, 1984, was the United Nations' International Year of the Family.

The rapid development in day surgery had put the spotlight on parents to provide good post-operative care at home. John McNee was confident that, with sufficient education and support, parents were capable of home care for children with a wide range of conditions. In 1981, he had spoken of 'third-generation' hospitals. First- and second-generation hospitals, he said, treated diseases, but not the underlying causes, many of which were lifestyle related and not well treated by current hospitals. Third-generation hospitals would reach out into the community, perhaps by offering visiting medical services, home help, childminding and courses on good health.[34] The Mater Children's Hospital had demonstrated one aspect of sensitivity to community needs in 1980, when an immunisation clinic was opened to cater for the large number of Aboriginal families in the area. Sister Mary Dorothea had found that many Aboriginal parents did not like the large, impersonal immunisation clinic at Brisbane City Hall.[35]

The nursing staff had new leadership in the mid-1980s. For the first time in the hospital's history, the director of nursing – succeeding Sister Mary Dorothea Sheehan RSM – was not a Sister of Mercy, but a married lay nursing sister, Rosalie Lewis RN.

ROSALIE MARY LEWIS was born in Brisbane and educated by the Sisters of Mercy at St Stephen's School and All Hallows'. In August 1960, Rosalie commenced her nurse training at the Princess Alexandra Hospital in Brisbane and completed her midwifery certificate at the Brisbane Women's Hospital in 1965. After working as a nurse educator at Princess Alexandra Hospital and, briefly, at the Royal Children's Hospital and on the part-time staff of the Mater Private Hospital, Rosalie Lewis was appointed to the registered midwifery staff at the Mater Mothers' Hospital in 1975. On 24 September 1986, she became director of nursing at the Mater Children's Hospital, a post she held until 1 November 1998, when she became project coordinator for the development of the new Mater

continued overleaf

> Children's Hospital. Rosalie Lewis continued her education during these busy years, completing her Graduate Diploma in Nursing Administration in 1983 and her Bachelor of Arts in 1991. She was a member of the Royal College of Nursing, Australia (RCNA) (now Australian College of Nursing) and was awarded the Mater's Clarice Mary Gately Distinguished Nursing Award in 1993 and, on her retirement, was made a life member of the Queensland Child and Family Health Nurses Association. In 2002, Rosalie Lewis was made a Member of the Order of Australia for her service to the nursing profession, particularly in the fields of paediatric care and hospital administration.

Many long-standing nurses remained in the early days of Rosalie Lewis's term as director of nursing. Sister Marie Fitzgerald RSM retired in 1988 after 23 years in senior positions. Several lay members of the registered nursing staff also stayed for many years. The McCarthy sisters, Libby and Cathy, for instance, had worked for a combined total of 30 years at the Mater Children's Hospital. They both held demanding positions: Cathy McCarthy RN was the charge sister of the intensive care unit and Libby was second-in-charge in casualty. As well as their professional work, both sisters devoted many hours to fundraising for the hospital.[36] Sister Brigid (Mary Ian) Hirschfeld RSM, who also had been on the Mater staff for several years, embarked on a new initiative when she began a grief counselling service. The Mater Children's Hospital staff included nurses from further afield when an exchange system with the children's hospital in Toronto, Canada, was in full swing during the 1980s.

Mater Children's Hospital nurses also travelled, not only to Canada, but also to South-East Asia, working in Kampuchea (now Cambodia) in 1979, in the aftermath of the Pol Pot regime. Mary McCarthy RN wrote of their experience running a triage system and dispensing medication and food in a crowded camp: 'The flies and the kids were neck and neck in the race for the milk'. She was grateful for the mosquito nets that she and Dr David Taylor had brought from Brisbane, but this was a small luxury. Their case load was enormous – as many as 100 patients each day. Trying conditions often forced them to examine their small patients on the floor. Seeing very young soldiers with rifles was only one of many disturbing sights. The Mater teams in South-East Asia included two Sisters of Mercy, Sister Patricia Kirchner and Sister Marie Therese Rosenberg.

As well as raising money for their colleagues working in South-East Asia, nurses in the wards at Mater Children's Hospital treated patients with serious conditions, as well as the routine illnesses of childhood.[37] Viruses, especially respiratory infections, were the most common reasons for admission, and there were outbreaks of gastrointestinal infections, including the nasty – and sometimes fatal – rotavirus.[38] Children with cystic fibrosis were frequent in-patients. Cystic fibrosis, the most common lethal genetic disorder, affected about one in every 2,500 children causing recurrent chest infections, malabsorption of food and nutrients, liver disease and diabetes.[39] Many children with cystic fibrosis died in late childhood from chronic pulmonary infection but, in the late 1970s, evidence was emerging that early diagnosis and management in specialised clinics greatly improved the outlook for patients with cystic fibrosis. With this in mind, Dr Ian Robertson assembled a multidisciplinary team and, in 1980, the cystic fibrosis clinic began seeing patients. Screening babies soon after birth, supervised by Frank Bowling, began shortly afterwards. The first patient detected by screening in Queensland was managed in the Mater Children's Hospital's cystic fibrosis clinic. More than 250 children with cystic fibrosis were clinic patients between 1980 and 2014. Understanding and treatment of this complex disease had advanced greatly, with corresponding improvements in survival.

Managing asthma and other acute and chronic respiratory diseases is always a large part of any children's health program. Chronic lung disease in small infants became a significant issue with the survival of more extremely premature infants. Measuring lung function is essential in managing respiratory diseases. Following visits to Sydney and Melbourne, Ian Robertson gained funding to establish and equip the Mater Children's Hospital respiratory function laboratory, located in the flyover between the children's hospital and the original adult hospital. The respiratory scientist Gordon Williams, an integral figure in the development and growth of the respiratory and sleep unit, was the first staff member appointed to the laboratory. Reliable funding for staff and equipment was a challenge. No government funding was received until 1982; medical staff gave their time generously. For some years, funding for the cystic fibrosis clinic was supplemented by money raised by an energetic group of parents running an opportunity shop opposite the hospital in Annerley Road.

Dr Brent Masters, the Mater Children's Hospital's first full-time respiratory physician, was a key figure in the subsequent development of the asthma clinic, the home oxygen clinic supporting premature babies, bronchoscopy services and the sleep studies unit. Kind friends of the hospital helped with equipment. The Asthma Foundation and Lions Clubs Australia donated 24 portable nebulisers in 1981 to support the hospital through the winter increase in asthma patients. The hospital allowed parents to borrow the machines so that asthma could be treated at home, reducing the length of hospital stays.[40] Asthma could be aggravated by allergic reactions. The Mater's Professor of Child Health, Yee-Hing Thong, established Queensland's first child allergy clinic at the Mater Children's Hospital[41] and, with Dr Brent Masters, wrote a guide for parents of children with asthma.[42]

Some children could not be nursed at home and had to spend long periods in hospital. In 1985, for instance, a little girl spent her first year in the hospital for surgical treatment of life-threatening congenital abnormalities.[43] Surgery in the 1980s achieved results once thought impossible. Professor Robert Jeffs visited Brisbane from the Johns Hopkins Hospital in Baltimore, USA, and operated on a child to insert an artificial muscle near his urinary tract to help control urine flow.[44]

Some childhood cancers also became more amenable to successful treatment in the 1980s. Many children were successfully treated at the Mater Children's Hospital for lymphoblastic leukaemia, once almost always fatal.[45] Cancer treatment was, however, long and arduous. Many parents relied heavily on the hospital's oncology nursing staff. In 1983, the Queensland Cancer Fund (now Cancer Council Queensland) and the Queensland Nurses' Union funded Sister Mary McCarthy RN, in charge of Ward 3 at the Mater Children's Hospital, to study cancer nursing in England, New York and Memphis, Tennessee.[46] In 1987, a song called 'Dignity' by Renee Laycock was recorded by a group of 17 Mater Children's Hospital patients with cancer. The proceeds of the record's sales were donated to the hospital.[47]

The loss of a young life from any illness is always tragic. Christine Riordan died on 7 April 1982, when she was 15. Her mother wrote about Christine in a very popular book, *Chris: A rose with thorns,* and dedicated the proceeds of book sales to a fund for terminally ill children.[48]

Multidisciplinary clinics, which had begun to emerge in the 1970s, developed strongly in the 1980s. Considerable organisation was needed to bring busy professionals from various disciplines and members of allied professions together as a team, but the clinics enabled specialists to collaborate efficiently and saved patients from multiple visits to the hospital to see various practitioners individually. Nurses and social workers were particularly important members of the teams caring for children with disabilities or lifelong illnesses. In 1981, multidisciplinary clinics at the Mater Children's Hospital cared for children with spina bifida, cystic fibrosis, diabetes, and craniofacial injuries and abnormalities.

The craniofacial clinic, opened in 1980, was the only clinic of its kind in Queensland and the second in Australia. The neurosurgeon Dr Leigh Atkinson and plastic surgeon Dr Tony Emmett had travelled to Toronto, Glasgow and New York to bring the most up-to-date skills to the clinic. In 1977, craniofacial surgeons at the Mater Children's Hospital made national news when they removed a massive, disfiguring tumour from the face of a four-year-old boy, Robert Hoge, in a 13-hour operation. Robert recovered well and eventually graduated from university with an honours degree in journalism.[49] Other patients travelled long distances for treatment. In 1985, for instance, a baby was brought from Papua New Guinea for the removal of a tumour protruding from his forehead and nose.[50]

The International Year of Disabled Persons in 1981 emphasised the importance of ensuring that people with disabilities reached their full potential. Children with spina bifida needed several different types of special care. Coordinated care in a clinic setting was particularly appropriate for this complex congenital disorder that involved the failure of some vertebrae, particularly in the lower spine, to fully form and completely enclose the spinal cord. The opening could be closed surgically, but damage to the spinal cord impaired movement and often affected the bowel and bladder. Treatment for children with hydrocephalus as well as spina bifida was complicated; shunts, which often became infected, were needed to drain fluid from their brains. The multiple needs of children with spina bifida put great strain on families, particularly in mobile populations, where assistance from extended families was not readily available.[51] The neurosurgeons Dr Geoff Toakley and Dr Leigh Atkinson worked with a community group to develop a support centre for children with spina bifida and their families.[52]

A general practitioner, Dr Jennifer O'Brien, coordinated the spina bifida clinic at the Mater Children's Hospital in the 1980s. She overviewed the care of patients who usually needed attention from neurosurgeons, orthopaedic surgeons, urologists and physiotherapists.[53] The paediatric urologist, Dr Ron Yaxley, was a very important member of the team, supported by Sister Marie Fitzgerald RSM and Sister Mary Winifrede Patterson RSM, who, in her official retirement, assisted parents in managing urinary appliances.

Even with coordinated care, there could be immense frustrations when necessary splints and other appliances were difficult to obtain. In 1979, the mother of a seven-year-old boy with spina bifida, hydrocephalus and cerebral palsy, who had been a Mater patient since he was born, wrote of her distress at the long waiting list for equipment her son needed. To buy the necessary appliances privately, instead of waiting for Health Department issue, would cost hundreds of dollars for a year's supply.[54] As Dr Yaxley commented, the hospital received 'many brickbats, very few bouquets' before the issue was resolved.[55]

Diabetes in children requires very careful management. At the Mater Children's Hospital in the 1970s, Dr Geoffrey Bourke established a multidisciplinary clinic to treat children with diabetes and to support them and their parents. It was Queensland's first team approach to childhood diabetes. By 1980, paediatricians Geoffrey Bourke and Michael Thomsett, dietitian Bernadette Wright, social worker Helen O'Brien, and nurse educator Amanda Coburn coordinated treatment for the 40 children enrolled in the clinic. As diabetes is a lifelong problem, educating the children and their families in managing the condition was an essential part of their work.[56]

Children with hearing impairments and their parents also needed support and education, particularly as they could become isolated and withdrawn in group situations. Heather Mohay, a psychologist in the University of Queensland's Child Health Department unit at the Mater Children's Hospital, developed a counselling service in the early 1980s, which developed into an out-patient clinic. In 1982, Heather Mohay was photographed by a local newspaper using Auslan sign language with a child who had been very alienated by the hospital setting as he could not communicate with the staff.[57]

Medical care in the clinics was essential in improving the lives of children with lifelong illness or disabling conditions, but parents and families at home had the hardest and most relentless work. Yet home could be a dangerous place for some children. About 27 per cent of admissions to the Mater Children's Hospital came through accidents; 60 per cent of these occurred at home, a phenomenon that was increasingly preoccupying paediatricians around the world.[58]

Road accidents were responsible for many admissions to the Mater Children's Hospital. In 1988, a Mater study revealed that road accidents caused about 25 per cent of injuries to children under the age of 14.[59] Some injuries were catastrophic. In 1981, Heath Pedley became a tetraplegic following a car accident; the daily press regularly reported his determination to use his mouth to manipulate pens, paint brushes and computer controls. Doctors at the Mater joined their colleagues everywhere in advocating properly fitted child restraints in cars and compulsory helmets for cyclists.[60]

A formal retrieval team, established in 1980, brought very ill or injured children to the hospital from all over South East and South West Queensland and northern New South Wales. In the late 1980s, the reach of the retrieval team extended more widely across Queensland, bringing children to the accident and emergency department and often to the intensive care unit where Dr Mansu Pabari was director.[61] As the medical superintendent, John McNee, had forecast, the hospital was reaching increasingly more broadly into the community and regarding itself as a resource for families. This direction became increasingly important when dealing with a particularly troubling phenomenon: child abuse.

Chapter 9
Dealing with Damage

Child abuse is a highly complex issue now assuming major proportions within all children's hospitals.

Annual Report, Mater Health Services, 1978

The construction of new buildings and the development of multidisciplinary clinics were not the only memorable features of the 1980s at the Mater Children's Hospital. Like children's hospitals everywhere, the Mater had to grapple with a very disturbing issue that grew in prominence in this era: child abuse and neglect. The team approach, working well in the multidisciplinary clinics that treated illness and disability, was also employed in developing ways of helping neglected and abused children and their families. Heightened awareness of child abuse demonstrated modern paediatrics' understanding of the relationship between a child's physical and emotional wellbeing and the surrounding social context. Dealing effectively with child abuse became a pertinent example of the strengthening links between children's hospitals and the communities they served.

Dealing with the damage caused by child abuse – the deliberate infliction of physical, sexual or emotional injury on a child and neglectful failure to provide adequately for a child's needs – was one of the most tragic and complex situations all children's hospitals faced in the final decades of the twentieth century. Although child abuse became a prominent subject in the public discourse, it was by no means a new phenomenon. Inquest records reveal an appalling catalogue of fatal injuries inflicted on children by adults in nineteenth-century Queensland.[1]

Literature in the English-speaking world, particularly the novels of Charles Dickens, highlighted some of the awful consequences for children when social and family stress, poverty and inadequate services combine. Yet the United Kingdom was slow to protect children, regarded as their parents' possessions, rather than people in their own right. Parents, therefore, were assumed to be entitled to treat their children in any way they chose. Intervention to protect children conflicted with an inviolate social tenet: the privacy of the home. The situation changed first in the United States. In New York in 1874, Mary Ellen McCormack was removed from the care of her abusive guardians when a court decided that Mary Ellen was a 'human animal' and therefore entitled to the protection given by 1860s legislation to prevent cruelty to animals.[2]

Legislation and organisations protecting animals – but not children – indicated the place of the child in nineteenth-century societies. Organisations protecting children developed in the United States and the United Kingdom in the 1880s and in Australia in the 1890s. In the 1920s, in the aftermath of the First World War, greater recognition that some families needed support and guidance in raising their children achieved little more than removing some children from their homes and placing them in orphanages. The United Nations Declaration of the Rights of the Child in 1959 stipulated that children are individuals with certain rights separate from adults.

In 1946, the American paediatric radiologist John Caffey published his observations of the association between long-bone fractures and chronic bruising in infants. Caffey believed that physical abuse was the cause, a finding that American paediatricians and radiologists described as 'deliberate' in the 1950s.[3] In 1962, Dr C Henry Kempe and his colleagues described the disastrous consequences of manhandling infants and violently shaking them.[4] The term 'battered baby syndrome' was coined from their work. Kempe published his landmark book *The Battered Child* in 1968. The Australian doctor Kim Oates, Professor of Paediatrics and Child Health at the University of Sydney, took up the cudgels in Australia.[5]

Child abuse was noticed more frequently in Queensland in the 1960s. In 1968, Sister Mary St Pierre McCormack RSM reported the admission of three children with nasty burns and noted that 'there seems to be some neglect attached to these accidents'.[6] Some injuries were very serious: two children needed extensive surgery after being injured by their father and, in 1970, a father was charged with serious assault after striking his infant child in the head.[7] Queensland police had also become increasingly aware of child abuse in the mid-1960s.[8]

In 1972, the Mater's director of medical services, Des O'Callaghan, set out firm guidelines in a memorandum: 'The management of the maltreated child'. All children thought to have been abused had to be admitted to the hospital immediately without communicating suspicions to their parents. The medical superintendent of the children's hospital, Dr Kerry Sullivan, was to be informed, extensive X-rays were to be taken and tests for nutritional deficiencies performed; all bruises were to be photographed.[9]

The first Australian conference on child abuse was held in Perth in 1975. Collaboration developed between police, child protection officers and health professionals in all Australian states. Agitation for mandatory reporting of abuse, promoted as necessary to protect children's rights to life and health, gathered strength. It was distressingly clear that the passage of any legislation for the compulsory reporting of child abuse would increase the number of children needing help and treatment. In 1977, South Australia was the first state to pass mandatory reporting legislation, followed by Queensland in 1978,[10] the Northern Territory in 1984, New South Wales in 1988, and Victoria in 1994. The Commonwealth developed a limited role in child protection with the passage of its *Family Law Act* in 1975, which removed divorce and child custody decisions from state courts to the new federal Family Court.

The 1978 and 1980 amendments to the Queensland *Health Act* made it compulsory for doctors to report cases of suspected child abuse and to refer the children to specialist teams.[11] The medical superintendent of the Mater Children's Hospital, Dr Barrie Heyworth, did not regard mandatory reporting as a perfect solution. He was concerned about threats to confidentiality as notification went first to Queensland's Director-General of Health; only in extreme urgency were children to be immediately referred to hospital. Parental objection to treatment could be over-ruled if two doctors agreed that treatment was necessary. Dr Heyworth supported the temporary custody arrangements, which placed a child in danger into the custody of the medical superintendent of either children's hospital in Brisbane, or to a regional hospital elsewhere in Queensland.[12]

The Mater's multidisciplinary team treating child abuse and its effects combined the skills of paediatricians, social workers, occupational therapists, physiotherapists, psychologists, psychiatrists and volunteer parent aides.[13] Although the Mater Children's Hospital described child abuse as a 'highly complex issue now assuming major proportions within all children's hospitals' in the late 1970s, the absence of accommodation for teenagers limited its comprehensive care of maltreated children.[14]

Child protection legislation generally recognised that resorting to the criminal law was not the only – or even the most effective – means of protecting children in abusive situations. Recognising the problem was always the first step.[15] In Queensland, as in many other parts of the world, the press supported the effort to prevent – or at least reduce – child abuse. As early as the 1960s, many researchers agreed that media coverage was perhaps as important as the research itself.[16] In October 1978, for instance, the *Courier-Mail* published an extensive article on 'shaken baby' syndrome. Barrie Heyworth was interviewed and revealed that he was one half of the Mater's child abuse unit; the social worker Susan Sellars was the other. Since October 1977, the hospital had dealt with 70 reports of child abuse, a huge increase from the ten cases reported in 1972. In 1978, occupational therapists watched children at play to pick up clues to a particularly nasty manifestation of maltreatment: sexual abuse.[17] In 1981, Barrie Heyworth reported that sexual abuse accounted for at least 10 per cent of all cases of child abuse.[18]

Press coverage continued. 'Heyworth fears baby bashing crisis' proclaimed the *Sunday Sun* in 1979, the *Sunday Mail* gave extensive publicity to a child abuse conference in 1981, and the *Courier-Mail* informed the public that abuse had become the third-largest killer of children after drowning and car accidents.[19] Some reports were particularly distressing. In 1983, there were six-year-olds in the Mater's child abuse unit reported as contemplating either suicide or setting fire to schools.[20]

In 1980, the Mater established its Suspected Child Abuse and Neglect Unit, always known as the SCAN unit. Similar units were established in many parts of the world. The Mater's child protection unit introduced a key Mater strategy: parent aides.[21] The concept was based on the idea that support for families was very important in preventing child abuse. The belief that 'intensive work in the early stages means fewer crises later' was very strong.[22] All parent aides were volunteers, coordinated by the social worker Janis Hinson, and trained to work with families where there had been abuse. In the first group, seven volunteer aides trained once a week for three months.[23] In 1978, the federal government funded Janis Hinson's part-time salary, administrative assistance and a mileage allowance for the aides for three years at $15,000 per year.

The 11-bed Mater SCAN unit was soon too small. Some children stayed for as long as seven months. As well as beatings, burns and sexual abuse – which increased to 25 per cent of admissions in the early 1980s – children were treated for many other forms of abuse, including deliberate poisoning and wilful denial of food. Many of the patients in the Mater unit were preschoolers. Their symptoms were serious: as well as damaging physical injuries, some were depressed, many were hyperactive or attention-seekers, and some were psychotic. There were also warnings of more subtle forms of maltreatment, such as forcing children into excessive training regimes for sport, or unduly long hours of study in the pursuit of success at school.[24]

The increase in numbers of children needing treatment and parents needing support began another round in the battle for resources. In 1985, the Mater was appalled by a newspaper headline, 'Major child abuse unit near collapse', leading to an article intimating that the Mater unit could no longer cope and might close. Even worse, the report was immediately followed by a letter from the minister to the Mater, defending his decision not to allocate further resources beyond the special grant for the unit in the 1984–85 financial year, even though the Mater's annual report had shown that admissions for child abuse had doubled in the previous year.[25]

The minister's comment that all hospitals were expected to live within their budgets, and his intimation that the Mater had somehow 'leaked' information about the child abuse funding crisis in order to coerce the government, prompted a forthright response from the Sister Administrator, Sister Angela Mary Doyle RSM. She was infuriated by the suggestion that a member of the Mater staff was responsible for the press leak. Rather, 'a public servant connected to the SCAN teams' had contacted the paper.[26]

Sister Angela Mary also made the Mater's position very clear in letters to the *Courier-Mail* and the *Catholic Leader*. She elaborated her defence with statistics: the number of patients had increased from 186 in 1981–82 to 600 in 1984–85, generating an obvious need for an increase in staff. The statistics included the number of families referred to the SCAN unit: 140 families and 186 children in 1981–82, 170 families and 217 children in 1982–83, 333 families and 474 children in 1983–84 and 383 families and more than 600 children in 1984–85.[27]

The population in the Mater's catchment was continuing to grow rapidly and the number of patients treated at the hospital for the usual wide range of conditions had not decreased. Consequently, staff could not easily be spared from other areas. In fact, since January 1982, the Mater SCAN team had functioned with one registrar, supplemented in 1983 and 1984 by three visiting specialist sessions each week for a total of nine hours.

The SCAN unit had never been funded for nursing staff, occupational therapists, social workers or clerical staff. These key members of the SCAN team had been redistributed from busy wards. The load was heavy: 678 child abuse cases had been referred in one year; three children had died.[28] It was thought unlikely that the actual incidence of child abuse had risen so greatly but, rather, the figures revealed an increase in families admitting that they needed help, more diligent reporting and greater public awareness.[29] The Mater Advisory Board was disturbed that the government had approved funding for positions lower down the Mater's priority scale than child abuse. The minister seemed to have forgotten a meeting in December 1984 with the Mater and the Royal Children's hospitals to discuss the great increase in child abuse notifications and the consequent need for increased resources for the 1985–86 year.[30]

The Queensland branch of the Australian Medical Association joined in the very public discussion. The President, Dr Lloyd Toft, said that funding was essential, as the numbers of patients in the child abuse units in both children's hospitals were increasing so rapidly. He also advocated sufficient resourcing to enable counselling for parents to continue.[31] Any rivalry between the Mater Children's and the Royal Children's hospitals, which may have existed in other areas, did not extend to child abuse services. Dr Simon Latham wrote indignantly from the Royal Children's Hospital that he regarded the press reports as a 'complete slur on the dedicated service that the Nuns have given over the years'.[32]

The situation became more alarming in August 1985 when the Health Minister indicated that Cabinet might decide to remove the SCAN units from Brisbane's two children's hospitals and place them in the community to be managed by social workers working in the Children's Services Department. Under this scheme, hospitals would treat only physical injuries.[33] This arrangement would destroy the unity of management of child abuse, which recognised that families and their circumstances, as well as the children, needed care and attention. In addition, psychological damage was often as serious in abused children as physical injury.

Ultimately, persistence in pleading the case succeeded. In the 1985–86 State Budget, the child abuse unit gained the highest number of additional staff approvals among all the many departments of the Mater hospitals: five additional paediatrician sessions; a social worker; occupational therapists, two full-time and one part-time; one registered nurse; and an administration assistant.[34]

Funding for parent aides was always insufficient. There were many public pleas for financial support, better accommodation for the program and additional volunteers, particularly by the mid-1980s when reporting of child abuse increased markedly. In this period, there was plenty of work for as many as 30 volunteers, but funding for the expenses of running the program could support only half that number.[35] The aides were so busy that there was little time for fundraising and they often dipped into their own pockets to pay for things for families. In 1988, the situation was very serious; government funding amounted to $12,000 but, ideally, the parent aide unit needed $100,000.[36]

By the mid-1980s, the Mater unit was recognised internationally; various overseas countries often asked for advice. The aides worked with families – only if they agreed – in their own homes for 12 months. A booklet about the unit included the story of a mother, with three children very close together in age, who was in danger of losing control through sheer exhaustion. She believed that her aide had intervened just in time.[37] The booklet was valuable in explaining the role of parent aides, as was a video, 'Break the cycle', launched in February 1990.

The aides reported considerable success in 1988: no child in a family with parent aide support had been re-injured since the program began in 1979. Education was an important part of the aides' work; some mothers as young as 15 had to be taught mothering skills. The aides had a demanding brief: to be 'mature, warm, stable and reliable with a good sense of humour'. The aides and their auxiliary continued their fundraising efforts and, in 1988 alone, raised $16,000.[38]

There were several crises when it seemed that the parent aide unit or the sexual abuse treatment unit – or both – would be disbanded and, once again, the government had to defuse alarming rumours.³⁹ Parent aides, indeed all members of the Mater Children's Hospital child abuse unit, also faced difficult ethical issues. Discussion of matters that contravened the church's teachings, such as contraception or termination of pregnancies, even those resulting from rape or incest, had to be handled delicately in a Catholic hospital.⁴⁰

Despite the challenges and the distressing nature of the work, several members of the Mater Children's Hospital child protection unit remained for many years. Annette Murphy and Irene Wilson, for instance, worked in the unit for more than 20 years.⁴¹ The paediatrician Dr David Wood was a tower of strength in the child protection unit and the SCAN teams. He was pointed in that direction by Dr Barrie Heyworth in the unit's very early days.

David Wood became well known in the press and in the wider community for his work in child protection. He refuted any belief there may have been in the public that child abuse was a problem confined to lower socio-economic groups by noting that people in the higher socio-economic groups were responsible for more emotional abuse than those in less affluent circumstances; professional people sending children to boarding school so that they didn't interfere with their parents' working or social lives was one example.⁴²

The statistics continued to be alarming. In 1988, for instance, sexual abuse of girls headed the list, followed by almost equal neglect of girls and boys. Emotional abuse was more common in girls than in boys, who suffered higher levels of physical abuse. In the late 1980s, the staff of the child protection unit had grown to three consultant paediatricians – Dr David Wood, Dr Maree Crawford and Dr Tony Leslie, who gained further experience in Canada – one registrar, one social worker, one registered nurse and one administration assistant. Funding to employ a psychologist, an occupational therapist and a speech therapist to work full-time in the unit was, however, urgently needed.⁴³

In the late 1980s, research in the previous couple of decades identified a phenomenon that workers in child protection had long suspected: abused children often became abusing parents and that poor living and parenting skills often crossed generations.⁴⁴ This was a growing social problem. After three years of planning, the Abused Child Trust (now Act for Kids) was formed in 1988 with David Wood on the inaugural board; he became chairman in 1991. The Trust's initial goals were day care for abused preschoolers, a research and evaluation program and a comprehensive program to work with parents and children in a number of centres.⁴⁵

Within its first few years, the Trust accumulated disturbing statistics. Physical abuse headed the list at 54.7 per cent, sexual abuse came next at 38.5 per cent, followed by emotional abuse at 4.7 per cent and neglect at 2.1 per cent. Some of the broader statistics were very thought-provoking: 70 per cent of prisoners in Australian jails had been abused as children, as had 43 per cent of psychiatric patients.[46] Children had particular difficulties in the legal system. Protect All Children Today (PACT), formed in 1985 by the Queensland government to support children and young people giving evidence in the criminal courts, became an advocate for all children.

Psychiatric disorders and behavioural problems could follow child abuse, but could also arise from a multitude of other causes and conditions. The model for the ideal children's hospital, considered by the Health Minister's Paediatric Advisory Committee in 1976, recognised that increasing numbers of children were presenting with behavioural problems or psychiatric disorders, a trend that continued to increase.[47] A submission to the McSweeny committee reviewing the Mater Children's Hospital in 1977 observed that the psychology clinic was probably the area with the most 'growth potential' and that a family therapist was badly needed.[48]

Dr Irene Apel, a visiting psychiatrist appointed to the Mater Children's Hospital in 1966, became a determined advocate of comprehensive care for children with behavioural problems and psychological disorders. She reported that, with an increasing incidence of broken marriages, the family clinic was increasingly in demand and should be extended beyond developmental paediatrics to an approach that included the whole family and the child's school.[49] The number of children treated in the Mater's psychological disorders clinic had grown from eight in 1975 to 51 in 1980.[50] Before extensions to the Mater Children's Hospital in the 1980s, there was no dedicated in-patient ward for children with major psychiatric disorders.

Dr Apel recommended the conversion of one of the houses the Mater owned in an adjoining street for work with children with learning difficulties or behaviour problems, particularly children from remote parts of Queensland and those who had been moved from foster home to foster home and had become disturbed and unhappy. In 1980, Barrie Heyworth supported the use of one of the Mater houses to cater for children who had been abused and children with behaviour problems. This, he thought, would be in tune with the developing emphasis on community outreach.[51]

The need for increased psychiatric services for children, beyond the specialist unit developed at the Royal Children's Hospital, was broadly recognised. Dr Helen Connell, a leader in child psychiatry in Brisbane, completed a survey of psychological disorders among children in Queensland primary schools in 1978.[52] Helen Connell's survey of children in isolated parts of Queensland was based on a method used in the United Kingdom. Answers to questionnaires issued to parents and teachers made sobering reading. The survey of teachers reported that 10.5 per cent of the 500 children in the survey scored above the 'Rutter level' indication that a disorder could be present. On full screening, this became 7.65 per cent, compared with 6.8 per cent on the Isle of Wight, where Sir Michael Rutter conducted the first survey. It was, Connell noted, very difficult for children in far western Queensland to access appropriate psychiatric help.[53] Increased facilities in the children's hospitals and a visiting service to isolated areas were urgently needed.

Psychiatric services at the Mater Children's Hospital gradually developed. A child psychologist was appointed to the visiting staff in 1978, as was a full-time psychiatrist, Dr Aidene Urquhart, in 1980. A dedicated unit at the Mater Children's Hospital was not established until the mid-1980s, even though paediatric practice recognised that child psychiatry was an integral part of a children's hospital, rather than a mere adjunct.[54] Emotional factors were known to play a significant part in all aspects of health and disease in children.

The 12 beds for children with psychological disorders in the former babies' ward were soon completely inadequate. The out-patient clinic in the old university unit struggled to the point that the child psychiatry unit concentrated on in-patients, well aware that it needed to serve the community more broadly. If World Health Organization (WHO) standards were followed, Queensland needed at least three 20-bed units, in addition to out-patient and day-patient facilities, to service its population. The flying psychiatrist service to the outback helped, but visits more frequently than once a month – or once every three months in some regions – were needed. Children who were too disturbed for out-patient or day-patient treatment stayed in hospital for as long as six weeks. This caused considerable difficulty at the Mater Children's Hospital because the government had not formally recognised the unit; its staff, therefore, had to be borrowed from other areas.

The Mater service, the unit at the Royal Children's Hospital, the community-based units in Ipswich, Toowoomba, Townsville and the Gold

Coast and the ten guidance clinics in Brisbane could see only a fraction of the children who needed help. Research revealed that 10 per cent of all children could suffer from a recognised disorder, yet the Mater could accept only 1 per cent of these children.[55] The opening of the dedicated out-patient building in 1987 at last began to relieve some of the strain, but psychiatric services were developing a broader remit, which reflected the damage a disturbed world could inflict.

Psychiatrist Aidene Urquhart found that some of her patients had been exposed to trauma and torture in their countries of origin, thus attending to their medical needs alone was insufficient.[56] She developed the Mater Children's Hospital torture and trauma unit, known as TRUSTT (Treatment and Rehabilitation Unit for Survivors of Torture and Trauma).

Psychological problems and a wide range of physical conditions can impede healthy child development. Developmental paediatrics became a rapidly growing area in the 1980s. Dr Michael O'Callaghan led the child development unit at the Mater Children's Hospital. As he described it, developmental paediatrics was concerned with the maturation process from viability to full growth in all children. There were three essential goals: to promote optimal physical and mental health, to ensure early diagnosis and treatment of handicapping conditions of body, mind and personality, and to discover the cause of handicapping conditions and means of preventing them. Development could be affected by both biological and environmental factors and, therefore, the focus was always on the child within the context

> MICHAEL O'CALLAGHAN, MBBS, MSc, MD, FRACP, graduated in medicine at the University of Queensland in 1971 and was a resident medical officer at the Royal Brisbane Hospital before beginning his post-graduate training at the Royal Children's Hospital, Melbourne. Between 1976 and 1979, Michael O'Callaghan developed his interest in developmental paediatrics at the Nottingham Children's Hospital in England. He joined the staff at the Mater Children's Hospital in August 1979. As well as his clinical responsibilities, Michael O'Callaghan chaired the Paediatric Staff Society in the 1990s. He retired from the Mater in 2012.

of the family and the community.⁵⁷ When he was appointed to the Mater Children's Hospital staff in 1979, Michael O'Callaghan was one of the few doctors in Australia fully trained in developmental paediatrics.⁵⁸

The child development clinic was one of the Mater Children's Hospital's growing range of multidisciplinary clinics. In 1980, for instance, this team included an occupational therapist, Cathy Croft; a speech pathologist, Kerrin Finch; and a physiotherapist, Cathy Bagley. Referrals to the clinic came from preschools and general practitioners.⁵⁹ The clinic's work evolved into involvement in three main areas: multidisciplinary services to children with serious or complex disorders of development, a rehabilitation service for children with acquired brain injury and neuromuscular disease, and children with autism spectrum disorders. Like all Mater Children's Hospital services, the child development clinic had its wish list. In 1985, a full-time respiratory technician was urgently required,⁶⁰ as were a social worker, a psychologist, an occupational therapist, a physiotherapist, a speech pathologist, an audiologist and a nurse to undertake the formidable task of coordination.

In 1988, a report by Dr Ken Mitchell noted that resourcing the SCAN teams had delayed the development of adolescent units and child development units at both children's hospitals in Brisbane. Nevertheless, the Mitchell investigation found that the SCAN units should be maintained and better resourced.⁶¹ Balancing urgent needs, both old and new, against resources delayed the implementation of long-delayed plans. Rationalisation soon became an all-consuming topic.

Chapter 10

We Shall Not Be Moved

Commonwealth and state governments agree that most specialised facilities and services should be concentrated in large units, rather than dispersed among smaller units.

Commonwealth of Australia, Report on rationalisation of hospital facilities, 1979

In 1970s Australia, health budgets in all states were affected by the increasing presence of the Commonwealth government in health policy. Health care became a major factor in changing the balance between state and federal power. Under the Australian constitution, the states were responsible for health care, but the federal government had the money, largely due to the power to tax incomes, which it had exercised since the early stages of the Second World War.[1] Pressure to manage health costs increased at the same time as new techniques and technologies offered enticing vistas of new, more effective patient services. Two immense forces – population increase and escalating costs – deposited health care and its financing into the centre of political debate in Australia. All public hospitals were caught up in the furore.

Higher standards in health services were benefits of twentieth-century science and social concern, but they were not gifts. Health grew almost eightfold from 0.38 per cent of Australia's gross domestic product in 1900–01 to 2.68 per cent in 1969–70, and more than doubled to 6.3 per cent in 1981–82.[2] The Commonwealth government's share of expenditure on health care grew from 19 per cent in 1975–76 to 39 per cent by 1982.[3] Most of the money was spent on the treatment of illness, rather than on its prevention, which largely had to wait while debate raged on reducing costs in the most expensive sector of health services – the acute-care hospitals.[4]

'Rationalisation' – a basket of strategies aimed at achieving the most efficient distribution of health services and facilities – became the order of the day. At the Mater Children's Hospital, rationalisation set the scene for vigorous discussions on the whole future of the hospital. In the early 1990s, the Mater Children's Hospital faced an acute rationalisation dilemma: being asked to move from its existing home to an entirely new location. This controversial situation had a long gestation.

The situation in which the hospital found itself in the 1980s and early 1990s is best understood in the context of the policies and funding models that prevailed. While rationalisation was embraced by government policy makers, it was regarded by hospital administrators and clinicians occasionally with enthusiasm but more often with scepticism, even dread. Reducing the duplication of clinical services, an apparently economically sensible notion, was often extremely difficult to implement.

In March 1977, the government's Paediatric Advisory Committee was asked to investigate the possibility of rationalising paediatric services between Brisbane's two children's hospitals, a compromise on the real need – a single tertiary-level children's hospital. Many major world cities – London, Boston, Paris and Toronto among them – had single children's hospitals. The suggestion that there should be one Institute of Child Health in Brisbane recurred at various times since University of Queensland's Professor of Child Health, John Rendle-Short, suggested it in 1970. In 1976, for instance, the Paediatric Advisory Committee considered administrative and clinical integration of Brisbane's two children's hospitals. In this model, the two campuses would continue, but tertiary services would be divided between them.[5]

Pressure to provide services as close as possible to those who needed them accompanied the emphasis on rationalisation and put a spotlight on one of the elephants in the room: the Queen Elizabeth II Jubilee Hospital (QEII) at Mt Gravatt on Brisbane's southern outskirts, which opened in 26 September 1980. This new hospital – the first on Brisbane's south side since the South Brisbane Hospital (now the Princess Alexandra Hospital) opened in 1956 – symbolised a major shift in Australian health-care planning.[6] The nation's major public hospitals were located in the centres of cities, rather than in outlying suburbs where the great postwar suburban sprawl had placed most of the population. Hospitals in growing areas were to redress this demographic imbalance. Simultaneously, a movement towards health care in the community – rather than in expensive acute-care hospitals – would relieve budgetary pressure.[7] If a children's hospital were to be included on the Mt Gravatt site, it would have sophisticated equipment and able to share some of the up-to-date facilities of the main hospital. However, such a move would mean that development at either of the existing children's hospitals was unlikely.

In the mid-1970s, the Australian Universities Commission recommended that a teaching unit in obstetrics be established at Mt Gravatt.[8] This idea did not augur well for the Mater Mothers' Hospital as a major university teaching hospital, or for the Mater Children's Hospital, which received new babies requiring further treatment. The University of Queensland's Dean of the Faculty of Medicine, Professor Eric Saint, thought that the Mater Children's Hospital, where a new Department of Child Health building had been funded, would be 'the only string left in the bow' for the Mater if a major new maternity hospital eventuated at Mt Gravatt.[9] There was an element of *déjà vu* in this situation. In the late 1950s, the Princess Alexandra Hospital opened close to the Mater, rather putting the Mater Adult Hospital in the shade. The Princess Alexandra Hospital symbolised the Queensland government's reluctance to fund capital works at the privately owned Mater Adult Hospital.

Some of the recommendations of a committee investigating teaching hospitals on Brisbane's south side in 1977 appeared to improve the outlook for the Mater Children's Hospital. An orthopaedic unit could be useful at Mt Gravatt, provided that the treatment of scoliosis remained at the Mater Children's Hospital. A neurosurgical unit for adults should remain at the Princess Alexandra Hospital and one for children at the Mater. The Mater Children's and Royal Children's hospitals could share nephrology services, but open-heart surgery should remain at The Prince Charles Hospital on the other side of the city at Chermside.[10]

Good nutrition and modern medical care had also imposed a new burden on the health system at the other end of the age spectrum. All acute-care hospitals treated aged patients who would be more appropriately cared for in nursing homes, but places were inadequate.[11] The Mater regarded this problem as urgent, ranking far ahead of the need of another acute-care general hospital.

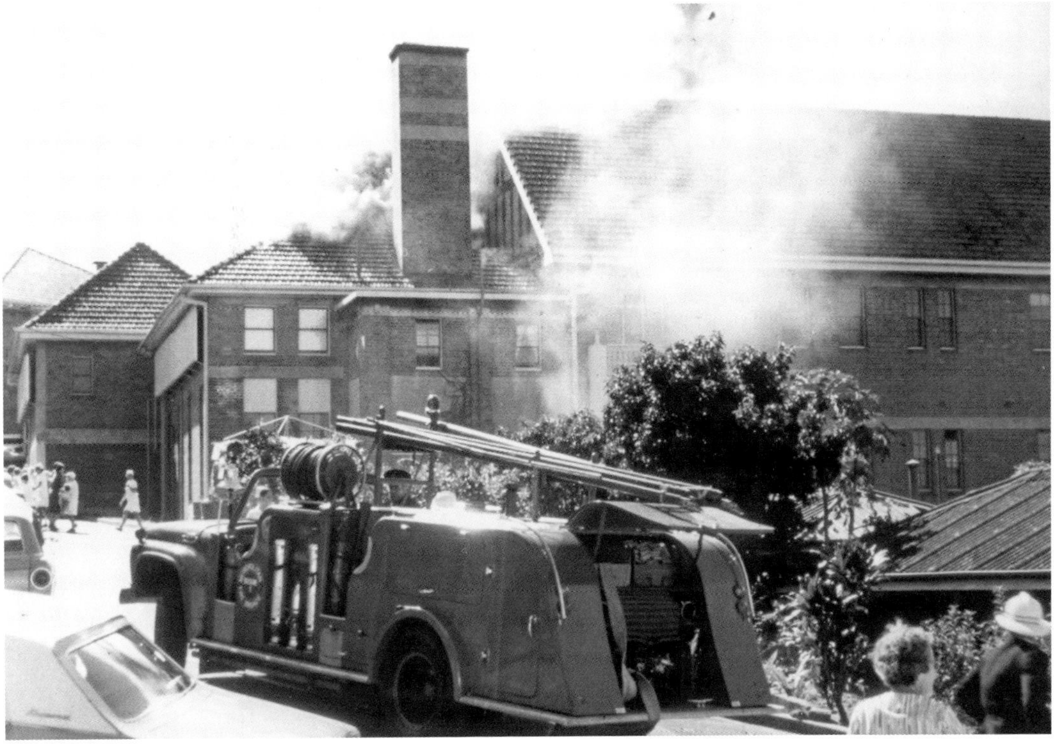

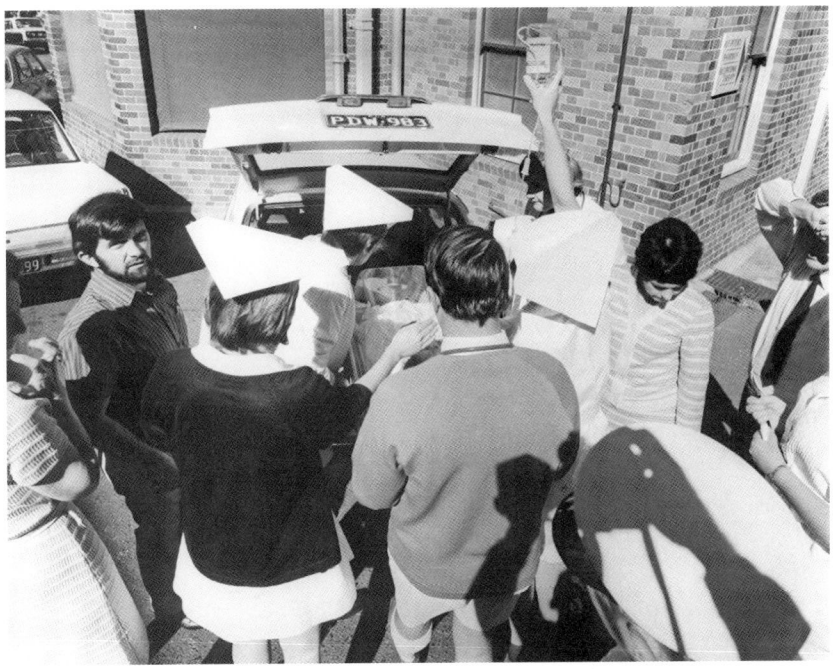

Smoke billowing from the roof of the Mater Children's Hospital during the fire in 1971.

A very difficult situation: evacuating a tiny baby during the fire emergency. The surgeon Dr Des McGuckin is at far left.

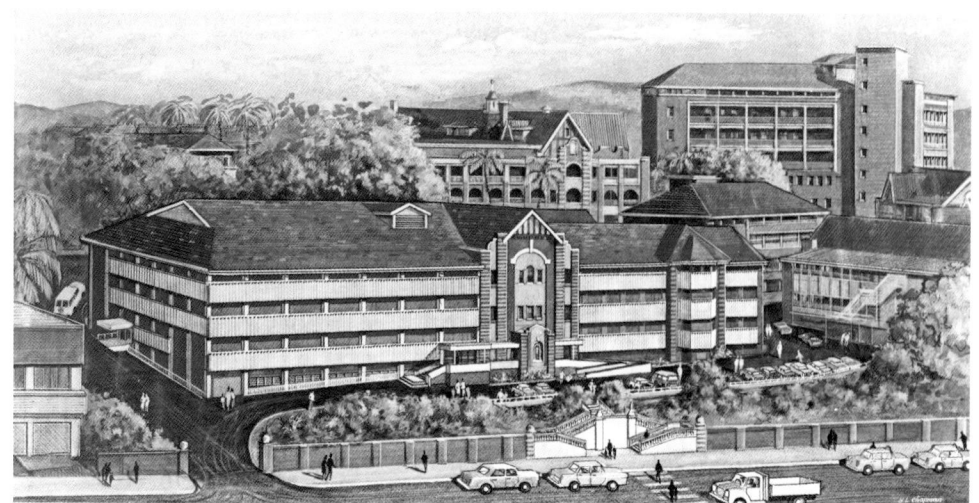

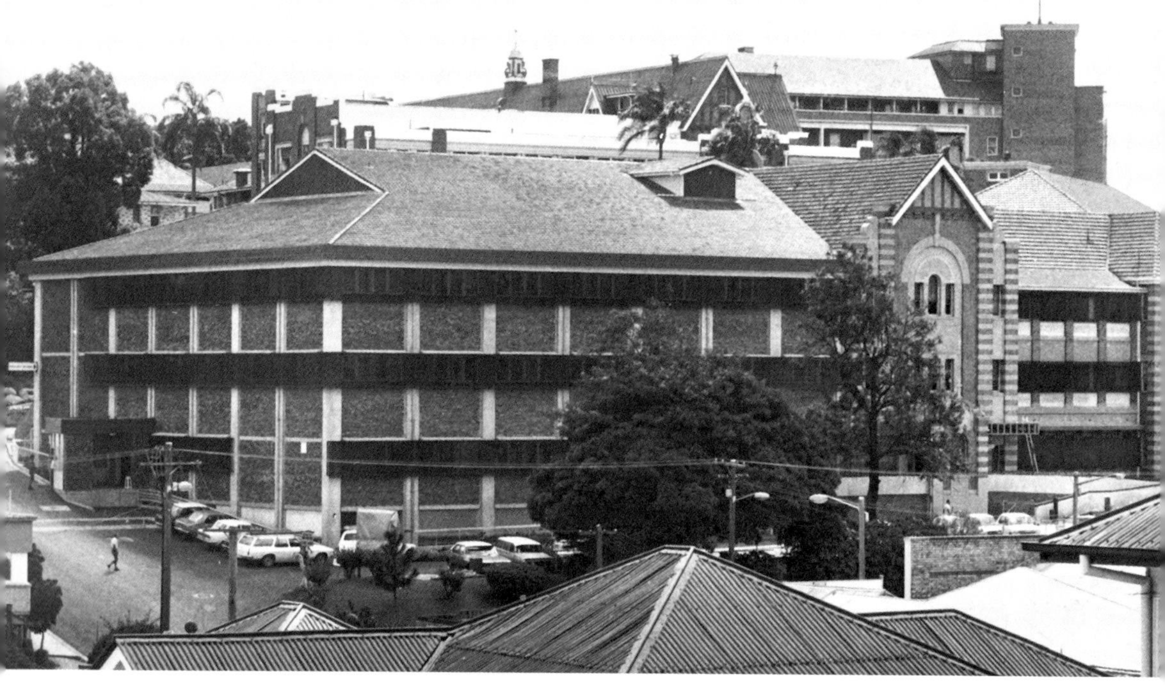

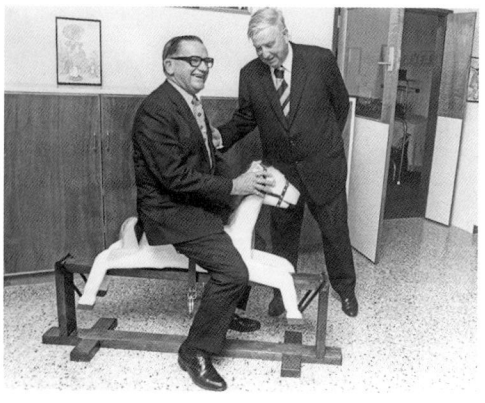

TOP: The second wing as planned in the early 1970s.

ABOVE: The second wing in reality in 1976.

LEFT: Hijinks after the opening of the second wing: the Queensland Treasurer, Gordon Chalk, tests out a rocking horse, watched by JP Kelly.

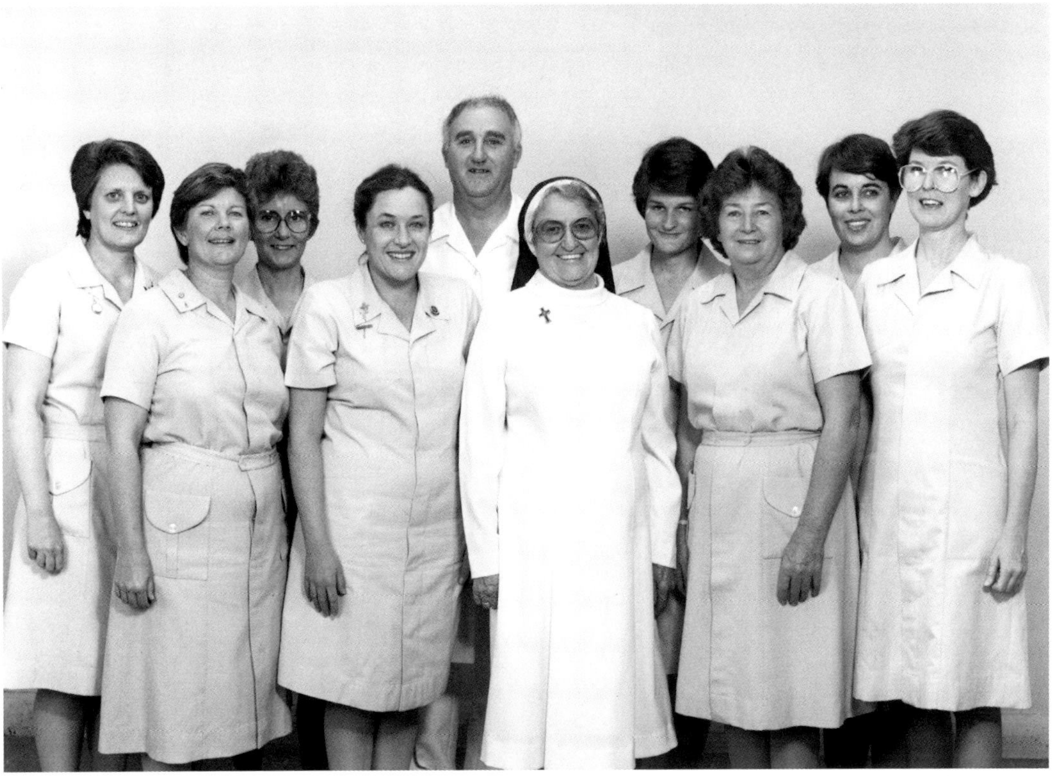

Sister Mary Dorothea Sheehan in 1986 with senior members of the Mater Children's Hospital nursing staff, from left to right: JA Denne, DT O'Neill, J Hemy, SM Norman, Mr W Howgego, Sister Mary Dorothea, MC O'Neill, M Welsh, M McCarthy, MM Hart.

RIGHT: Dr Kerry Sullivan photographed in 1975 with (from left to right) Sister Mary Colette Anderson, Sister Mary Dorothea Sheehan and the hospital secretary, Josey Holyer.

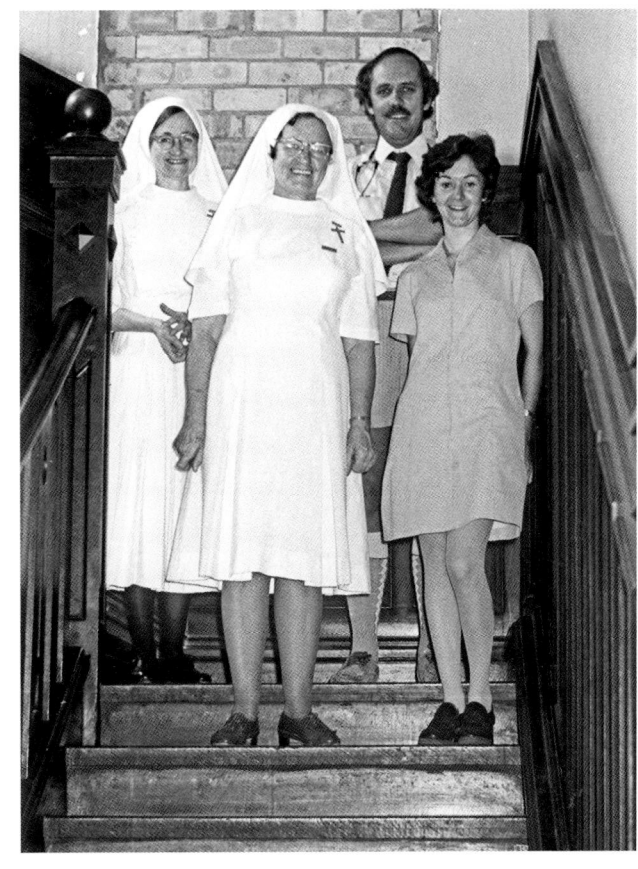

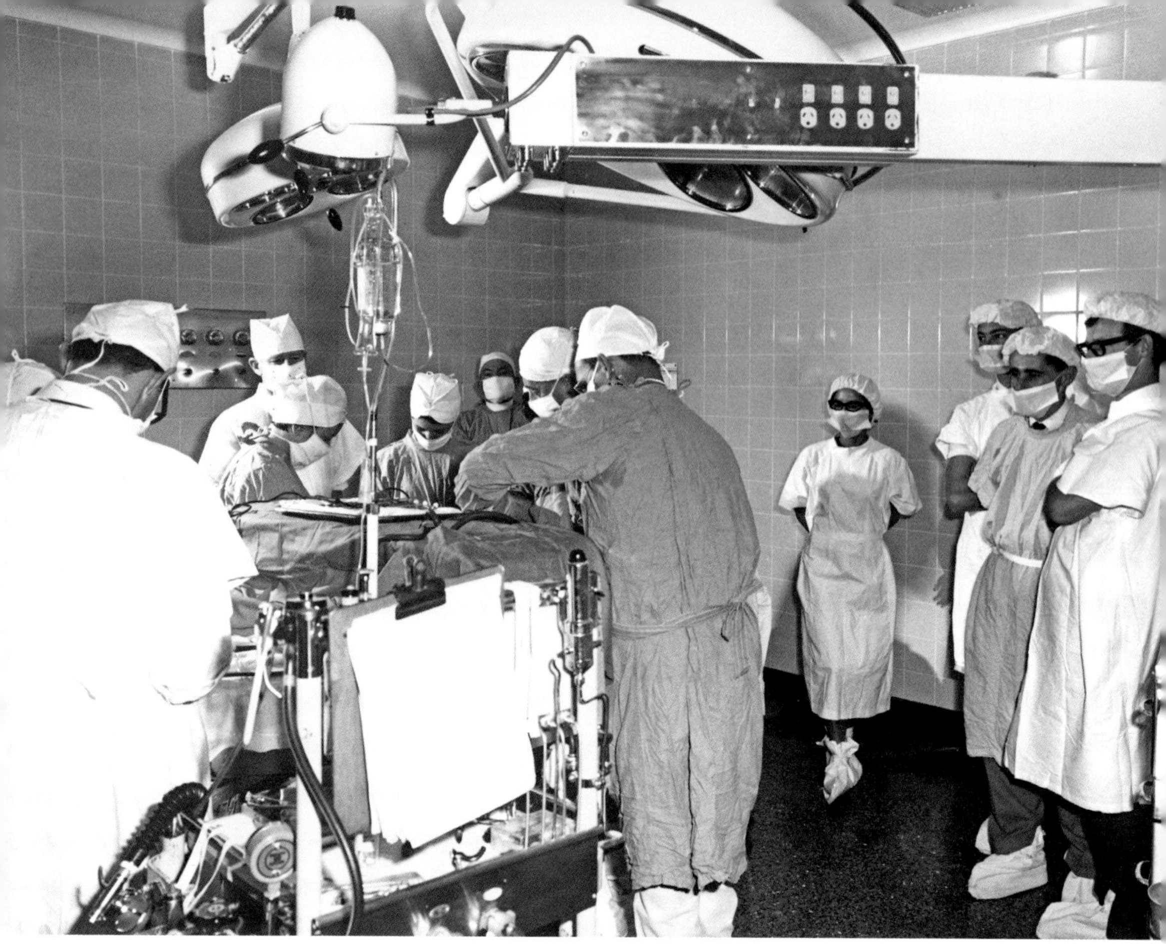

Dr Len Marriott and Dr Des McGuckin hard at work in the new operating theatres in 1986.

Linda Blackwell and Dr Des O'Callaghan watch 1970s hydrotherapy treatment with physiotherapist Cathy Bagley.

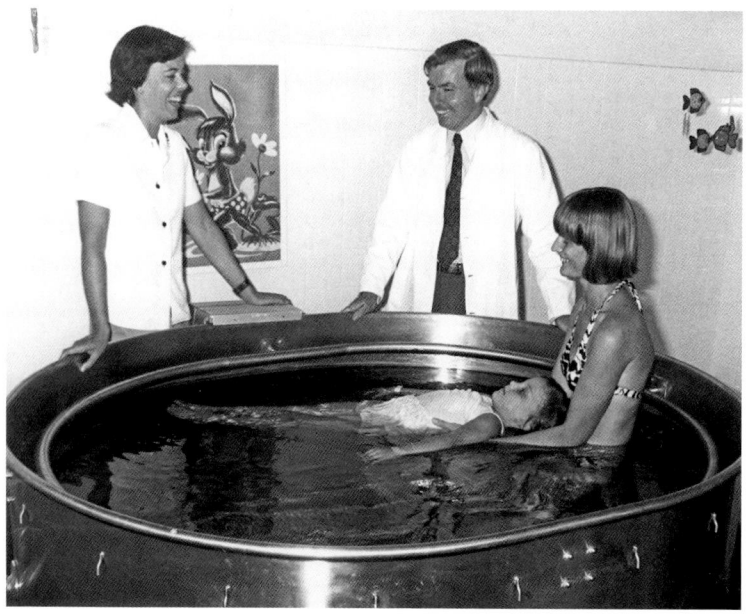

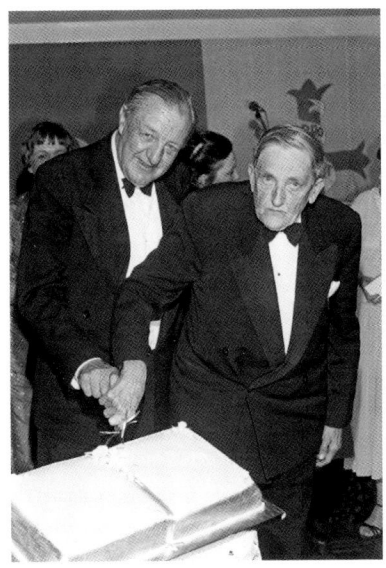

Dr Tom Carroll (left), the Mater Children's first resident medical officer, and Dr George Taylor, pathologist, at the Golden Jubilee dinner dance in 1981.

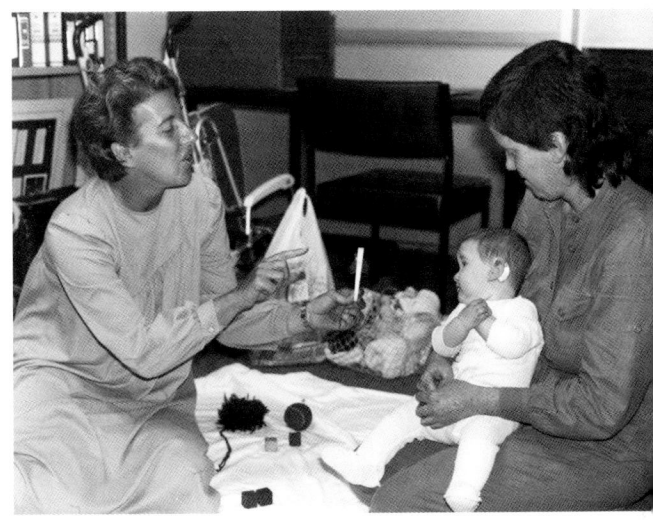

RIGHT: Heather Mohay, psychologist, working with a mother and baby in the 1980s.

The Mater Children's Hospital's successful float at the Warana (blue skies) Festival in 1981.

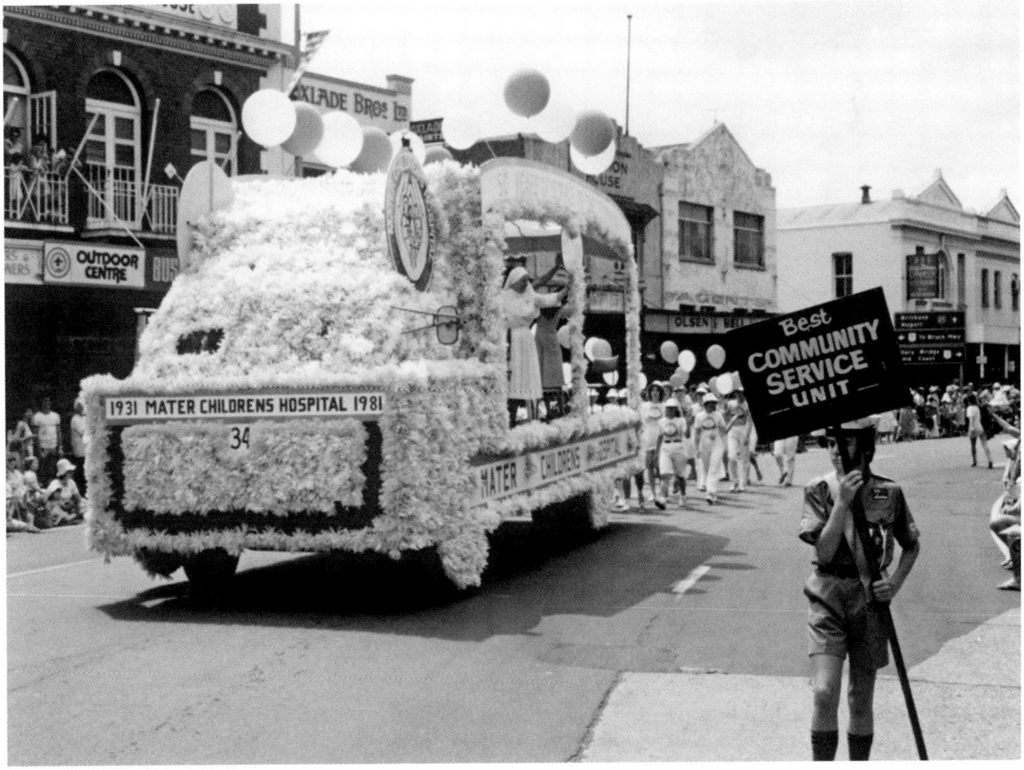

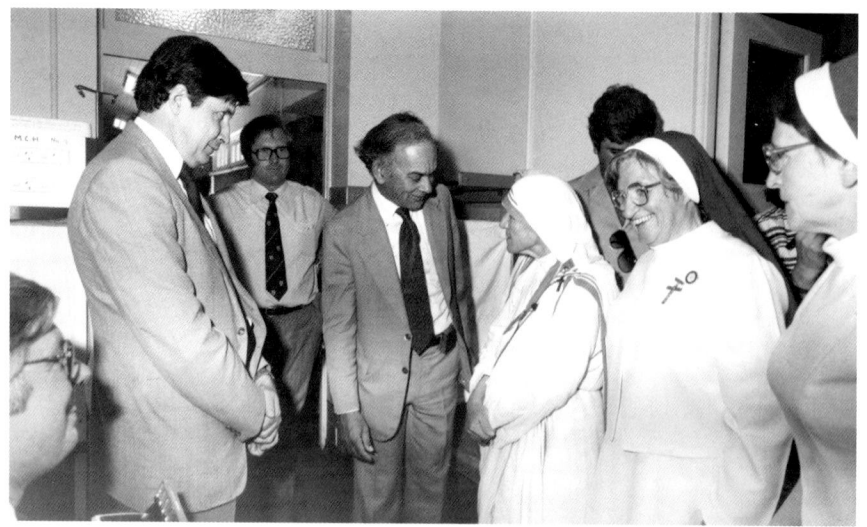

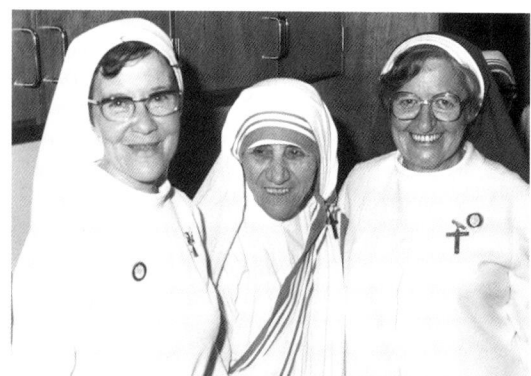

Mother Teresa with (from left to right) Drs Leigh Atkinson, John Vance and Geoffrey Bourke.

LEFT: Mother Teresa with Sister Marie Fitzgerald (left) and Sister Mary Dorothea Sheehan (right).

Mother Teresa engaging the attention of a small patient.

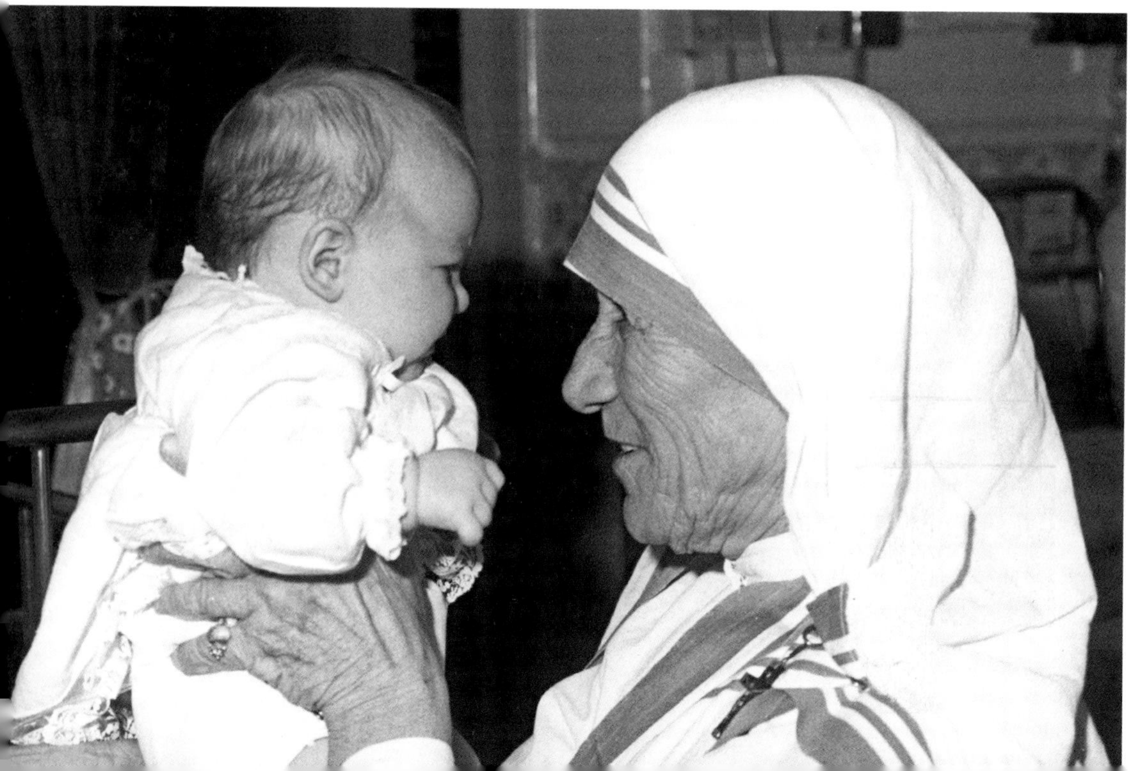

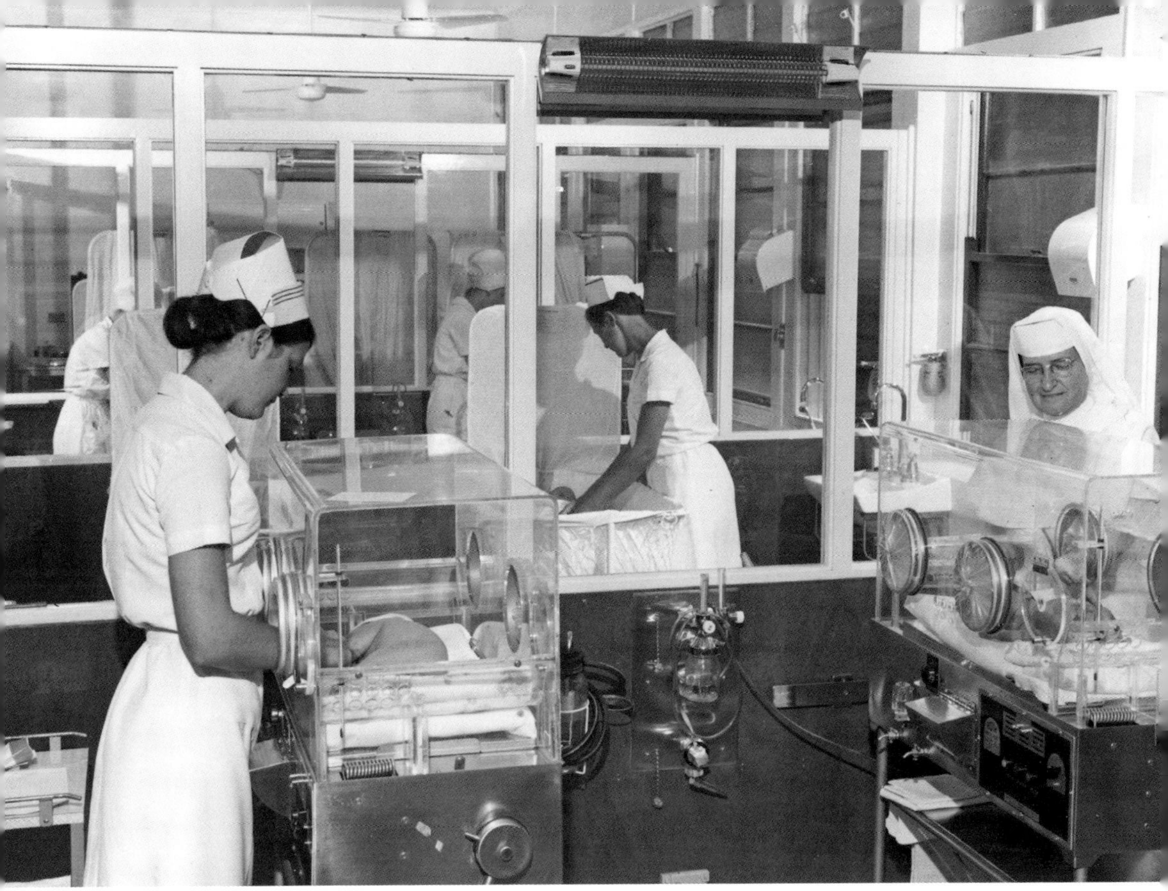

The much larger babies' ward with Sister Mary Dorothea Sheehan and several nurses attending to patients in intensive care cots in 1986.

Lessons underway in the schoolroom before the new school opened in 1983.

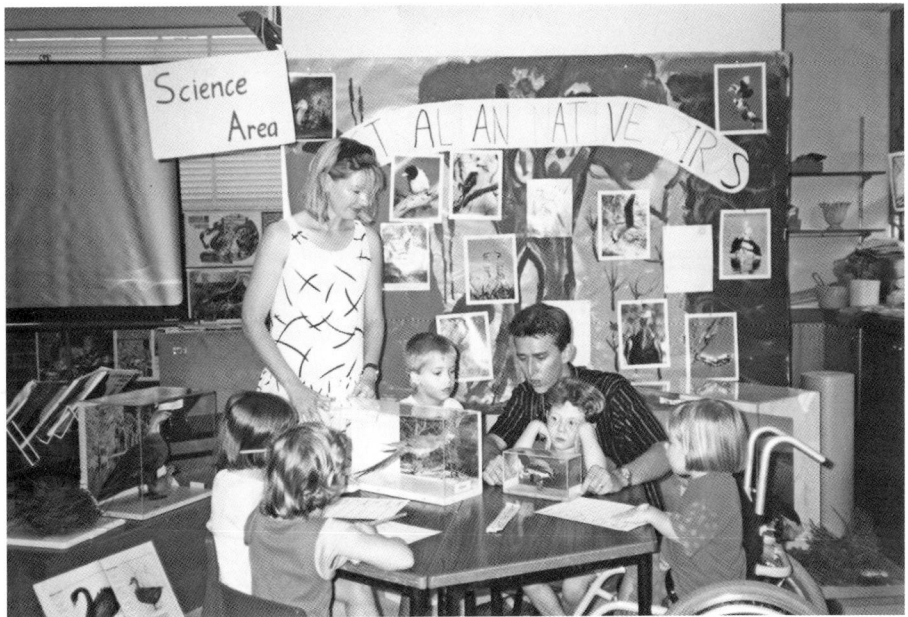

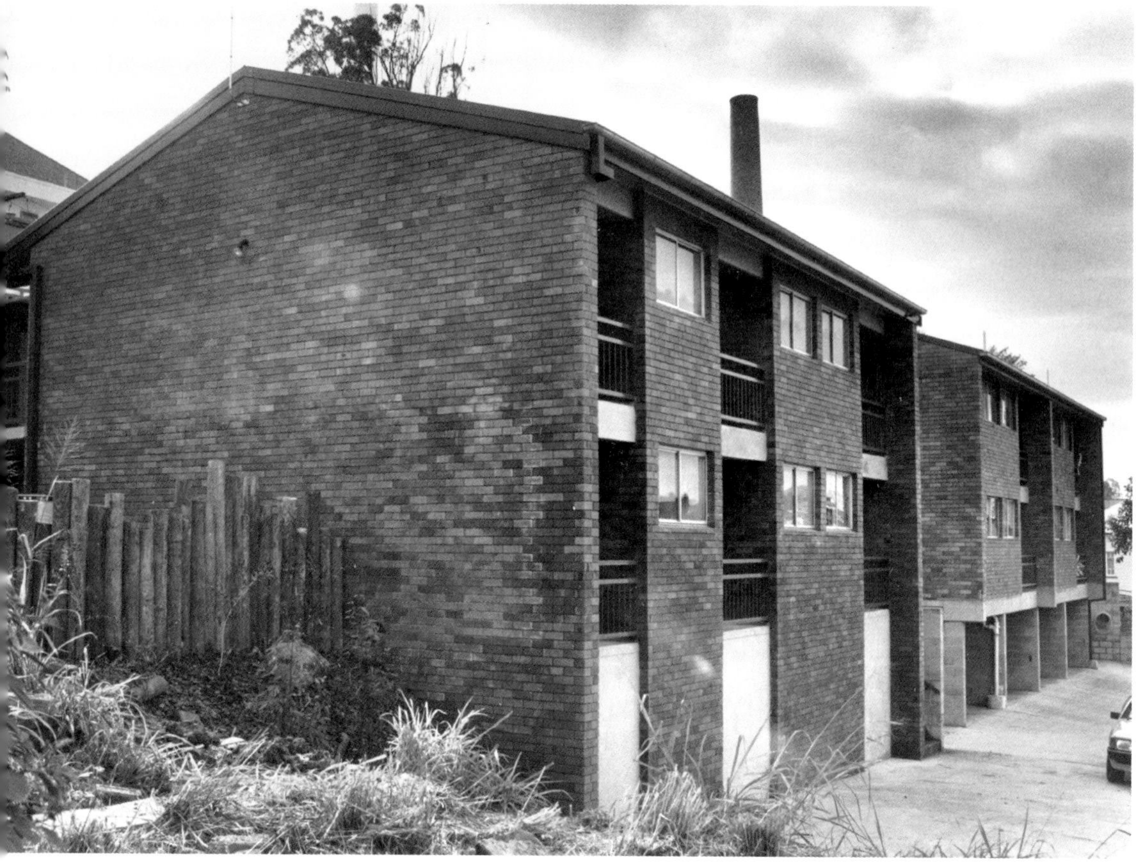

The Reg Leonard units after an extension in 1980.

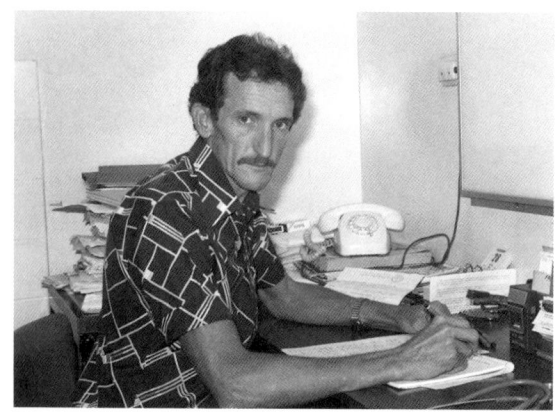

Dr John McNee working at his desk in 1981.

RIGHT: Rosalie Lewis RN was appointed director of nursing in 1986.

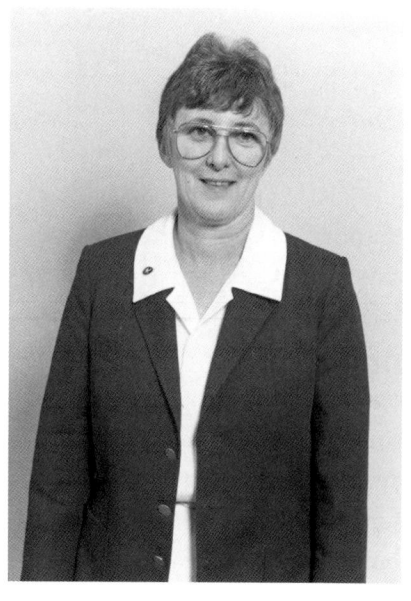

The intensive appraisal of the Mater Children's Hospital by the McSweeny committee in 1977 took place against the background of discussions on rationalisation.[12] This committee could see benefit for the Mater Children's Hospital in sharing staff with the Princess Alexandra Hospital in neurosurgery and improved contact with the Royal Children's Hospital. Discussions with the Royal Children's Hospital, the McSweeny committee recommended, should include the concept of an Institute of Child Health to be situated 'on neutral territory'.[13] However, the committee accepted 'that the die is already cast for the continuance of two teaching children's hospitals in the City of Brisbane, each complete in its own right'.

In 1978, Queensland's Health Minister, Dr Llew Edwards, produced a White Paper on rationalisation of health services.[14] Sister Angela Mary Doyle, Sister Administrator of the Mater hospitals, was dissatisfied with some aspects of the paper. She wrote:

> The expanding field of paediatrics has not been developed at length and we would welcome inclusion in any committee which may be established to study the future of paediatrics.[15]

Sister Angela Mary was frustrated that discussions about rationalisation had made no progress when the costs of hospital services were escalating rapidly. Services could be organised economically, even if that meant that the Mater complex would not necessarily retain every service or specialty. She reminded the minister that the Mater Children's Hospital expertise in neurosurgery allowed it to be the only Queensland hospital undertaking craniofacial surgery.[16]

This was an era of considerable pressure on children's hospitals. In 1970, an article in the *British Medical Journal* drew attention to the ever-diminishing number of specialist children's hospitals in Britain. Paediatricians, the article said, felt oppressed and longed for improved services for children.[17] In this context, a combined Mater burns unit for adults and children was inappropriate. A paediatric burns unit would need a play therapist and an occupational therapist, as well as other highly specialised staff. At that time, the Mater Children's Hospital was caring for 40 patients with burns each year. Some patients stayed for only a few days and returned to the hospital for dressings, but live-in facilities were necessary for children referred for burns treatment from other parts of Queensland.

Great upheaval at the Mater followed another response to the Edwards paper. The medical superintendent of the Mater Children's Hospital, Dr Barrie Heyworth, who had strongly promoted the development of subspecialties at the Mater, was a member of the Queensland Coordinating Committee on Child Abuse, the Queensland Standing Committee on Paediatric Training and the Health Minister's Paediatric Advisory Committee. Dr Heyworth had attended a meeting with Dr Edwards and Professor Rendle-Short to discuss improved links between the two children's hospitals. In December 1978, in commenting on the Edwards paper, Dr Heyworth emphasised that coordination should be the first priority and that the Mater Children's Hospital should further develop particular specialties such as craniofacial surgery, respiratory medicine, endocrinology and gastroenterology.[18]

By 1982, Dr Heyworth was annoyed that, in the four years since Dr Edwards issued his paper, there had been 'no rationalisation, no coordination and no joint administration' of the two hospitals, which had continued to develop as rivals. Instead, the government's goal should be to provide Brisbane with a centre of paediatric excellence. This would save about $20,000,000 – the estimated cost of renewing the Royal Children's Hospital – enabling the government to rationalise adult services, particularly rehabilitative and geriatric services.[19]

Between the Edwards paper in 1978 and Dr Heyworth's personal response in 1982, the Commonwealth government's rationalisation investigation reported in 1979 that both Brisbane's children's hospitals were too small.[20] The Commonwealth believed that state governments would agree that most specialised facilities and services should be concentrated in large units, rather than dispersed among smaller units, because a large population was needed to support tertiary services, especially in neurosurgery, thoracic surgery, radiotherapy, plastic surgery and expensive diagnostic services.[21]

Dr Heyworth pointed out that the Mater Children's Hospital had expanded rapidly in the four years since Dr Edwards' paper and was caring for more in-patients, more casualties and an equal number of out-patients, even though it had only 140 beds compared with 250 at the Royal Children's Hospital. The difference was explained by a lower average length of stay at the Mater Children's Hospital: an average of 3.5 days compared with 6 at the Royal Children's Hospital and a higher daily occupancy rate: 75 per cent compared with 50 per cent.[22]

Even though the areas south and west of Brisbane were expanding more rapidly than areas to the north, Dr Heyworth did not believe that rebuilding the Mater Children's Hospital was justified. Developmental paediatrics, adolescent medicine in Brisbane generally and improved psychiatric services on the south side were pressing needs, but the present system would mean that both hospitals would have to have them. This, he thought, could be avoided. Staff salaries comprised 70 per cent of the budgets of the two children's hospitals; staff duplication should, therefore, be eliminated.

The Commonwealth's promotion of preventive medicine rather than curative medicine was, in Dr Heyworth's view, a further reason for rationalising paediatric services in Brisbane.[23] The answer was a Queensland Institute of Child Health aimed at health promotion, clinical excellence, research and education. Dr Heyworth claimed that Professor Rendle-Short, the Australian College of Paediatrics and prominent paediatricians all agreed.

Though it was his personal view, Heyworth's position as medical superintendent of the Mater Children's Hospital made the next stage of his paper even more controversial: the Mater Children's Hospital should be closed, as no further development was possible on its present site and, further, 'the management of that hospital is inefficient and not geared to modern paediatrics'. The Royal Children's Hospital should also be closed as the re-development of that site would be very expensive. The two hospitals should be combined on one site as central as possible in Brisbane.

The site of the Mater Adult Hospital would, Dr Heyworth said, be appropriate. The QEII hospital at Mt Gravatt was too far from the northern suburbs and the Mater was better serviced by public transport than the Royal Children's Hospital. The South Brisbane site was the right size with full service facilities, and could accommodate 250–280 beds, considerably fewer than the 380 beds existing at the two children's hospitals, but day wards would allow a bed to be occupied multiple times, reducing overall bed numbers. Modern facilities such as day wards, family care wards, developmental paediatrics, adolescent facilities, child abuse and neglect teams and preventative and educational facilities could all be included. A central tertiary children's hospital would require secondary beds at various district hospitals under the direction of the Institute's board.[24] The Institute would be economically efficient, able to direct and integrate metropolitan community paediatric services and would require only one university Department of Child Health.

Dr Heyworth realised that there would be 'political ramifications' in taking over the Mater Adult Hospital and suggested that the Mater Children's Hospital building could become a centre for geriatric care and rehabilitation. Beds for acutely ill adults could be distributed among other south-side hospitals, in line with the Commonwealth government's emphasis on rationalisation.[25] Dr Heyworth suggested that the proposed Institute be staffed by senior clinicians from both children's hospitals.[26]

Barrie Heyworth's paper was intended only for the minister's advisory committee, but Sister Angela Mary Doyle RSM, Sister Administrator of the Mater hospitals, became aware of it at a meeting of the Standing Committee on the Rationalisation of Health Services. It was claimed that the paper had emanated from the Mater.[27] She was horrified and wrote immediately to the Health Department stating that she had been completely unaware of the paper and that it most certainly did not represent the views of the Mater's administration, which was hoping for state support to renew the Mater Adult Hospital.[28] She also wrote to Dr Heyworth that his opinions 'do not represent the views of the Sisters' and that she expected him to resign, as his views were 'completely contrary to those held by the administration of the Mater, ... and since you are strongly critical of the Hospital and of its management'.[29] The request for Barrie Heyworth's resignation was eventually withdrawn, and he left the hospital voluntarily and became professor of paediatrics at the National University of Malaysia.[30]

The 1980s notion of combining Brisbane's two children's hospitals into one Institute of Child Health was – for the time being – vanquished, disappointing many clinicians.[31] There were, however, niggles at the political level. In 1983, a Sunday newspaper published the views of a parliamentarian, Rosemary Kyburz, which seemed to draw on inside knowledge. Brisbane's two children's hospitals, Ms Kyburz maintained, were 'fighting' over which hospital should be allocated funding for specialist doctors and equipment and there was 'no sharing' of either doctors or equipment. To make matters worse, she believed that the Department of Health could not decide which hospital should be funded, so made no decision at all. Her conclusion, although not new, was accurate: both children's hospitals were antiquated and Brisbane needed one excellent hospital, instead of two outdated and inadequately equipped hospitals.[32]

Although the two children's hospitals were not to be amalgamated, the Joint Children's Hospitals Coordinating Committee (JCHCC), comprising senior representatives from each hospital, was formed in 1984. The committee's brief was to investigate the coordination and rationalisation of services. The situation in which children with disabilities found themselves was one illustration of the problem. In 1985, Trevor Parry, senior developmental paediatrician in the Western Australian Department of Health, visited Brisbane and commented on its scattered services.

The Royal Children's Hospital cared for children with physical disabilities, and the Mater Children's Hospital specialised in the continuing care of low birth-weight infants with disabilities. Psychological services for children were community based, rather than located at either children's hospital, and services for children with intellectual disabilities were supervised by a separate department, often with the involvement of the children's schools, but with little medical input. Non-government organisations involved in the care of children in both groups included Montrose Home (now MontroseAccess) and the Xavier Home for children with physical disabilities, the centre at New Farm for children with cerebral palsy and the Endeavour Foundation for children with intellectual disabilities.

Dr Parry suggested that a multidisciplinary centre of excellence could be located at one place where children with developmental problems could be assessed and recommendations made for their management.[33] This centre could also be a referral centre for paediatricians, an educational base, and a centre to coordinate research. Rather than anoint one or other of Brisbane's existing children's hospitals, the government's child health facility in St Paul's Terrace was suggested as a base for the developmental assessment unit. The establishment of such a centre would enable the two children's hospitals to focus on rehabilitation and the follow-up of at-risk infants.[34]

Dr Simon Latham, acting superintendent of the Royal Children's Hospital, suggested that, if this model was followed, the clinic for spina bifida, head injury, and other severe traumatic and neurological problems could be located at the Royal Children's Hospital, as the Australian College of Paediatrics had recommended in 1976.[35] This plan may have created efficiencies, but would have required considerable reorganisation, if not outright rejection. Both a spina bifida clinic and neurosurgical services were well established at the Mater Children's Hospital. Conversely, the JCHCC's clinical sub-committee on intensive care services recommended that the two children's hospitals should retain their intensive care units.[36]

The Health Department was frustrated at the JCHCC's lack of progress. The Mater Board rejected any suggestion that the two children's hospitals be united under a single board. Such a move, the Board decided, would 'interfere with the autonomy and smooth running of the Mater complex'.[37] Energy-sapping competition between the two children's hospitals continued, irritating paediatricians in rural and regional Queensland who looked to their colleagues in the hospitals to provide leadership and education.[38]

The medical superintendents of the two children's hospitals agreed, however, that the government was mistaken in believing that rationalisation and integration would save millions of dollars, as most tertiary services depended on other tertiary services. Evidence all over the world had shown that multidisciplinary approaches saved money by, for example, including physiotherapy, occupational therapy, general paediatrics and psychology with neurology and neurosurgery. In other fields, such as gastroenterology, there would be no savings in staff or equipment if procedures were confined to one hospital, as the same specialists worked in both.[39] In any case, correction of cleft palates, craniofacial surgery and faciomaxillary surgery were already rationalised between the two hospitals.

The government seemed not to be following its own rationalisation policy in proposing a short-stay paediatric ward at the QEII hospital, likely to duplicate services already available at a higher level at both children's hospitals.[40] Gaps in services were equally worrying. There were no beds anywhere in Brisbane for adolescents in the 14–20 age group.[41]

Rationalisation of health services was high on the agenda of the Queensland Labor government elected in December 1989. The new government reorganised health administration by creating health regions. Included in the new Brisbane South region, with Dr John Golledge as regional director, the Mater could no longer rely on direct access to the Director-General of Health, or to the minister. The Paediatric Society of Queensland was concerned that there was no requirement for paediatric expertise – or even medical representation – on the governing authorities of the various health regions.[42]

In July 1991, Dr Golledge attended a meeting of the Mater Board and announced that child health would be a very important program in the region, and that it was hoped that a strategic plan would be completed by March 1992.[43] In May 1992, Dr Golledge made a startling suggestion: the Mater Children's Hospital should consider moving from South Brisbane to the under-used QEII hospital at Mt Gravatt. The official capacity of the QEII hospital was 240 beds, but one floor had been vacant ever since the hospital opened in 1981.[44] Demand for adult services at QEII was expected to fall further when the second stage of the new hospital further south in Logan City was completed in 1993.[45] Dr Golledge later revealed that he had always been opposed to the construction of the QEII hospital on its Mt Gravatt site.[46] He recalled his approach to the Mater:

> I decided that I would ring up Pat Maguire, the Chief Executive Officer at the Mater, and bounce an idea off him. I ... said 'Pat, what would you say if we suggested the Mater Children's Hospital move out to QEII. We have a very nicely built facility out there, it would bring you closer to where the kids are, there's always been this open-ended talk about whether Brisbane needs two paediatric hospitals or only one and I think it would lock you into paediatrics coming up from the South Coast and from Logan where it's all developing.' He said, 'We would be quite interested in that, I'll sound people out'.[47]

At that time, the Mater board was dealing with advice from its Medical Advisory Committee that 'if the Mater Children's Hospital is going to survive on this site, we need to have a major injection of more first-class people not buildings' and that the various subspecialties needed five or six additional full-time staff doctors who could be trained in clinical research and afforded the opportunity to continue their research.[48]

The Mater insisted that the proposal to move the children's hospital be closely examined. Ross Dunning, deputy chairman of the Brisbane South Regional Health Authority, chaired the steering committee appointed to conduct a feasibility study. The members of the steering committee were Sister Angela Mary Doyle RSM, as senior director of health services for the Sisters of Mercy; Pat Maguire, her successor as chief executive officer at the Mater; Peter Read, executive director, policy and planning at Queensland Health; Dr John Golledge, Brisbane South regional director; and Grace Grace and John van Leent, representing the unions whose workers would be affected by any relocation. A core project team was appointed to direct the research: Dr Amanda Smith, assistant regional director, Brisbane South; Dr Greg Wuth, medical superintendent of the Mater Children's Hospital; Dr Julie Hudson, medical superintendent of the QEII hospital; and

Ermanno Nobilio from the project management section of the Queensland government's construction section, QBuild.

The study team first had to absorb some critical facts and figures. In the early 1990s, the Mater Children's Hospital appeared to fulfil the Brisbane South region's expectations that the hospital offering sophisticated tertiary-level services for the region should be close to the paediatric population it served.[49] The catchment was huge: south from the Brisbane River to the New South Wales border and west from Moreton Bay to the western border of the Darling Downs Health Region. Patients also came from remote parts of Queensland, the Northern Territory and northern New South Wales. The Mater Children's Hospital's share of the region's child population was predicted to grow to 44 per cent by 2001.[50] Based on the New South Wales guideline of 1.14 paediatric beds per 1,000 children up to the age of 14 with 23 per cent of the beds to be at tertiary level, Brisbane would need 503 paediatric beds, including 152 tertiary beds by 2001.[51]

The prediction for the years ahead, however, indicated that the greatest rate of population increase would occur between 15 and 40 kilometres from the inner urban area where the Mater Children's Hospital was located.[52] The QEII hospital, some 13 kilometres south of the Mater, would be closer to the centre of the paediatric population. The southern part of the catchment contained 56 per cent of the total paediatric population, which was predicted to rise to 58 per cent by 2001 when planned major housing developments were fully populated.[53]

There was a major difficulty with a scheme based solely on predicted population. The study also found that many consultants would resign if the new hospital was situated in the south of the region, affecting a core principle of rationalisation: joint appointments with the Royal Children's Hospital in the smaller subspecialties.[54] In addition, there was likely to be greater demand for tertiary services at the Royal Children's Hospital if the Mater Children's Hospital moved too far south.[55]

The feasibility study considered four options:
- Redevelopment of the existing Mater Children's Hospital;
- Conversion of the QEII hospital to a tertiary paediatric hospital to be the new Mater Children's Hospital;
- A new stand-alone hospital adjacent to stage 2 of the Logan Hospital;
- A new stand-alone hospital on a 'greenfield' site.[56]

The Mater Children's Hospital was described as a 139-bed tertiary paediatric hospital, defined by the study team as 'a specialised paediatric hospital which, while providing primary and secondary paediatric services to its local community, provides state-wide tertiary inpatient and outpatient services'.[57] Accommodation varied from an original Nightingale ward to a new medical ward designed for contemporary treatment. There were, however, insufficient consulting rooms in the out-patient department and too little space for multidisciplinary clinics.[58] The study estimated that level 5 paediatric services required support services including a level 6 operating suite, level 5 pathology, pharmacy, X-ray, nuclear medicine, intensive care and anaesthetic services, and level 3 coronary care. Level 6 paediatric services, the most sophisticated, would require even more support.[59]

Even though research funding at the Mater Children's Hospital was scarce, some staff members were world authorities in areas such as sleep studies, child protection, emergency medicine, and growth and development. The Mater had also appointed Australia's first director of ambulatory paediatrics, an important contribution to the efficiency of the hospital's services. More than 50 per cent of surgical patients were day patients, reflecting the Mater's pioneering work in day surgery in the early 1970s.

The QEII hospital was described as a 'modern community general hospital' located close to Griffith University and several retirement villages. The hospital was equipped with a full emergency department, a day surgery area, a maternity unit, a dental suite and support services such as pathology, pharmacy, diagnostic radiology, nuclear medicine and anaesthetics, but only 178 beds were in use. On the other hand, the intensive care unit, the coronary care unit and the operating theatres – very expensive facilities – were not considered to be sufficiently satisfactory to support a tertiary paediatric hospital'.[60] The newer Logan Hospital, situated even more centrally in the region south of Brisbane, had 83 beds and was due to expand in January 1993 to 200 beds including a 25-bed paediatric unit. The usual diagnostic services and a psychiatric service were already functioning at Logan.[61]

Analysis of the four options revealed that the most obvious advantage of option 1 – redeveloping the Mater Children's Hospital on the Mater campus – was the economy of scale created by including three hospitals on the same campus offering a continuum of care from neonatology to adult medicine and enabling expensive diagnostic services to be shared.

Redevelopment would have the least impact on the current staff, a matter of no small concern to the unions.[62]

The greatest advantage of the QEII site was its convenience for people in the region south of Brisbane. Redeployment of QEII staff to the Logan hospital would save costs, but would be resisted by the staff and their unions. Mater staff valued good access to the hospital and were concerned about the distance they would need to travel to potential relocation sites.[63] A move to the Logan hospital would have the greatest impact.[64] Transport was also very important to patients, 80 per cent of whom came to the Mater by car; road access and parking were essential.[65] The public transport connections between Brisbane and Logan City and any other likely site for a stand-alone hospital were even poorer than for the QEII hospital.

The relocation of the QEII's adult services to other hospitals was vocally and publicly resisted by the local community, led by the president of the QEII auxiliary, Clem O'Keeffe, who was frequently quoted in the local papers. Even the local Labor member of Parliament, Len Ardill, opposed the move.[66]

Economies of scale and the support provided by tertiary-level ancillary services on the Mater site were not available at QEII, increasing the likely costs of moving to QEII. The capital cost of redeveloping the Mater Children's Hospital on its original site was estimated at $35,100,000 with annual operating costs at $40,400,000.[67] In contrast, the costs of creating a children's hospital at QEII were likely to be $48,800,000 with annual operating costs at $43,200,000. However, a net present value analysis posited the QEII option as the only option to achieve a positive value, even though this would not be achieved for six years.[68] This result was, however, dependent on redeploying Mater staff to QEII and some QEII staff to Logan, a transition that many resisted.

The Mater was preparing its own strategic plan for the whole campus while the feasibility study was gathering its data.[69] The strategic plan recommended that the complex should 'think as one institution' and 'increasingly adopt a continuum approach to health, including appropriate community outreach'. The Mater's four greatest strengths were found to be children's health; mothers', babies' and selected women's services; neonatology; and oncology.[70] The Mater's Director of Strategic Planning, Chris Geckeler, reminded the board that 'the children's hospital is a pawn in a much larger health-care rationalisation game' and that the QEII proposal was likely to be a short-term solution to problems in the Brisbane South region by closing beds without appearing to do so.[71] Using capital letters to communicate his vehemence, Geckeler was of the view that:

> Relocation of the MCH may be seen as short term expediency by the Region/Qld Health, but WE should view it in the broader perspective of RATIONALISATION of ALL SERVICES in the Region ... Thus, in my view, the children's hospital is but one part of a much larger tapestry.[72]

Geckeler suggested that a nexus between the Mater at South Brisbane and the new Logan Hospital could become a leading model of health care into the twenty-first century.

Ideas and suggestions also came from other quarters. Dr Robert McCrossin from Queensland Health, a medical administrator and paediatric endocrinologist, contributed his personal view. He thought that the population, from the New South Wales border to Noosa in the north, needed two children's hospitals, but in 'cooperation, not suicidal competition'. He also thought that stand-alone paediatric hospitals were very expensive as they could not share services such as pathology and radiology with other hospitals. It was also productive for subspecialists to be able to mix clinically within their craft groups at adult hospitals. Dr McCrossin recommended that that the Mater Children's Hospital continue at South Brisbane until Logan Hospital became the 'Westmead of Brisbane', a reference to the relocation of Sydney's Royal Alexandra Hospital for Children from Camperdown to the large Westmead general hospital campus.[73]

Several Mater doctors wrote to the Brisbane South region in June and July 1992 opposing the move.[74] The Mater's Head of Pathology, Dr John Bell, once ambivalent about relocation, had come to oppose it as 'all elements of Mater care are dependent one on the other'. It would be very expensive to develop top-level pathology services in a stand-alone hospital. He also noted that in the United States, stand-alone children's hospitals were no longer being established.[75] The Director of Neonatology at the Mater Mothers' Hospital, Dr David Tudehope, suggested that moving obstetrics from the The Townsville Hospital to a women's hospital in the suburb of Kirwan in 1984 had not been successful. In Brisbane, the separation of pathology at the Royal Children's Hospital from the Royal Women's Hospital was unsatisfactory, contrasting with the single pathology section at the Mater. Separating the Mater Children's Hospital from the Mater Mothers' Hospital would be 'devastating'.[76]

David Tudehope believed that subspecialties, such as paediatric respirology and cardiology, had developed close links between the Mater Mothers' and the Mater Children's hospitals. Moving the Mater Children's Hospital would, therefore, involve the duplication of expensive testing services already developed on the Mater site. It would also be very difficult to manage the multidisciplinary growth and developmental clinic on another site as so many different disciplines were involved. Neonatal surgery was yet another difficult issue: if the Mater Children's Hospital moved, it would have to be performed at the Mater Mothers' Hospital, further congesting its operating theatres.[77]

The psychiatrist Aidene Urquhart emphasised the need to be close to educational support units, which were very important in assessing children. Speech therapy, occupational therapy and audiology also needed to be easily accessible to mental health services. Rehabilitation services for survivors of torture and trauma also needed to be centrally located. In this respect, the Mater campus was ideal. It was close to the most multicultural part of the city and public transport was excellent. The Mater's 'needs-based' model, with sharing of resources to provide services and programs, was very cost effective, but had never been studied or assessed.[78]

Consultation during the feasibility study yielded varying results. Doctors and the ambulance service favoured the South Brisbane site. General practitioners wanted access to secondary paediatric beds in all sectors of the region and took the opportunity to say that parents liked the Mater Children's Hospital, but thought it should be upgraded.[79]

Chris Geckeler stressed that the Mater should ensure that negotiations equipped it to play an important evolving role in health care. A multi-campus Mater – with a presence in the Redlands and Logan City as well as at South Brisbane – would provide cost-efficient care, enriching careers and strengthening the Mater into the twenty-first century. Geckeler suggested that the Mater should offer to staff the Logan and Redlands paediatric services from the Mater and seek permission to establish a private children's hospital. This would establish very important links to the growth areas to the south and on the shores of Moreton Bay, connections that should be developed further by the Mater Adult Hospital and the Mater Mothers' Hospital.[80]

Medical concerns mounted. The New Life Centre at the Mater Mothers' Hospital, opened in 1991 as the tertiary referral centre for all babies in the catchment area, could be imperilled if the children's hospital moved. There were also risks in not moving: the drift of young population to the outer suburbs could threaten both the Mater Children's and the Mater Mothers' hospitals; the regional health authority could develop a paediatric retrieval hospital at QEII independently of the Mater; and there could be strenuous efforts to make the Royal Children's Hospital the major paediatric hospital for the city.[81]

Mater paediatricians preferred the current links with other facilities on the Mater campus and said that, if a move to QEII meant that the hospital would be only a secondary unit, 'they would rather remain on this current campus and risk an uncertain future'.[82] Clinicians believed that the Mater Children's Hospital existed as a tertiary hospital only through its access to tertiary services on campus and, if it moved without the allocation of costs for the extra services, children would lose.[83] Aboriginal and Torres Strait Islander people who lived near the Mater also resisted the move because of the public transport issue.[84]

Ear, nose and throat surgeons liked the 'one-stop shop' advantages of the South Brisbane site and thought that the Mater Children's Hospital had 'the potential to be the full-blown 'American dream' with private, intermediate and public patients, new consulting suites and an improving socio-economic local environment and, possibly, a south-side medical school. Moving the hospital would 'kill' the cross-campus *esprit de corps*.[85] There was limited capacity for surgical expansion at QEII. Only five operating theatres would be available at QEII, but 63 operating theatre sessions would be needed each week by 2001 – requiring seven theatres.[86]

Meanwhile, Queensland's Department of Health was proceeding with its plans. In October 1992, government lawyers prepared a lease for the Mater to manage QEII as a children's hospital. It appeared that the government wanted to make the announcement before Christmas.[87] The Mater, however, decided to show its strategic plan to the government on the grounds that, if the Mater did not take steps to determine its own future, the future would be determined for it.[88] It was also determined that the second stage of the feasibility study should be completed before any announcement was made.[89]

The second phase of the feasibility study, originally intended to determine the precise location of secondary-level beds and their clinical emphases, became, in the government's eyes, an implementation strategy.[90] The Mater had strong views. A Mater Children's Hospital at Mt Gravatt would be a tertiary referral teaching hospital operating within the Sisters of Mercy's mission and philosophy; all staff would be employees of the Sisters. There would be 150 beds for primary, secondary and tertiary patients, including provision for private beds, and with outreach to community health centres.[91] Further, the state would make the total capital investment for the new hospital, fund the consequent changes on the Mater campus and supply recurrent funding. The name should be the Mater Misericordiae Children's and Community Hospital, Nathan Campus.[92] The government dismissed these stipulations as an 'ambit claim'.[93]

The medical superintendent of the Mater Children's Hospital, Dr Greg Wuth, did not believe that the Mater should agree to the move 'as I believe we run the risk of being in the same situation Logan Hospital is now, where a bright, shiny new facility is available without staff or equipment to allow utilisation of the facility for the benefit of patients'.[94] Draft plans for QEII did nothing to comfort him. The emergency department, the respiratory unit, the out-patient department and the day-patient ward looked small and there did not seem to be a procedure room.[95]

Despite the Mater's statement that acceding to the second stage of the feasibility study did not mean agreement, the Brisbane South regional authority prepared a draft 'Heads of Agreement' for the relocation. There was one clause that would never be acceptable to the Mater: managing the QEII children's hospital 'for the authority', which meant that the government's regional health authority, and not the Mater, would be in control.[96] The Mater's tradition of providing public hospital services under the control of the Sisters of Mercy was not to be yielded. Fortunately, the Mater had a card up its sleeve. In May 1992, the Health Minister had assured the autonomy of the Mater within the Queensland health structure under section 5.8 of the *Health Services Act 1991*.[97]

The pressure intensified. The Mater staff was told about the proposed move on 12 October 1992. Dr John Golledge said the move was 'highly likely' to go ahead in the middle months of 1994.[98] The QEII hospital auxiliary was enraged, and stated that there was already a backlog of 1,800 orthopaedic operations at QEII. The auxiliary was also offended that its donations of equipment worth $1,000,000 appeared to have been overlooked.[99]

Even though the Health Minister had reiterated his commitment to creating a world-class tertiary paediatric hospital at QEII, the Mater was considering broader factors.[100] Queensland was moving to a more competitive model of health care, which would require better coordination between hospitals and community health services in the interests of integrated care. A community health centre on the QEII site, offering primary care and therapy services, was a more acceptable option. The Sisters had several options to consider: withdrawal from health care, re-using the Mater property or perhaps disposing of it; reducing acute care to concentrate on community services with a limited number of integrated tertiary services; developing several campuses and expanding into management of health care through ownership, management contracts, partnerships and other cooperative arrangements to provide broad-spectrum, managed health care.[101]

Ultimately, the Sisters accepted the board's recommendation that they refuse to move the Mater Children's Hospital, with 're-development to be further considered as our preferred and more viable option'.[102] The government abandoned the proposal late in March 1993. A recession in the Australian economy in the early 1990s put pressure on government budgets and the money the government could offer for the operating costs of a children's hospital at Mt Gravatt had fallen. Any savings the government might have made from changing the function of the QEII hospital had to be redirected to the new Logan Hospital. Moving the Mater Children's Hospital was no longer viable.[103] As Greg Wuth expressed it, the original proposal for a full tertiary hospital had been reduced to merely a 'basic paediatric facility'. Nevertheless, the government was said to have been so certain the relocation would occur that it had approached Buckingham Palace for permission to remove the Queen's name from the title of the hospital.[104]

In the aftermath of the Mater board's decision, several significant issues were revealed. The *Courier-Mail*, disclosed that Dr Golledge believed that the QEII should never have been built on the Mt Gravatt site. The advent of the new Logan Hospital had put even more pressure on finding a role for the QEII.[105] Government sources also revealed that the government had advocated the proposal to move the Mater Children's Hospital against the advice of its own Health Department planners, who thought that a study supporting the move was biased towards the government to save the political embarrassment inherent in closing the under-used QEII hospital.[106]

The whole troubling issue focused Mater minds on future needs. The possible relocation of the Mater Children's Hospital highlighted the efficiencies, inter-dependence and economies of scale gained by the group of Mater hospitals operating on a single site.[107]

Chapter 11

Making Do

Selected areas should be further developed to excellence – national and international ...

Dr Michael O'Callaghan, 1989[1]

Rejecting the proposal that the Mater Children's Hospital should leave South Brisbane focused Mater planners on immediate needs, an essential step if the hospital was to have any hope of coping with the demands made upon it. In the early 1990s, it remained a 139-bed tertiary hospital, but its range of services introduced many more patients than bed numbers indicated. Big dreams were limited only by space and funding. Many needs were generated by advances in paediatric care, but financial stringency and changes in governmental funding formulae were uncomfortable companions to medical developments. Nevertheless, tertiary services expanded, research intensified, liaisons between hospitals firmed, and outreach into the community broadened.

The move towards keeping children in hospital for the shortest possible time accelerated in the 1980s. As early as 1980, the average length of stay in the Mater Children's Hospital had fallen to 2.9 days;[2] the 'hospital at home' was becoming a reality for more children; and the *Health Services Act 1991* foreshadowed the 'hospital without walls' through the development of ambulatory care, day surgery and short-stay observation wards.[3] Treatment of the serious disease diabetes was a case in point. In 30 years, hospitalisation for the assessment and treatment of a child with diabetes had dropped from one month to one or two days.[4]

Reducing hospitalisation for children with serious conditions relied considerably on educating patients and families. By 1990, the clinic that instructed parents on how to administer oxygen to children at home had cared for 400 children in five years. Before that, many infants who could otherwise go home were kept in hospital because they needed oxygen.[5] Technology had made a great difference. At least 45 infants each year needed Continuous Positive Airway Pressure (CPAP) ventilators at home to manage their complex problems. By the late 1990s, a child who had always been dependent on a hospital ventilator was able to live at home with special new equipment and carefully trained parents.[6]

Children dependent on technology formed only a small proportion of children treated in hospitals, but the cost was very high. About 0.2 per cent of all patients were children dependent on technology, but their treatment cost about 4 per cent of the total operating incomes of major paediatric hospitals – a considerable issue when hospital budgets were continually trimmed. Treatment on a ventilator, for instance, cost as much as $250,000 per patient annually and parenteral nutrition cost $100,000 annually. A survey of major Australian children's hospitals in April and May 1991 examined the numbers of patients, the cost of treatment – and how it was funded – and whether children could be nursed at home and, if not, identified the reasons.[7]

Treatment at home was better for the child's growth and development, but some parents did not have sufficient support for home care, or adequate access to trained carers for essential advice; others could not fund the cost of home care without assistance.[8] The focus on family-oriented care and on the role of psychological and emotional factors in enhancing clinical care extended to surgery. A new ward, opened early in 1992, catered for children who did not need to stay overnight after their operations. In its first year, 1,000 children passed through this ward.[9] Solomon, the hospital-wise owl, took children and their parents on a tour of the hospital to reduce their anxiety and the 'Hello Hospital' program in primary schools was designed to defuse fear of hospitals.[10]

The advent of the endoscope increased the range and complexity of day surgery and, in other instances, greatly shortened the length of hospital stays. By 1996, the Mater claimed that its paediatric surgeons, among them Dr Peter Borzi and Dr Athol Mackay, worked at world standard in paediatric endoscopic surgery across a wide range of procedures, including splenectomy; appendectomy; nephrectomy; heminephrectomy, removal of part of a kidney; orchidopexy, surgical correction for undescended testes; and fundoplication, a procedure to strengthen the valve between the stomach and oesophagus.[11] The number of day-surgery patients continued to grow and, in the mid-1990s, the day ward was moved closer to the operating theatres.[12] A fourth operating theatre was constructed during Easter 1996.[13]

Decreasing the length of hospital stays also reduced costs, which had continued to rise: the daily average cost of maintaining a child in the Mater Children's Hospital trebled between 1980 and 1990.[14] Technical and medical advances saved children who would once have died, but many needed long stays in hospital. Conversely, advances that enabled day surgery reduced pressure on hospital beds, but increased the pressure on other services. There was an ever-growing demand for multidisciplinary specialist clinics and the ambulatory services area – once known as casualty and out-patients – treated more and more patients in the 1980s and 1990s. Many families who would once have consulted a general practitioner or a paediatrician in private practice found the rising costs of private health insurance and the falling numbers of doctors who charged only the fully rebatable 'common fee' put private medicine beyond their reach.[15]

Out-patient clinics had been relocated to the lower floors of the new Potter Building on the corner of Clarence Street in 1987. The remaining floors offered great promise for future development.[16] Whether one or two floors could be brought into service depended on how much could be achieved for $1,800,000, the amount the government allocated to fit out further floors and to construct a link to the main children's hospital building. One floor was certainly possible. It could have a nursing station, 27 beds configured as three six-bed wards, three two-bed wards and three single rooms – the old Nightingale wards were fading from view.[17] The new medical ward on level D4, and the link to the second floor of the main Mater Children's Hospital building – one of many bridges over roadways that became a feature of the Mater campus – were opened in April 1992.[18] The next stage, a new babies' ward with live-in facilities for parents and shared bathrooms, was opened on 28 July 1994.[19]

Bringing floors of the newer building into service was part of a suite of major developments on the Mater campus in the early 1990s. The New Life Centre opened at the Mater Mothers' Hospital in 1991, the new Mater Private Hospital opened in 1993 and a new Mater medical research facility was planned.[20] The laboratory for paediatric respiratory medicine, funded largely by $500,000 from the government's Golden Casket lottery, opened in November 1994 with Professor Brian Hills as director. It was the first laboratory within the Mater Medical Research Institute and was soon productive.[21] A paper elucidating the action of surfactant by Dr Brian Hills, paediatrician Dr John O'Duffy and respiratory physician Dr Brent Masters was published in the *Lancet*, the English medical journal, in 1993.[22] Research on surfactant continued and, by the late 1990s, was thought to be an alternative treatment to the insertion of grommets for the common childhood condition 'glue ear'.[23]

Top of the wish list in 1994 were an in-patient unit for psychiatric patients, a ward for the adolescent age group and improved capacity for cardiology and cardiac surgery. Some division of tertiary services between Brisbane's two children's hospitals was both necessary and inevitable. Bone marrow and liver transplants and the treatment of burns would remain at the Royal Children's Hospital, while the Mater Children's Hospital would concentrate on areas such as craniofacial surgery and sleep studies.[24]

The former babies' ward beneath the University of Queensland's Department of Child Health unit became the only paediatric sleep studies unit in Queensland, an innovation relieving families of the need to go interstate for investigations and treatment.[25] Sleep studies were important in investigating many conditions, including upper airway obstruction, muscle and neurological problems, and potentially life-threatening events such as the mysterious and tragic condition of sudden infant death syndrome (SIDS).[26] Mater researchers' identification of a post-mortem marker for SIDS attracted worldwide attention.[27] By 1997, Brent Masters also coordinated an outreach service to the Redland Hospital and a special clinic for children with severe asthma.[28] Obstructive sleep apnoea diagnosed in the unit was associated with the type of developmental and behavioural disorders managed by the Mater's specialist in child development, Dr Michael O'Callaghan.

Preventing or treating serious illnesses and saving many more premature babies was one side of the paediatric medical coin; ensuring that children whose health remained impaired could achieve their full potential was the other. Multidisciplinary clinics – teams of doctors, nurses, physiotherapists, speech pathologists and social workers – became even more important. Coordination between hospital and community services was a reprise of the debates over rationalisation, but also consolidated the movement towards broader outreach. In the single year 1995–96, 1,134 children were assessed at the child development clinic at the Mater and 209 in the school function clinic; 463 children regarded as being at high risk were also assessed in the growth and development clinic. Speech and language difficulties and behavioural problems were the most common reasons for referral to the child development clinic.[29]

Liaisons with community organisations were essential to the child development clinic, with its focus on supporting the optimal health and development of the child within the family. Clinical liaison and networking also led to many referrals to other Mater Children's Hospital specialist clinics. The child development team visited five regional centres and developed strong links with the clinic at the Logan Hospital. Quarterly child development symposia became important educational tools; a symposium in 1993 on the origins and management of aggression in young children attracted 100 delegates. Strong relationships with community health nurses and liaison with school guidance officers were essential.

Research was an important aspect of the child development clinic's work. A long-term follow-up study of the children of 8,556 women who had their babies at the Mater Mothers' Hospital between 1981 and 1984 examined the physical, psychological, emotional and educational development of their children as they grew. The study was originally funded by the National Health and Medical Research Council, but, in 1995, a group of investigators in America obtained a large grant from the United States National Institutes of Health to research the same group of families in conjunction with the continuing Mater study.[30]

Brain damage as a result of disease or injury can impede children's development. A multidisciplinary team cared for children with head injuries and, in July 1993, the rehabilitation and neuromuscular clinic was established as a pilot project with Medicare funding.[31] The clinic, known as ROBIN (Rehabilitation of Children with Acquired Brain Injuries and Neuromuscular Disorders), became permanent, treating children with many debilitating conditions and coordinating their transition into the community after their hospital stays. The community supported the clinic: a volunteer group coordinated by Dorothy Stringer raised more than $100,000 for equipment.[32]

New appointments fostered the development of subspecialties. Dr Cameron Ward's paediatric cardiology service thrived. An additional paediatric cardiologist was high on the urgent wish list.[33] Some cardiac surgery could be performed at the Mater Children's Hospital: correction of coarctation (narrowing of the aorta), failed closure of a major fetal blood vessel after birth and creation of Blalock-Taussig shunts to improve pulmonary blood flow.[34]

Oncology, pioneered at the Mater Children's Hospital by Dr Peter O'Regan, became more prominent in 1996 when Dr Ram Suppiah was appointed as the first full-time director of paediatric oncology and haematology. He wanted more of his patients to be treated at home by a multidisciplinary team rather than as in-patients. A new anti-nausea drug, ondansetron, reduced the time children spent in hospital for cancer treatment. The day care centre for child cancer patients opened in January 1997, avoiding the need for many patients to stay overnight for treatment.[35] The appointment of case managers to support not only the patients, but also their families, was an important step. The oncology unit introduced sibling support and bereavement workshops to support families. Ram Suppiah emphasised the importance of integrated care for his patients and dreamt of co-locating in-patient and out-patient services, perhaps in an under-used ward in the Mater Adult Hospital. The first paediatric stem cell transplant was performed a year or so after Ram Suppiah's arrival.[36]

Treating children in home, school and community settings became a goal of the paediatric endocrinology unit. The number of patients with diabetes, treated by Dr Mike Thomsett and Dr Geoffrey Bourke, increased noticeably in the 1980s and 1990s.[37] Nurses with special training were very important in supporting patients newly diagnosed with diabetes and their families. Encouraged by Helen Kearney, an educator at the Mater Children's Hospital, Jill Morris wrote *Dido has diabetes*, featuring a diprotodon – a talented athlete – who was navigating his way through the risks of a birthday party as he learnt to live with diabetes.[38]

Helen Kearney's successor, Jill Stillman, visited children with diabetes at their schools to assist them to manage their diabetes.[39] This was barely a stitch in time – the number of school-age children and adolescents with diabetes increased by 50 per cent in three years. An outreach service to children in rural Queensland commenced in 1997. Dr Andrew Cotterill, appointed in 1996, attracted considerable research funding, including a prestigious Juvenile Diabetes Fellow Scholarship from the United States.[40]

Craniofacial surgery exemplified the team approach increasingly highlighted in both medicine and surgery. In 1991, the craniofacial surgery team was coordinated by the plastic surgeon Dr Michael Lanigan, who had trained in Toronto.[41] The neurosurgeon Dr Leigh Atkinson and the plastic surgeon Dr Tony Emmett had pioneered craniofacial surgery at the Mater. They remained key members of the team, which included the ophthalmologist Colleen Boreham, the geneticist Christine Oley, the radiologist John Masel, the anaesthetist Mansu Pabari, and the periodontist Rodney Auer. Meeting a large team of doctors was intimidating for some patients and the clinic decided that, whenever possible, each doctor should see patients individually before the children faced the full team.

Craniofacial surgery had an international dimension. Children from the South West Pacific, including two boys from Fiji, were brought to Brisbane through the plastic surgeons' organisation, Interplast, which began work in the Asia–Pacific region in the 1980s.[42] In 1996, Dr Richard Lewandowski, a University of Queensland medical graduate, came to the Mater and expanded the international reach of the craniofacial unit. Dr Lewandowski was a co-founder of Operation Smile Australia, having been involved in the original Operation Smile, founded and based in Norfolk, Virginia, in the United States, where he had trained in plastic surgery. A child from the Philippines was Lewandowski's first international patient.[43]

Ironically, some Queensland patients were funded by the Department of Health to travel away from Brisbane to the Adelaide craniofacial clinic pioneered by Dr David David.[44] In 1982, Leigh Atkinson wrote that craniofacial surgery should not be confined to just a few special units around the world; families would need multidisciplinary teams much closer to home. There was no need for patients with craniofacial disorders to leave Queensland,[45] but in 1991, the Mater's craniofacial clinic made an exception for Marie Matejic, who flew to Dallas in the United States for her surgery. The patron of the internationally recognised Dallas unit, the singer Cher, met Marie on a visit to Brisbane and arranged her trip, which included a visit to Cher's home in Los Angeles.[46] Commercial sponsors also helped to fund Marie's visit to the United States. Fundraising was very important to the craniofacial clinic, as the surgery – wherever it was performed – was expensive. The Mater regularly applied to the government for funding for the clinic, but there was always a shortfall.[47]

Alayne McDowall and her Friends of the Craniofacial Clinic committee arranged numerous raffles and events to raise funds for essential equipment.

The committee held its first function at the Commonwealth Bank in Queen Street in November 1989.[48] In 1990, the clinic needed a 3D computerised scanning program costing $32,500 and a $15,000 device to fix miniature plates in tiny skulls and jaws.[49] Countless letters bearing a butterfly motif, signifying the emergence of new life, went to potential donors and invitees to events. By 1997, the Friends had raised $150,000 for instruments and technical aids for craniofacial surgery, such as the modelling method developed by neurosurgeon Dr Paul D'Urso, which assisted surgeons to plug holes in skulls precisely and to make accurate plates for the gaps when faces or skulls were rebuilt.[50]

Social workers and psychologists were needed to help children with disfigurements to overcome problems with people who were disconcerted by their appearance. The Mater's first child psychiatrist, Irene Apel, advocated improved psychological and psychiatric services in the 1960s, but mental health services at the Mater Children's Hospital had never been able to match the need. Children with behavioural problems and mental illness were admitted to general wards, testing the nursing staff, and sometimes frightening other children and their parents. The need for specially trained nurses and better in-patient care for children with mental illness was urgent.[51]

Government action had a large impact on mental health services. The national reform of mental health services closed the large psychiatric hospitals, creating the need for in-patient wards in general hospitals for acutely ill patients. The Queensland government moved community mental health services, including the child guidance clinics, into the hospitals. The Mater Children's Hospital became the base for the Child and Youth Mental Health Service (CYMHS) in the Brisbane South region.[52] The World Health Organization (WHO) recommended that staffing levels for any community should be one full-time child psychiatrist with a multidisciplinary team for every 100,000 people. Brisbane South had only two psychiatrists, well short of the seven stipulated by the WHO formula.[53] It was unsurprising, therefore, that the 1993 report of the national inquiry into the human rights of people with mental illness criticised the level of services in Queensland.[54]

A former general practitioner who had trained as a psychiatrist, Dr Michael Beech, was appointed the Mater Children's Hospital's director of child and youth mental health service in 1996 and, through an arrangement with Queensland Health, was also deputy director of the south-side unit.

With the psychologist Erica Lee, Michael Beech developed the hospital and community care model so that it was applied more broadly. By 1998, the Mater service had been integrated with the Inala, Yeronga and Greenslopes services to form the South Brisbane CYMHS.[55] The move towards home and community care of children with mental illnesses included treating as many patients as possible as day patients. The Mater also established a 'Kidz Club' for children of parents with mental illnesses.[56]

In the mid-1990s, the CYMHS extended its reach to an area of long-felt need: adolescent mental health.[57] This became an important area where community outreach grew as the years passed. The community participation model developed by the mental health service at the Mater Children's Hospital was adopted by other services. The model depended on management by parents. A parent who coordinated the early meetings at the Mater Children's Hospital became a member of the staff.[58]

Although the staff did not increase as rapidly as the child and youth mental health service had hoped, there were important initiatives in the late 1990s. Music and art therapies – non-threatening media enabling young people to express their feelings – were developed for children with mental health problems, those with developmental delays and children who had been abused. Art became more prominent as the 1990s progressed. In 1998, Anna Bligh, as Minister for Families, Youth and Community Care and Disability Services, opened the CYMHS art show, the first time young people on a recovery program had organised a show themselves. Making decisions and taking responsibility supported their recovery.[59] With developmental medicine, cardiothoracic medicine, sleep medicine, craniofacial, orthopaedic and neurosurgery, child and youth mental health was defined as a core area for the Mater Children's Hospital in the mid-1990s.[60]

Community engagement, essential in mental health services, took on an international dimension with Operation Smile in craniofacial surgery and in orthopaedics through the Nadezhda project. Vera Derevtsov coordinated the relationship between the Mater, Brisbane's Russian community and clinicians in Russia. Several Russian children were sponsored to come to Brisbane for essential surgery and a Mater team – orthopaedic surgeons Dr Terry McGuire and Dr Bill Ryan and physiotherapists Cathy Bagley, John Gilmour and Rosemary Forster – visited Russia to work with clinicians there. In August 1997, for instance, they examined 80 children and selected eight for surgery in Russia, all with good outcomes; a further 30 children had intensive physiotherapy treatment. The team was delighted when an eight-year-old girl with cerebral palsy walked across the room after surgery to release some of her contractures.[61]

Treatment of children recovering from complex surgery, or acutely ill from other causes, was an important marker of the hospital's transition to tertiary patient care. The Mater Children's Hospital became the Queensland centre for paediatric kidney transplantation in 1996.[62] An intensive care unit – larger and more sophisticated than the original unit at the end of the surgical ward – was essential.[63] Dr Bruce Lister, director of paediatric intensive care, was supported by a second intensivist, Dr Phil Sargent, appointed in 1996.[64] Some seriously ill children were 'retrieved' from the country, often by helicopter. The paediatric intensive care unit educated staff in regional and rural hospitals on the best ways to stabilise a child's condition before the trip to Brisbane.

Some of the intensive care unit's patients initially presented at the accident and emergency department directed by Dr Rob Pitt, with Marie Hand as clinical nurse consultant. Many of Rob Pitt's patients needed treatment for asthma, which, in 1991, was recognised as the most common cause of admission to children's hospitals throughout Australia.[65] The aim to discharge emergency patients as soon as possible to the care of families and general practitioners required very careful, effective triage. A study of the Mater Children's Hospital's emergency department in 1993 revealed that 27,531 children – 60 per cent with urgent or semi-urgent conditions – were examined in the department, but only 5,412 were admitted as in-patients.[66] Rob Pitt developed the software MacPaED to help manage his department and continued the training program in emergency medicine, which was the earliest to be established in Queensland.[67]

Assessment of injuries, preparation for surgery, investigations of many medical conditions – indeed most tertiary services – relied on modern radiology, but this was an area of difficulty in the 1990s. Like other specialties, techniques and technology in radiology developed considerably in the 1980s and 1990s. Ordinary X-rays retained a place in modern medicine, but innovations – computerised tomography (CT) scans and magnetic resonance imaging (MRI) among them – offered insights into the body beyond the reach of earlier methods. But keeping abreast of developments in radiology was very expensive.

The Mater Children's Hospital needed to expand its staff and upgrade the radiology equipment and its accommodation. Dr John Masel, director of radiology at both children's hospitals since 1978, was frustrated at the deficiencies in the department, as was the staff radiologist, Dr John Ratcliffe. There were delays in procuring new radiology equipment while the proposal to move the Mater Children's Hospital to QEII ran its course.[68] Some visiting radiologists had been so distressed at the condition of radiology at the Mater Children's Hospital that they had withdrawn their services. There was also concern that the recently appointed director of paediatric radiology, Dr Tony Lamont, might not wish to stay.[69]

The incorporation of paediatric radiology with the CT scanner at the adult hospital was one suggestion to put the Mater generally in a better position to establish its own nuclear medicine facility and MRI capability.[70] At last, in January 1995, the Health Department offered $2,600,000 for new equipment and building modifications at the adult hospital, with some temporary improvements for the children's hospital.[71]

Finance was always an issue, not only for radiology. The Mater Children's Hospital auxiliary had been essential since the hospital's beginnings in the 1930s and, in 1990, raised almost $50,000 for equipment and $5,000 for the Sister Dorothea Jubilee Fund for post-graduate nursing education.[72] Some newer services, such as the respiratory group and the craniofacial unit, had their own fundraising committees.[73]

Fundraising fashions were, however, changing. Telethons, which had been very important in earlier times, were less successful and the ever-reliable children's hospitals' appeals run by the *Courier-Mail* were drawing to a close. There was one unexpected, magnificent windfall: a bequest of $1,300,000 in the will of the antique dealer Cecilia McNally in 1996.[74] Newer fundraising methods included the Mater Children's Hospital Art Union but, by the late 1980s, its proceeds were steadily eroded by growing administrative costs and the traditional repatriation of about half the profit to the Sisters of Mercy to support the work among people with intellectual disabilities.[75]

By 1986, better research facilities, equipment and funding, beyond the capacity of the fund established in memory of the long-serving Advisory Board chairman, JP Kelly, were badly needed. Supported by John McNee, long-standing Mater Children's Hospital visiting paediatricians Dr Peter O'Regan and Dr Ian Robertson proposed a fundraising foundation for the

Mater Children's Hospital.[76] Despite the doctors' enthusiasm, the Mater Executive and the Board found many obstacles. Creating a foundation under the *Hospitals Foundation Act 1982* required Cabinet approval. A foundation created under either the 1982 Act or the Commonwealth *Companies Act 1981* required its own board with powers that could affect the management of the Mater, which, at that time, continued to be owned and managed by the Sisters of Mercy. Either way, establishment costs would be considerable and there were no guarantees that a foundation would be sufficiently successful to warrant the expense.[77] There was to be no Mater Children's Hospital Foundation; the Royal Children's Hospital Foundation raised more than $200,000 in its first two years, 1986–87.[78]

The idea of a foundation did not lapse, but re-emerged in 1989 as the Mater Trust (now called the Mater Foundation), developed to support research and clinical services across the Mater campus. The Mater Children's Hospital was not overlooked. In the early 1990s, celebrities such as swimming stars Hayley Lewis and Kieren Perkins and basketball player Leroy Loggins lent their names and their presence to the Trust's fundraising efforts for the children's hospital.[79] The professional foundation reduced the profile of hospital auxiliaries, whose generations of members had worked so hard.

The capacity of the Mater Trust to support services in the Mater hospitals became even more important in the 1990s when the Commonwealth government, through the Medicare agreement with state governments, imposed a new methodology, casemix funding, based on diagnosis related groups (DRGs), which organised funding for patients according to similar clinical features with similar costs.[80] Casemix funding was introduced in Queensland on 1 July 1995. Funding based on historical costs became a thing of the past; contemporary patterns of demand established the new benchmark.

Although tertiary-level hospitals with their more complex services were sometimes disadvantaged by casemix funding, the Mater Children's Hospital found that the new methodology gave improved recognition to the importance of specialist nurses in some of its key areas: diabetes, oncology, stomal therapy, growth and development, rehabilitation, cystic fibrosis, child protection, mental health services and sleep studies.[81] The new model's focus on patients and their illnesses accorded with the Sisters of Mercy philosophy of patient care. On the whole, however, a review by the accounting firm Deloitte Touche Tohmatsu found that casemix funding had underfunded the

Mater hospitals by $4,500,000. The new model increased the pressure to do more with less, and widened the discrepancy in funding between Brisbane's two children's hospitals. This was particularly galling to the Mater, which had a long history of cost effectiveness.[82]

Differences between the two children's hospitals were startling. Treating a child with bronchitis and asthma, for instance, cost $1,383 at the Mater and $2,537 at the Royal Children's Hospital; treatment for pneumonia and pleurisy cost $1,676 at the Mater and $2,553 at the Royal Children's Hospital. The report also demonstrated that casemix funding was unsuitable for intensive care and most specialist tertiary services. Research grants awarded to Mater staff earned additional casemix funding, but this was little comfort when funding for essential services was tight.[83]

Analysis of costs per DRG demonstrated that the Mater Children's Hospital was efficient, largely due to the hard work of the nursing staff. A study by the Australian Association of Paediatric Teaching Centres (AAPTC) revealed that nursing hours per patient were well below the national average. There was an important caveat on looking for further efficiencies in nursing: any decrease in nursing staff could jeopardise care. Mater Children's Hospital staff shed many tears at the idea of reducing activity to avoid a budget overrun; they had worked so hard to ensure the best possible care for every child.[84]

Unusual situations did not fit easily within the casemix funding model. At the Mater Children's Hospital, for instance, three patients with haemophilia needed special drugs, which cost between $460,000 and $555,000 each year.[85] Routine surgery was another illustration. Children with no other health problems would leave hospital very quickly, but children with complex conditions, such as cystic fibrosis, could need days of pre-operative preparation and post-operative care. Casemix funding categorised the surgery, but took no account of additional care in more complex circumstances. The Royal Children's Hospital also found that the casemix model was particularly difficult for tertiary hospitals, even though its additional state funding demonstrated at least some government understanding of the difficulties of highly specialised areas.[86] Working within the casemix system improved relationships between the two children's hospitals and encouraged a more productive approach to complementary services, rather than wasteful competition.[87]

Chapter 12

Reaching Out

Efficiency comes from the very hard work by nurses ...

Minutes, Mater Board, 27 March 1996

Outreach, innovations and major developments in the 1990s – as well as dealing with the demands of casemix funding – relied greatly on the efforts of the entire staff. This was anything but an easy decade. The nursing staff was, as always, the front line of clinical care. Nurses were usually the first people patients and families saw when they entered wards or clinics, and the last people they saw when they left. In the 1990s, paediatric nurses needed a wide range of skills. They worked as team members in clinics as well as in wards and were visible in children's homes and communities, as well as at their bedsides.

Rosalie Lewis remained director of nursing at the beginning of the 1990s. Her deputy, Linda Bognar, completed her training at the Mater and, like many nurses of her era, completed a university degree as well as her midwifery and maternal and child welfare certificates.[1] A great change in nursing at the Mater came in 1992 when the last nurses graduated from the Mater nurse training school, which, in 80 years, had educated thousands of nurses. University education was only one of the innovations for nurses in the 1980s and 1990s. Improving career structures was another. Nursing in Queensland hospitals was re-structured to create four streams: clinical, education, management and research. At the Mater Children's Hospital, four assistant directors of nursing were appointed: Linda Bognar, management; Irene Howgego, education; Margaret Murphy, clinical; and Dr Grace Croft, nursing research for the whole Mater campus.

By the mid-1990s, the nurses' hard work was recognised as enhancing the hospital's efficiency.[2] This distinction did not come without cost. The new patient–nurse dependency system helped to match nurses to patient needs, but needed continual refinement.[3] The scope of appropriate nursing practice became the subject of a Queensland Nursing Council project; Margaret Murphy was seconded to the Council to work on the project for six months in 1996. She had studied the development of a professional nursing workforce on an overseas study trip and was particularly interested in the family resource centres she saw in Toronto, Canada, and at the Hasbro Children's Hospital in Rhode Island, USA.[4]

Liaisons among paediatric nurses were developing. Linda Shields from the Mater Children's Hospital's operating theatres became the first president of the new Queensland Paediatric Nursing Association (QPNA), linking nurses in hospitals and community services throughout Queensland. The QPNA eventually became the Australian College of Children and Young People's Nurses (ACCYPN).[5] Another outreach opportunity came when Jan Cattoni RN joined a UNICEF and Australian government documentary film project on child health issues in the Pacific.[6]

Highly trained, specialist nurses were always in great demand, especially in emerging fields. Clinical nurse consultants in areas such as diabetics, oncology, child protection, child development and respiratory medicine supported the development of subspecialties.[7] The oncology department, where Linda Ewing was clinical nurse consultant, developed a special course for nurses. As well as caring for in-patients, oncology nurses had a key role in educating parents to care for children with cancer at home.

There never seemed to be enough nurses. Hospitals tried all sorts of strategies to fill senior nursing vacancies. The Mater advertised internationally and further developed its own education and orientation programs, including a special program to integrate new university graduates into hospital life.[8] Establishing a pool of specialist clinical nurses to work between Brisbane's two children's hospitals in highly technical areas, such as intensive care, was seriously considered.[9]

There were other changes at the hospital in the early 1990s. Dr Greg Wuth, who had been medical superintendent since 1988, left the hospital to enter private practice and, in 1995, was succeeded by Dr Peter Steer.

PETER STEER, MBBS, FRACP, FRCPC, FAAP, was a University of Queensland graduate and registrar at the Mater Children's Hospital. He became a Fellow of the Royal Australian College of Physicians in paediatrics before training as a neonatologist in Ontario, Canada. Peter Steer returned to Canada in January 2003 to the newly created position of President, McMaster Children's Hospital. He also became Chair of McMaster University's Department of Paediatrics and in charge of paediatrics for Hamilton Health Sciences and St Joseph's Healthcare. The role of president was the first of its kind in Canada, bringing together clinical, academic and administrative leadership responsibilities and integrating all paediatric services provided by McMaster Children's Hospital.[10]

As did Rosalie Lewis in nursing, Peter Steer faced difficulties in filling all necessary medical appointments. The staff of registrars had grown to 35 including, from January 1995, two in intensive care. To complete their training, registrars needed supervision by specialists and the Mater also needed to appoint specialists in general paediatric medicine, cardiology, endocrinology and gastroenterology.[11] By the mid-1990s, Peter Steer had re-structured the hospital into two main sections: medicine under Dr David Wood and Dr Tony Leslie and surgery under Dr Geoff Hirst and Dr Athol Mackay.[12]

Organisational restructures and the continuing search for efficiency in a busy hospital were stressful for the clinical staff wherever they worked. The paediatric intensive care unit was always a high stress area. Accidents accounted for many admissions. Children tossed into the air were injured by ceiling fans, others fell off bicycles and skateboards or were hurt by inappropriate Christmas toys. An old Queensland problem, poisoning from the lead in the paint on ageing timber houses, still added occasionally to hazards at home.[13]

Increasing prosperity in the community was reflected in some childhood accidents. Although the deaths of children in drowning accidents in creeks and rivers were regularly recorded in Queensland in both the nineteenth and early twentieth centuries, the rapid increase in swimming pools in home gardens in the 1970s and 1980s greatly added to hazards for very young children. In the 1980s, campaigns to fence home swimming pools became a feature of actions to prevent child accidents.[14] Kitchens became even more dangerous with dishwashers using detergents laced with caustic soda. The paediatric gastroenterologist Dr Geoff Cleghorn recorded increasing incidents of serious damage from dishwasher detergent.[15]

Accidents often had tragic outcomes.[16] Reducing the toll of death and injury from preventable accidents became a very important platform for community outreach. Injury was the health issue most common in the young, yet attracted the least research funding; injury was also the most costly health issue for adults in their most productive years.[17] Information on factors leading to accidents was needed in order to prevent them; conventional statistical data was inadequate.

In the 1980s, the medical superintendent of the Mater Children's Hospital, Dr John McNee, and the director of emergency, Dr Rob Pitt, began to collect statistics and qualitative information on child accidents, which developed into Australia's first child-injury surveillance system. By late 1985, the Mater Children's Hospital had recorded the details of an alarming total of 10,500 injuries to children since July 1984.[18] In 1986, the Commonwealth announced that it would fund two studies in two different states based on the Mater Children's Hospital system. Queensland and South Australia were chosen to be the pilot states for the National Injury Surveillance and Prevention Program (NISPP).[19]

Gordon Williams provided the essential computer expertise to analyse the data.[20] It was not long before alarming information emerged. In 1988, for instance, the top ten causes of child injuries were ingestion of dangerous substances; car accidents; falls from monkey bars; injuries involving sticks, branches and trees; bicycle accidents; foreign bodies; skateboards; stairs; bites and stings; and football. Injuries from playground equipment such as monkey bars declined when impact-absorbing materials were installed on the ground.[21]

About 40,000 accidents were analysed each year in the late 1980s and early 1990s.[22] Statistics collected by the Queensland Injury Surveillance and Prevention Program (QISPP) were vital evidence in the campaign for the compulsory installation of fences around backyard swimming pools. Queensland had acquired an unwelcome distinction: the swimming-pool drowning capital of the world.[23] QISPP statistics demonstrated that drowning was the main cause of death of children under four years of age and also exacted a high toll of very serious injury. Many children who survived near-drowning were affected by brain injuries for the rest of their lives. Between 1985 and 1990, 100 children arrived at the Mater after accidents in domestic swimming pools.[24]

Legislation to compel pool owners to erect fences was introduced into the Queensland parliament, despite opposition from many pool owners.[25] QISPP data demonstrated that none of the 98 toddlers who fell into domestic pools in the previous six years had climbed pool fences or opened gates.[26] The *Local Government (Swimming Pool Fencing) Amendment Act 1991* requiring that domestic swimming pools be fenced was proclaimed on 14 September 1991. This was not the end of the battle. Campaigns for a national register of child drownings and a revision of the Australian standard on swimming pool fences came next.[27]

Success in improving children's playgrounds and introducing the compulsory fencing of domestic swimming pools demonstrated the value of QISPP statistics. It was, therefore, galling that QISPP had to go 'begging' for funding to various government departments when a solid five-year funding commitment was necessary to develop proactive, effective strategies in design improvement, education and legislation.[28]

Newspapers became conscientious partners in distributing the child accident prevention message. QISPP also distributed frequent bulletins, such as one in 1994 that focused on injuries in soccer games and in falls from wheelchairs.[29] A large, furry creature – a human in a bear suit – became the mascot of the educational effort. The 'Matt the Mater Bear Show' toured schools carrying the accident prevention message. Matt calendars – sponsored by a mining company – were distributed to schools and preschools in Central Queensland.[30]

Within months, Matt was controversial. He was attacked as being 'zoologically inaccurate', as he resembled a koala, which is not a bear. Ironically, the furore increased newspapers' attention to the Matt campaign. One paper claimed that the issue had thrown into 'limbo a program which has saved lives' and another likened the 'thought police' action to insisting that Mickey Mouse and Donald Duck be removed from Disneyland. Matt was reborn as Matt the Mater Koala.[31]

Despite QISPP's efforts, children continued to be injured in accidents and often spent long periods in hospital. The Queensland-wide reach of many Mater tertiary services placed the families of very sick country children in a difficult situation. The Reg Leonard units accommodated parents of in-patients, but there was a growing need for accommodation for country children having day treatments and for their families. The American icon Ronald McDonald, a clown with bright red hair, yellow trousers and very large shoes, visited Brisbane in 1987, the first intimation that the Mater might have the first Ronald McDonald House in Queensland.[32]

The world's first Ronald McDonald House opened in Philadelphia in the 1970s, inspired by the efforts of a football player, Fred Hill, whose daughter was treated for leukaemia at a Philadelphia hospital, a long way from the Hill family home. The Hill family recognised the need for accommodation for country families at the hospital; the McDonald's restaurant in Philadelphia was enrolled to help.

Brisbane's Ronald McDonald House was announced on 30 November 1987. The Mater donated land in Allen Street, not far from the Mater Children's Hospital, and the Queensland Governor, Sir Walter Campbell, laid the foundation stone, which was sufficiently large to be a comfortable seat for parents and children.[33] As in Philadelphia and the other American cities where Ronald McDonald Houses were established, a great deal of fundraising was necessary in Brisbane. Support came from many quarters.

A telethon at Seaworld on the Gold Coast in February 1989 was very successful, the Variety Club donated $150,000, the Mater Art Union contributed $50,000, fundraising in Bundaberg added to the coffers, as did the auction of a slouch hat from the world-champion swimmer Hayley Lewis, the Ronald McDonald Ball in July 1990 and the sale of pens and calendars. Advertising and news reports kept Ronald McDonald House in the public eye; an offer from the dairy foods company Queensland United Foods to advertise the house on a panel of its milk cartons was gratefully received.[34] At the end of 1989, fundraising had yielded $418,501.84, but a further $271,498.16 was needed to complete the house. The generosity of building companies saved almost $250,000. Construction began in October 1989 and plans to manage Ronald McDonald House firmed. Families of children with serious long-term illnesses, such as cystic fibrosis and cancer, and parents of premature babies, were to be given priority.[35]

On 15 July 1990, the Queensland Premier, Wayne Goss, opened Ronald McDonald House entirely free of debt.[36] Even better, licensees of McDonald's restaurants, through Ronald McDonald House Charities, covered many of the running costs. With solid community support, the Mater's Ronald McDonald House joined the growing world group of 'houses that love built' and admitted its first three families in its opening month.[37] The house continued to be very busy in the final months of 1990 and included a child from Papua New Guinea and her family. The little girl had been very seriously injured in a fall through a plate-glass window.[38]

There were, however, teething problems. The rooms were hot in Brisbane's subtropical summer, but a shortfall in earnings not only put air-conditioning at risk, but also cast doubt on the business plan forecast that the house would be self-funding within three years. The house could accommodate 24 people at any one time in its eight rooms, but in early 1991, occupancy had fallen to 40 per cent. By the end of the first year, with an operating loss of $50,000, economising was essential, a considerable task for the managers, Ailsa and Colin Jensen, who succeeded Marijke Haeren and her husband, Leo.[39]

Ronald McDonald House supported children and their families who needed to be near the hospital. Another innovation enlivened the experience for children during their stay as in-patients. Paediatric care was steadily becoming more child and family focused. The needs and interests of the children were the entire *raison d'être* of Radio Lollipop, an idea that came from England, where a station had been opened at Queen Mary's Hospital in 1979. Perth was the only Australian state to have introduced Radio Lollipop before stations opened at the Mater Children's and the Royal Children's hospitals in Brisbane.[40]

Radio Lollipop went on air at the Mater on 2 December 1990. The studio was enlivened by murals painted by children from Woodridge State High School.[41] Radio Lollipop soon attracted an avid audience and was supported by its patrons, the sporting stars Grant and Lisa Kenny, local radio stations, a telephone company and many other businesses, and dozens of volunteers. Senior members of the staff also recognised the value of 'in-house' entertainment.[42]

The Mater Children's Hospital special school also offered a welcome break from hospital routine treatments. The school was even more important in offering the opportunity for sick children to keep pace with their healthy peers in the mainstream education system. It was, therefore, an important link between the hospital, the patients' homes and their communities. Teaching in a hospital school was quite different from mainstream schools.

The pupils were enrolled for varying lengths of time. Many needed to have time out of the classroom for treatments; children who could not leave the wards were taught in bed. Individual programs for each child were essential. The whole child – not the patient encased in plaster or attached to a drip stand or oxygen cylinder – had always to be at the forefront of the hospital teacher's mind. The emphasis was on health and normality rather than sickness.[43] The staff in 1992 – the principal, Vicki Sykes; ten teachers; an administrative assistant; four part-time teacher aides; a janitor–groundsman; and a cleaner – were always busy; many were overjoyed in 1991 to be part of a staff syndicate that won $1,500,000 in a lottery.[44]

As well as the usual requirement to discuss the children's progress with their parents, hospital-school teachers also had to liaise with the child's usual school and needed to be thoroughly aware of the children's conditions. This requirement often meant attending hospital clinic sessions and discussing special needs with the clinical staff. Devising suitable programs for children to follow at home became increasingly necessary with the move towards the shortest possible hospital stays for sick children, no matter how serious or enduring their illness.

The labour-intensive 'home' program had been running successfully since 1987. It seemed ironic that, at the same time as the Health Department was encouraging the care of the child at home with the family, or in a community setting, the Education Department's drive for economy appeared likely to weaken this important link by reducing the school staff. Like the Health Department, the Education Department had been 'regionalised'. The Mater Children's Hospital was in the Brisbane South health region, but in the Metropolitan East education region, along with the Royal Children's Hospital special school.

A review of hospital schools was announced in October 1992. The terms of reference made no bones about the expected outcome: significant savings in staff salaries.[45] The review came at a very tense stage in the negotiations about the proposal to move the Mater Children's Hospital to Mt Gravatt. Nevertheless, the school's staffing was defended by the senior echelons of the hospital and by teachers and parents.

The challenges of education in a hospital school were many. The pupils ranged from very, very sick children to those who were relatively well, and covered the full range of mobility.[46] The story of Nick, a little boy who had swallowed battery acid, highlighted the hospital view. Nick had been in hospital for almost a year enduring repeated surgery and painful procedures. The physical activity at preschool and the educational 'exploration' program helped his overall development. The company of children at school helped him in the difficult process of learning to eat again. The school was also very important for children who had been traumatised by child abuse.[47]

The Mater was appalled at the suggestion that nurses in the wards could supervise distance-education lessons supplied by the Education Department. Quite apart from not having appropriate teaching qualifications, the nurses were far too busy. The notion that education should be offered only to those in hospital for more than one week was just as surprising, displaying a lack of understanding of modern tertiary paediatric hospitals, which admitted children for the shortest time possible.[48] Children with chronic illnesses were, therefore, admitted frequently for short periods, but required long periods of recuperation, and would have little opportunity for education if home-care teachers were not available.[49] Advances in medical treatment enabled more children to survive serious illnesses, but they were often affected by some degree of disability. Diseases of the central nervous system, for instance, often had serious implications for that child's educational progress, as well as requiring regular hospital admissions.[50]

In the 1980s and 1990s, more and more children were admitted to the Mater Children's Hospital with psychological or behavioural problems. A close relationship between the child psychiatry service and the school began at the hospital in the 1960s and continued when Dr Aidene Urquhart became staff psychiatrist in 1980.[51] As many of the patients had physical, mental and emotional disabilities, adequate school staff was essential.

The teachers also had a broader role in their relationship with the child development clinic; they needed to know the child's developmental stage for educational purposes and were able to reciprocate with significant insight into a child's learning difficulties.[52] Nurses and medical specialists were equally disturbed at the proposition that teachers should not attend interdisciplinary meetings about individual patients. They regarded the move from ward to school and back to the ward as a continuum, integral to the Mater Children's Hospital philosophy of holistic care; therefore, the meetings were important for the child, both educationally and medically.[53]

The director of nursing, Rosalie Lewis, was surprised at the department's view that children from private schools should not attend the hospital school as, under Queensland law, all children were entitled to state education whether or not they sought it. In Rosalie Lewis's view, the school was essential in making a patient's day as normal as possible and in enhancing social interaction. To emphasise her views, Rosalie Lewis referred to the United Nations Convention on the Rights of the Child. Article 3 said that a child was entitled to 'such protection and care as is necessary for his/her wellbeing' and Article 24 guaranteed the 'right of the child to the enjoyment of the highest attainable standard of health and to facilities for the treatment of illness and rehabilitation of health'.[54]

The review found that the schools at the Mater Children's and Royal Children's hospitals were 'an integral part of the region's quality educational provision', but reduced the size of the teaching staff. The Mater Children's Hospital school lost two teachers and the larger Royal Children's Hospital school lost four teachers.[55]

In some instances, shortages in community services increased the demand for Mater Children's Hospital services. Many of the school's pupils were patients of the Child and Youth Mental Health Service (CYMHS) or undergoing rehabilitation in the special clinic for victims of torture and trauma, most of whom were refugees. Community child psychiatry services and the day program on the Mater campus were expanded, as were community services in centres such as Inala in Brisbane's south-west.[56]

Coping with daily demand did not divert the mental health team from developing new services. Refugee children and their families had been a particular interest of the Mater Children's Hospital's Department of Psychiatry since October 1985, when a refugee family sought the Mater's help to deal with the effects of traumatic experiences in their home country. Coordinated through the Department of Psychiatry, the Treatment and Rehabilitation Unit for the Survivors of Torture and Trauma (TRUSTT) at Mater Children's Hospital became the first such service in Queensland and treated 1,500 people in its first nine years.[57]

There were referrals from many parts of Queensland, but the Mater's location in South Brisbane placed the service where about 30 per cent of the population were from non-English speaking backgrounds.[58] In 1994, about 21 per cent of families treated at the Mater's Children's Hospital's

Department of Psychiatry did not speak English as their first language. Fifty of those families had been affected by torture or trauma.⁵⁹ They came from many different world trouble spots including Bosnia, Kurdistan, Ethiopia and various parts of Latin America. In the mid-1990s, it was estimated that one-third of the refugee population had been victims of torture and trauma, including 10,000 adults and children in Queensland.⁶⁰ This was a large burden for the small TRUSTT budget.

The Commonwealth government also had a keen interest in the health of refugees and was prepared to fund rehabilitation services, but wanted the service to be available throughout Queensland and to be based in the community, rather than at a hospital.⁶¹ The Mater was also reminded that the children's hospital was a paediatric service, rather than a service for adults and children, as was the TRUSTT practice. Dr Urquhart secured some funding from the United Nations to manage TRUSTT in a new location where services for adults as well as children could continue.⁶²

Another new program reached an often-overlooked age group: teenagers. The Adolescent Drug and Alcohol Withdrawal Service (ADAWS) was formed to address very difficult issues in adolescent health. A pilot program began in 1999, with five beds in a house owned by the Mater, and conveniently close to the campus but not actually part of it. A grant of $1,450,000 from Queensland Health funded ADAWS in its early stages.⁶³ The program was officially opened with the Health Minister's recognition that it was 'the first service of its type in Queensland'.⁶⁴ The state government allocated funding over three years to develop and staff the program and to refurbish the accommodation provided by the Mater.

Each participant spent two weeks in the ADAWS program. It was a 24-hours-a-day service, with supervision by specialist nursing staff and specially trained youth workers; a range of specialist medical staff and counsellors were available during the day and on-call after hours.

Demands for the Mater Children's Hospital child abuse program also grew. In a single year, 1990, referrals to the parent aide unit increased by 30 per cent. By 2000, there were 400 new cases referred to the Suspected Child Abuse and Neglect (SCAN) unit.⁶⁵ The pressures on the parent aide unit were somewhat relieved by funding from the Department of Family Services and Aboriginal and Islander Affairs.⁶⁶ In 1998, funding from the government's Golden Casket lottery enabled the SCAN unit to offer a fellowship in child protection and child development.[67] Dr David Wood, who had been a pioneer in child abuse services and a founder of the Abused Child Trust (re-named Act for Kids), was appointed to the government's new Child Protection Committee in 2000.[68]

Reaching out to the community to prevent child accidents, accommodating country families at Ronald McDonald House, services such as TRUSTT and CYMHS, when combined with the services that supported patients in their homes, spread the Mater Children's Hospital's influence even more broadly into the community. Each of these services needed a 'home base' at the hospital, the hub from which community services radiated and the centre for increasingly complex tertiary care services. But there was a problem: there was very little room at the inn for existing services, let alone expansion.

Chapter 13

Plans and Preparations

There is a momentum and an excitement within the staff of the children's hospital currently. It would be a tragedy if we could not build on this enthusiasm.

Dr Peter Steer, August 1996

A great deal had been accomplished within the ageing fabric of the Mater Children's Hospital – boosted by expansion into the Potter Building, as the ambulatory services had become known – but the hospital resembled an old patchwork quilt. Its sections were connected, but some contrasted with others, and the connections were fraying. In the 1990s, proposals for a new Mater Children's Hospital ranged from the troubling idea of re-locating to QEII to the possibility that the hospital would be rebuilt on the South Brisbane campus. Excitement mounted as hopes became plans and plans became reality. By the end of the decade, it was not merely one new hospital, but two: a shiny new building to accommodate the Mater Children's Hospital and a new addition to the Mater family – Australia's first children's private hospital.

Accommodation for fee-paying patients was by no means a new idea. The Mater Children's and Mater Adult hospitals had admitted 'intermediate' patients for decades. As intermediate patients, children were accommodated in the same wards as public patients, but their parents could choose the specialist who treated them.[1] In the mid-1990s, there was clear evidence that, to some extent, patients were voting with their feet. Parents with private health insurance were taking their children to the emergency centre at an adult hospital, the Mater Private Hospital, rather than seeking admission as intermediate patients at the Mater Children's Hospital. Paediatricians continued to believe that children should not be admitted to adult hospitals and were concerned that nurses at the Mater Private Hospital might not have expertise in paediatrics.[2]

At first, the Mater Board was not enthusiastic about the prospect of a children's private hospital and suggested that there could be provision for private patients in public areas when additional wards were opened in the Potter Building, but a survey of parents in February 1994 indicated that there was a demand for a private hospital.[3] As an interim measure, the medical superintendent of the Mater Children's Hospital, Dr Greg Wuth, suggested that paediatricians be accredited to the emergency department at the Mater Private Hospital. The Mater would then have Brisbane's only private emergency service for all age groups.[4]

Although there was no legislation preventing the establishment of a private emergency service for children, the Commonwealth government's Health Insurance Commission, which administered the government's health insurance program, Medicare, did not like the proposal.[5] The possibility that a children's private emergency centre might earn valuable revenue for the Mater was not the Commission's concern. It was much more worried that doctors in public hospital emergency departments might refer patients to their private practices, a way of shifting costs from the state health budget to the Commonwealth, which paid a rebate on fees charged by private medical practitioners. The Commonwealth was reassured that there would not be a private practice paediatrician in the public emergency service at the Mater Children's Hospital.[6]

By 1997, the Mater Board was contemplating expanding its private hospital interests and considered applying to co-locate Mater private hospitals on the campuses of the new Caboolture and Noosa state hospitals.[7] The Board's view of the children's private hospital proposal had changed. A feasibility study, which included consultation with Mater parents, staff and clinicians who referred patients to the Mater Children's Hospital, showed that a private hospital with 29 beds – 19 in-patient beds and ten day beds – could operate economically with a 45 per cent share of private paediatric patients from Brisbane's southern suburbs. It was even possible that sufficient cash flow could be generated in just over two and a half years to recoup the cost of the private hospital: about $2,235,000.[8]

At 89 per cent, surgical patients – with ear, nose and throat patients the largest group – were predicted to dominate day admissions. The average stay for an in-patient would be two days for surgery and 2.5 days for medical patients. The private hospital could also fulfil a long-held wish: accommodation for the adolescent age group, as a private hospital could admit patients up to the age of 18.[9]

Licensing private hospitals was the business of state governments. It was a considerable relief to hear that the Queensland Department of Health would not oppose the proposal. But there was a sting in the tail: the fear – later proved to be groundless – that the government could reduce the number of beds in the existing Mater Children's Hospital when the private hospital was licensed.[10] The children's private hospital could also accommodate fee-paying patients from overseas without attracting the complications that often arose when overseas patients were admitted to the public hospital. Only Australian residents were entitled to treatment free-of-charge in Australian public hospitals.

The key to success for the Mater Children's Private Hospital was differentiation from other private hospitals that maintained children's wards. The Mater, however, had an edge over other Brisbane private hospitals with children's wards: none of them could offer the support of a level 5–6 paediatric hospital, including sophisticated paediatric intensive care and modern accident and emergency services. The Australian Council on Healthcare Standards (ACHS) was concerned that private adult hospitals could not offer appropriate facilities or sufficient specialised nursing to support paediatric surgery.[11]

The Sisters of Mercy showed their confidence in the viability of the children's private hospital by financing it to the tune of $2,000,000, a loan that would be repaid when the private hospital became profitable. Although the Sisters always exercised their option to serve the poor first and foremost, they recognised that all sick children needed access to hospital facilities, and options like a children's private hospital needed to be made available.[12] The private hospital opened in March 1998.

The fourth floor of the Potter Building had been transformed. It was bright and cheerful, decorated around a seaside theme.[13] There were 25 beds, eight of which were in single rooms with ensuite bathrooms – and double beds for parents – and two six-bed wards that could be reconfigured for high-dependency nursing. Several play areas were included and the children had access to that necessity for a modern child: a computer. Another computer was available for parents who needed to keep in touch with work. Jennifer Pitt RN from the Mater Private Hospital was seconded to manage the new hospital through its early stages.

There were some teething problems. It was difficult to attract sufficient numbers of paediatric nurses to either children's hospital and there was a degree of tension between the staffs of the two children's hospitals. It was not easy to persuade the existing staff that the children's private hospital could enhance the whole Mater complex.[14] Convincing private general practitioners and paediatricians to refer patients to the private hospital was constrained by slow, tense negotiations with the private health insurance funds; insured families would expect their funds to refund part of the cost of their children's hospitalisation.[15] The concept of sharing the intensive care unit and operating theatres with the Mater Children's Hospital was one sticking point. A thawing in the health funds' attitudes by July 1998 marked an upturn in the private hospital's fortunes, even though its capacity to admit patients for day surgery was somewhat limited by the availability of the shared operating theatres.[16]

In December 1998, nine months after it opened, the Mater Children's Private Hospital recorded a profit and its highest occupancy at 82 per cent of its target. The plan to accommodate children brought from overseas – through Operation Smile – for craniofacial surgery was fulfilled in the first year and plans were made to host a surgeon from the Philippines.[17] More importantly, the new hospital had made an impact on the private paediatric hospital market. The Royal Brisbane Hospital had decided not to proceed with a co-located private hospital and it appeared that the large Wesley Hospital had slowed its plan to develop a large paediatric facility.[18]

The private hospital in the Potter Building was an opportunity to test state-of-the-art models of care in preparation for an entirely new Mater Children's Hospital. The first proposal for a new hospital, in 1992, involved a new building on the site of the old Clarence Court building, which faced Clarence Street close to the Potter Building. The new hospital would loop around the school to a new building on the site of the former registered nurses home further up the hill.[19] The vacant site next to the Princess Theatre on the opposite side of Annerley Road was also a possibility, but a bridge or tunnel would be necessary to connect the hospital to existing services. Although the Potter Building had been designed to allow it to expand above Clarence Court – an older building facing Clarence Street – it would not be large enough. Sufficient space for expansion was the chief advantage of the option to extend the hospital up the hill beyond the school.[20]

This plan was replaced by a much bolder scheme: a new hospital on the other side of the campus close to the Mater Adult and Mater Mothers' hospitals, so that the two children's hospitals could share expensive diagnostic services with the other Mater hospitals. The benefits of shared services had been frequently mentioned in various Mater quarters over the years, but were given official imprimatur in the 1996 Mater Hospitals' Master Plan Review.[21] The Mater Mothers' Hospital included private patients; babies born in the Mater Mothers' Private Hospital needing further treatment could be admitted to the Mater Children's Private Hospital. Co-location of the Mater Mothers', the Mater Adult and the Mater Children's hospitals emerged as the preferred option for the future development of the campus.[22]

Planning to build an entirely new Mater Children's Hospital close to the other Mater hospitals proceeded apace. It was badly needed. For some years, the ageing fabric of the old hospital and cramped conditions had attracted a rising tide of complaint. Some of the hospital's long-standing specialists were becoming increasingly frustrated. The orthopaedic surgeon Dr Terry McGuire, who had been associated with the hospital for 28 years and was loath to refer patients elsewhere, reported that some of his surgical patients did not want to stay at the Mater Children's Hospital. The ward for orthopaedic patients had changed little since the 1930s.[23] The urologist Dr David Winkle was concerned that ward CM1 was so crowded that only one person at a time could reach beds in the corners – dangerous in emergency situations. In addition, wheelchairs could not enter the toilets or bathroom. Renovations, such as attending to workplace health and safety issues, renovating wards and bathrooms in the original building, and even the sleep centre's $1,000,000 upgrade, could only be stopgap measures.[24]

The intensive care unit was in a particularly difficult situation. There were equipment deficiencies and a shortage of medical and nursing staff to the extent that it failed an assessment by the Australian and New Zealand College of Anaesthetists Faculty of Intensive Care (now the College of Intensive Care Medicine). The Mater Children's Hospital could not offer intensive care training, making it more difficult to attract high-quality staff.[25] The difficulties of fitting many services into old buildings was also highlighted by the speech pathology department, which had moved five times in little over ten years and, by 1994, was in the decrepit Clarence Court building.[26]

Developmental paediatrics and respiratory medicine were two of the Mater Children's Hospital's flagship areas in need of improvement. Michael O'Callaghan recommended increasing the number of staff subspecialists in areas such as gastroenterology and urology and advocated integration of hospital and community services in developmental paediatrics. Following up high-risk infants and improving the rehabilitation opportunities for children with various neuromuscular disorders was also recommended.[27] The respiratory physicians were particularly frustrated with difficulties at the Mater Children's Hospital. They were also concerned about the government's approach to paediatrics generally and, therefore, about the long-term viability of tertiary paediatrics at the Mater. There were, however, opportunities for the development of subspecialty paediatrics in a private hospital.[28]

Consultation with Mater staff helped the project team to define the specifications for a Mater Children's Hospital appropriate to twenty-first-century demands. It would need 150 beds or, in other words, one bed per 1,000 people in the catchment area; 25 per cent of those beds would be tertiary beds. The 2001 hospital would need 12 general consulting rooms, 12 specialised consulting rooms and two multidisciplinary areas, as well as a child and family psychology unit. Adequate spaces would be necessary for physiotherapy, speech pathology and occupational therapy. Emergency diagnostic investigations should be readily available, but more sophisticated services, such as magnetic resonance imaging, could be shared with the other Mater hospitals. Further, facilities for education and research, particularly in respiratory conditions, neurology and injury prevention, would be essential.[29] The steering committee also recommended that tertiary paediatric hospitals should have formal links with peripheral hospitals and community health agencies to facilitate care as close as possible to the child's home.

In 1996, the Mater administration pressed on with plans and preparations. The purchase of properties in Stanley Street was essential if the new children's hospital was to be co-located with the Mater Mothers' and Mater Adult hospitals. Some of these shops – Christie's coffee shop and Salon Zizzanie among them – had been familiar fixtures in the landscape for Mater patients and the staff.[30] While these negotiations were progressing, impatience was mounting at the existing Mater's Children's Hospital:

> ... there is a momentum and an excitement within the staff of the children's hospital currently. It would be a tragedy if we could not build on this enthusiasm.[31]

Planning the new hospital was not smooth sailing; there were some nerve-wracking moments. In 1996, the Health Minister, Mike Horan, announced a ten-year capital works program for health facilities, but did not mention the Mater.[32] The Health Department hastened to mend the fence by informing the Mater that the capital component for the Mater would be funded 'off budget', once a program had been settled.[33] The board wasted no time in notifying the minister that it was working to a master plan and that its priorities were the Mater Children's and Mater Mothers' hospitals and that the Sisters of Mercy had already acquired properties on Stanley Street in preparation for construction of the new children's hospital to begin early in 1997.[34] Queensland Department of Health could offer only $50,000,000 for the children's hospital. Even though the board hoped that government funding would increase as planning progressed, plans were adjusted to devise a building able to be expanded later.[35]

All was ready for an announcement in January 1997 that a new Mater Children's Hospital would be built as part of a 20-year plan to redevelop the Mater site, which included a new Mater Mothers' Hospital, and refitting the top floor of the old Mater Private Hospital (re-named Aubigny Place), to accommodate the Mater Medical Research Institute. The announcement mentioned some of the hospital's newer services: the respiratory team's outreach service to Aboriginal and Torres Strait Islander communities, the first Adolescent Drug and Alcohol Withdrawal Service (ADAWS) for teenagers and a partnership with the University of Queensland to establish the world's first centre to study paediatric pharmacology.[36]

Plans for the private hospital in the new building were sophisticated and exacting. The business case for the private hospital amplified the original feasibility study with two scenarios. First was a 40-bed hospital, including ten beds for day patients. A hospital of this size could manage with two or three operating theatres but the second scenario, a 50-bed hospital with 20 day beds, would require four operating theatres, which could be reduced if time could be 'bought' in one of the public hospital's operating theatres. In either scenario, flexibility would be essential so that the bed configuration could be changed to cater for the predicted continued rise in single-day admissions; day surgery was predicted to rise from 47 per cent in 1996–97 to 68 per cent in 2004 and 76 per cent in 2009. As full a complement of admissions as possible would be necessary to achieve the business-plan goal of offsetting the cost of the new Mater Children's Private Hospital within ten years.[37] The various specialties were generally well represented in the interim private hospital, but it needed to attract more patients in several areas, including ear, nose and throat, oncology and ophthalmology.[38]

The business case contemplated cost efficiencies, such as an intensive care unit shared by the two Mater children's hospitals. There was also the possibility of a private paediatric emergency service, which general practitioners were likely to support if they were sure that adequate day and night medical cover would be available. A private emergency service was unlikely to be profitable, but offered potential benefits in the admission of patients to the private hospital. It would also draw patients who had been presenting to the adult private hospital emergency centre, a disadvantage to the adult private hospital, which was a rare exception to the benefit of linkages across the Mater campus.[39] Containing costs was at the forefront of the suggestion that both children's emergency centres should be co-located.[40]

One very difficult area – a mental health service for adolescents – was excluded from the business case analysis on the grounds that there were likely to be very few private psychiatric patients. A private psychiatric unit would need between 12 and 15 patients each day to be viable, but more than five would be unlikely. Alternatively, teenagers could be treated as private psychiatric patients in an annexe to the proposed public psychiatric unit. The only other possibility would be a private psychiatric unit that could offer services to the government.[41]

The complexities of planning the two new Mater children's hospitals and bringing them to reality required a great deal of research. One principle stood out: family-centred care would be the foundation for services at both hospitals. Consultation with parents and clinicians during the planning process brought this principle to the fore again and again. In both hospitals, parents, with the support of expert nurses, would continue as the primary carers while their children were in hospital.[42]

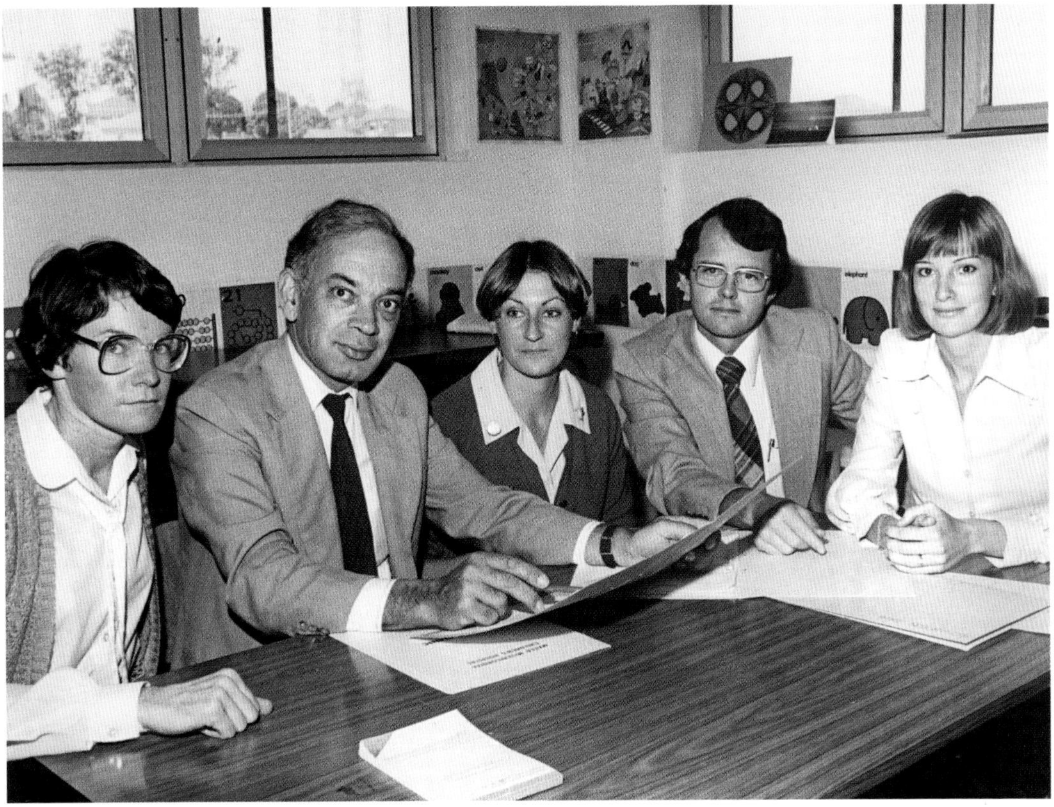

The team at the diabetes clinic in 1980, from left to right: Bernadette Wright, Dr Geoffrey Bourke, Amanda Coburn, Dr Michael Thomsett, Helen O'Brien.

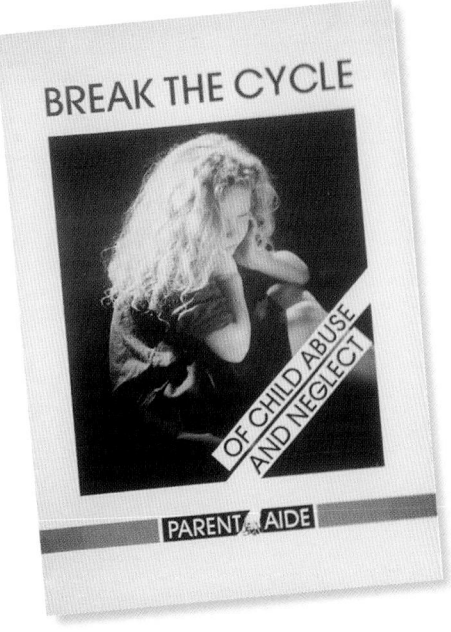

The Parent Aide Unit's 'Break the Cycle' booklet.

Dr David Wood with nurses
Vivienne Devine RN (left) and
Mary McCarthy RN (right).

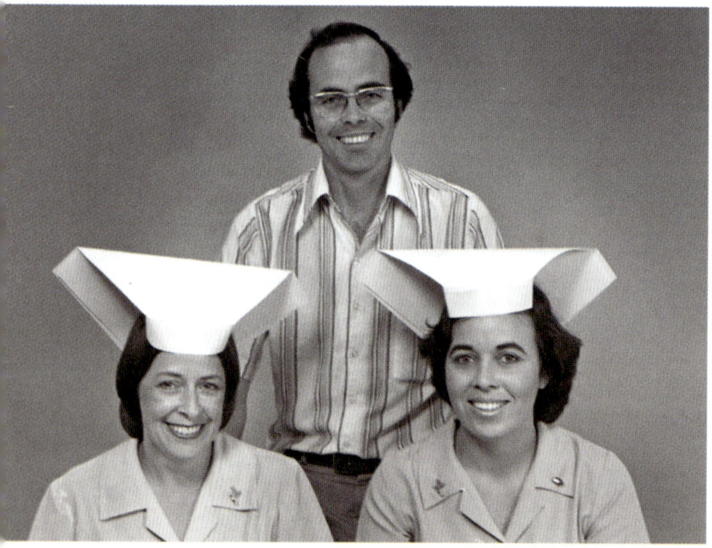

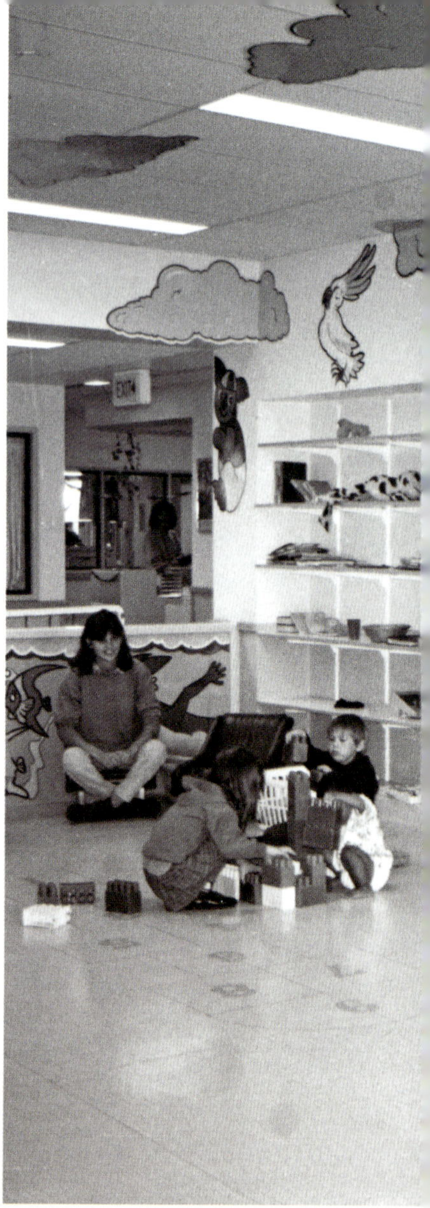

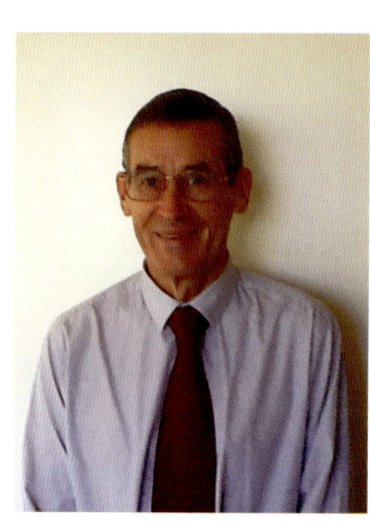

Dr Michael O'Callaghan.

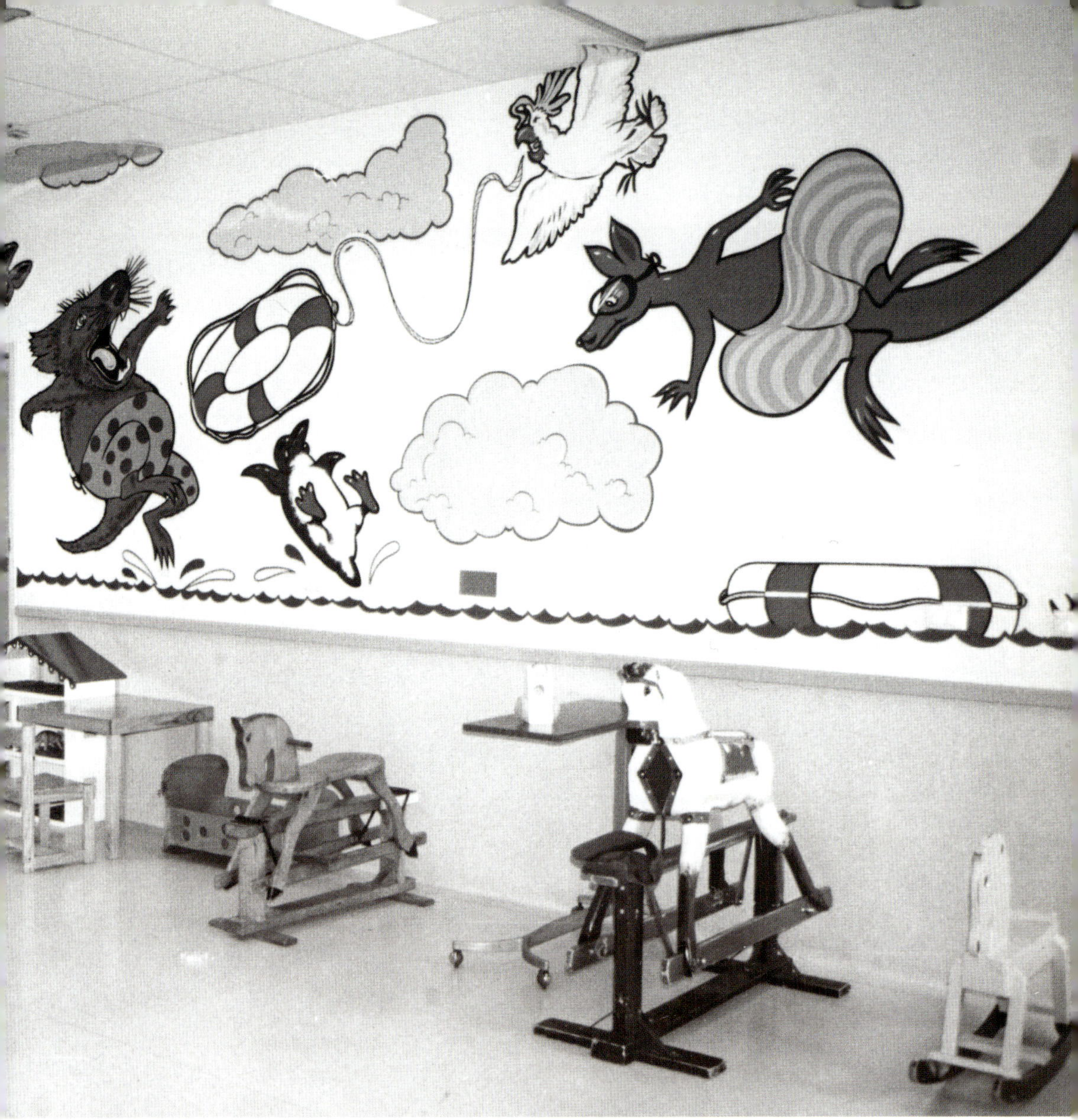

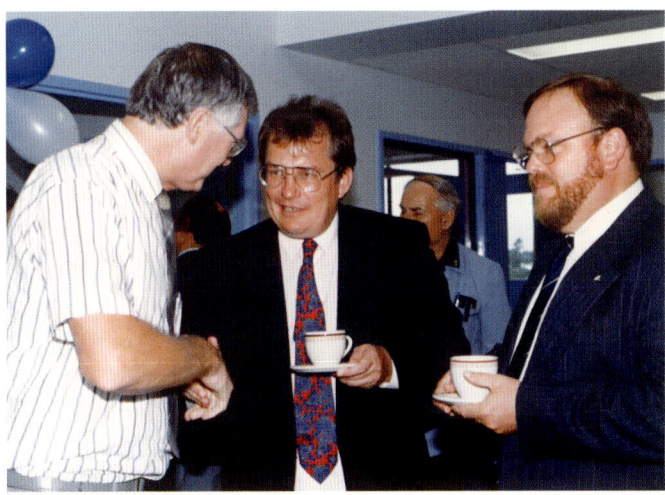

ABOVE: Colourful murals and toys in a play area at the Mater Children's Hospital in the 1990s.

Health Minister Ken Hayward (centre) at the hospital in the early 1990s, with Dr Greg Wuth (right).

FOLLOWING PAGES: Progress despite turmoil – the new intensive care unit in 1992.

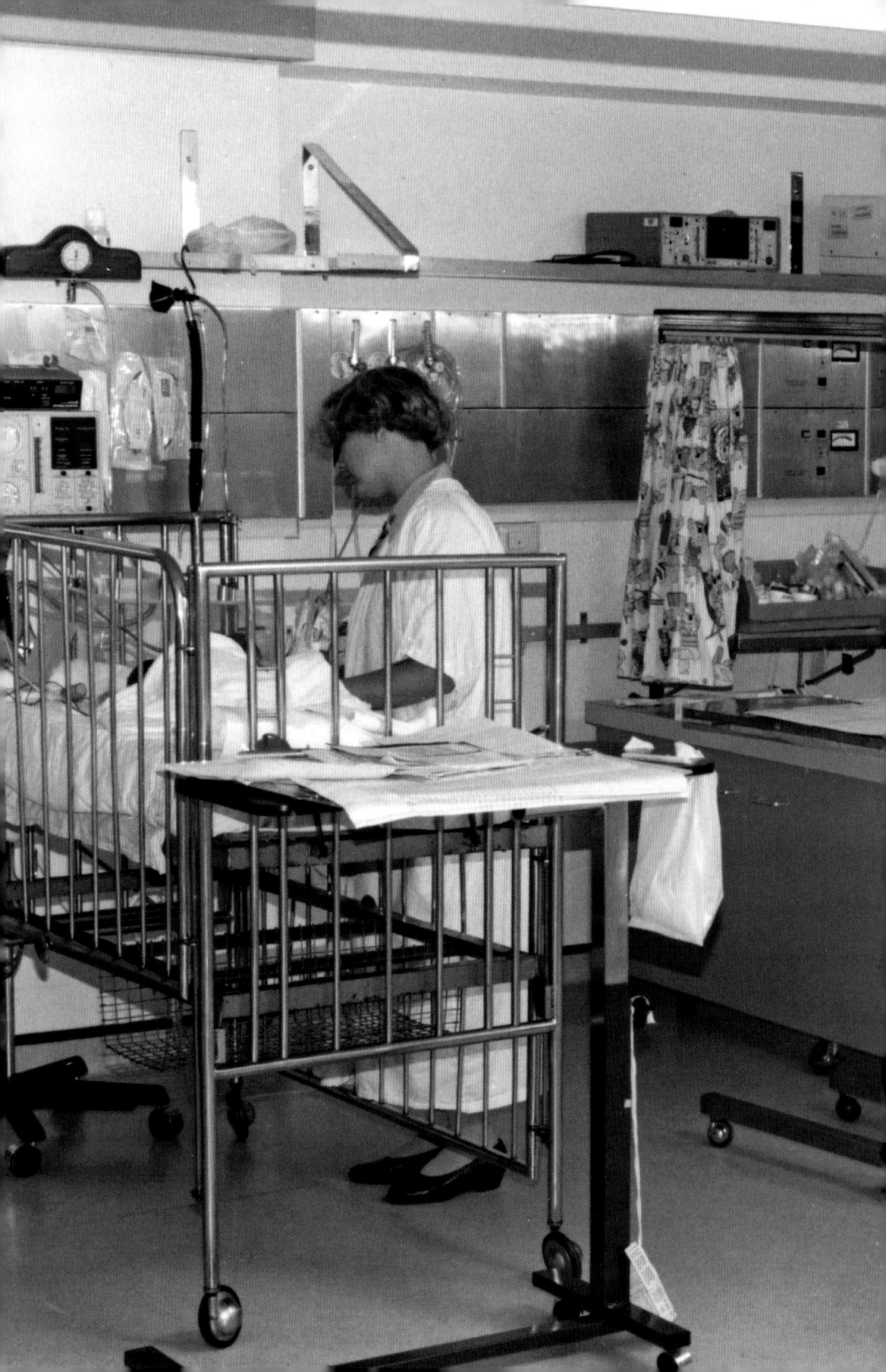

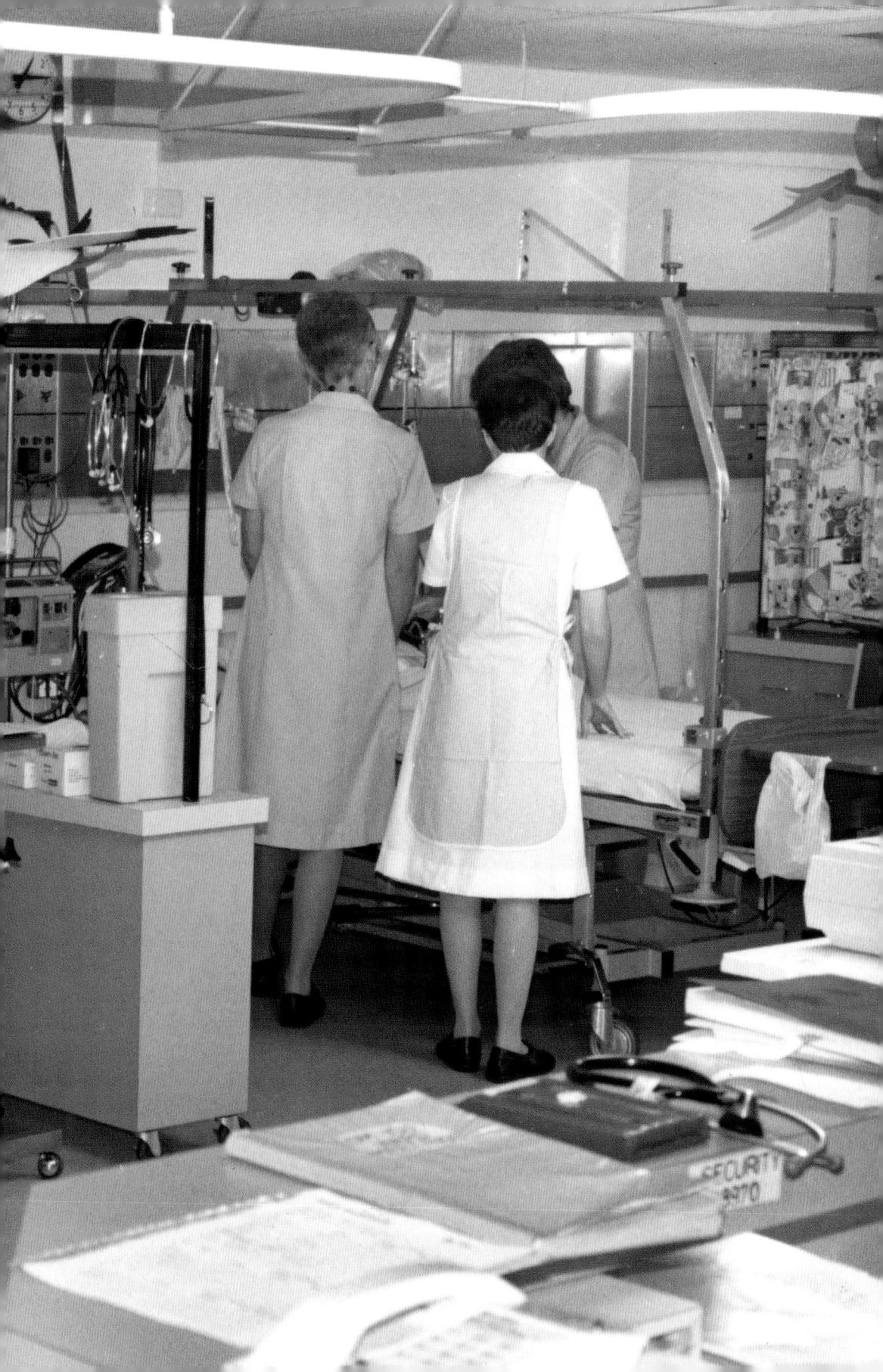

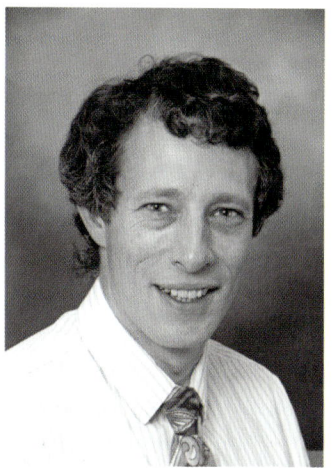

Dr Cameron Ward.

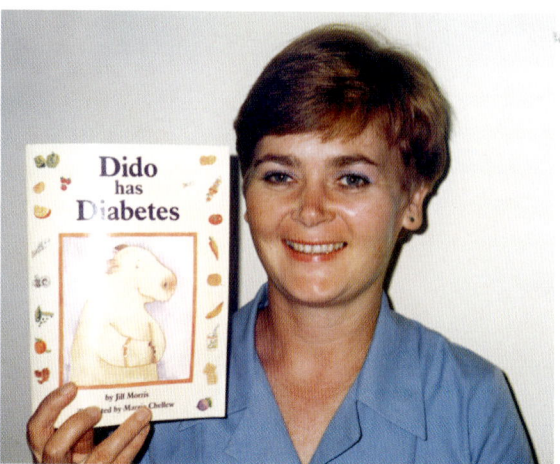

Helen Kearney RN with *Dido has diabetes*.

The craniofacial surgery team, (left to right) Drs R Black, Des McGuckin, Leigh Atkinson and Tony Emmett, examining an X-ray in 1985.

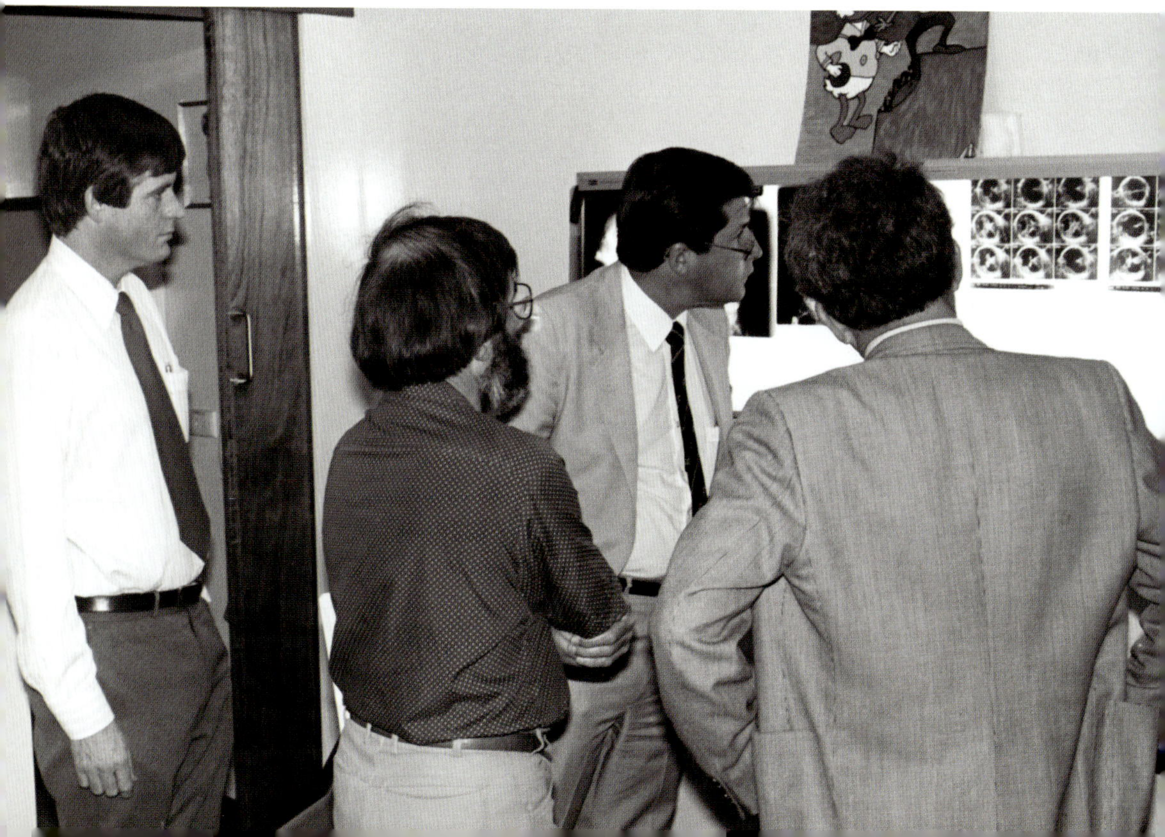

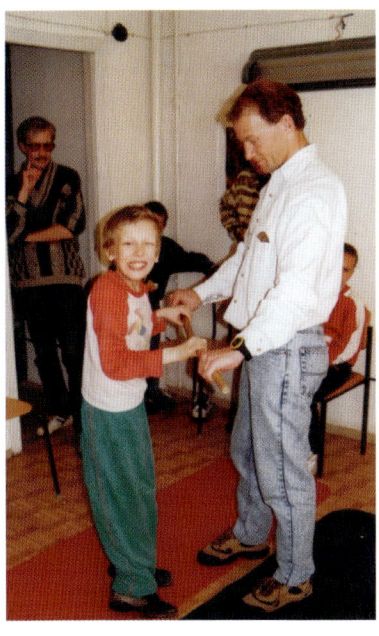

LEFT: Dr John Gilmour, physiotherapist, with a young patient, on a working visit to Russia in the 1990s.

Dr Robyn Brady, Dr Rob Pitt and Marie Hand RN with the certificate recognising the Mater Children's Hospital's accreditation to educate advanced trainees in emergency medicine.

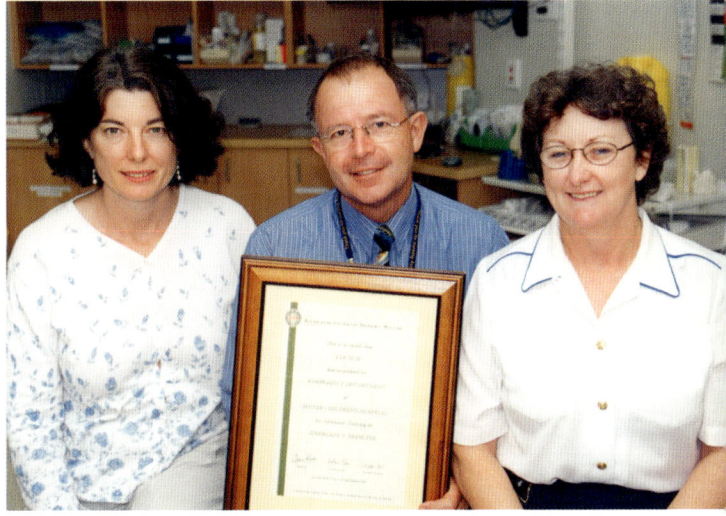

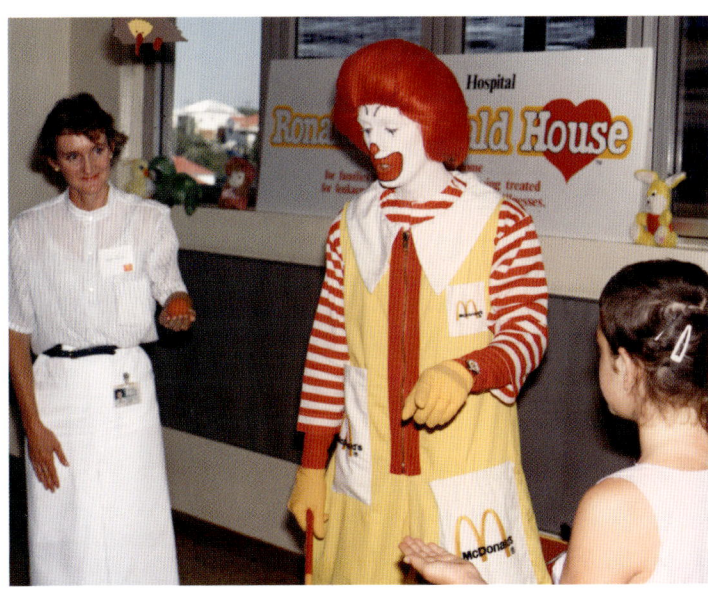

Ronald McDonald with Linda Boyle RN and an enthusiastic child at the opening of Ronald McDonald House.

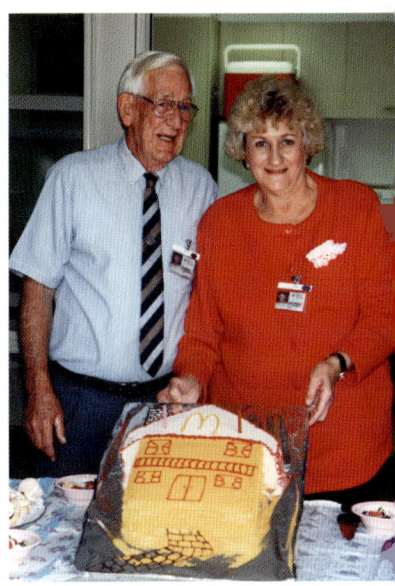

Colin and Ailsa Jensen at the second birthday party for Ronald McDonald House.

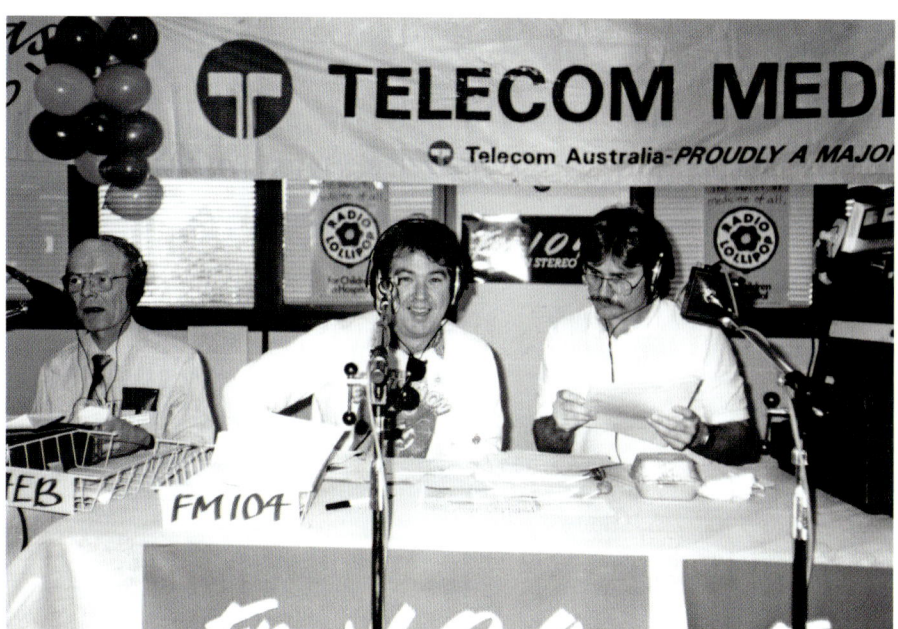

Brisbane radio personalities drumming up support at the radiothon for Radio Lollipop in 1989.

LEFT: Radio Lollipop on air.

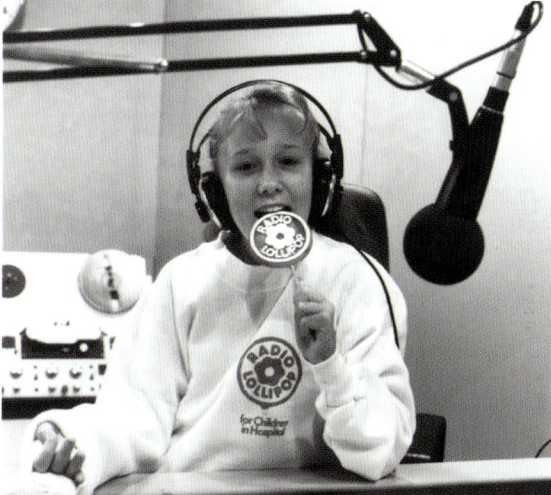

Breaking new ground: Dr Peter Steer at the opening of the new Mater Children's Private Hospital in 1998.

OPPOSITE PAGE: The new building in the 1980s.

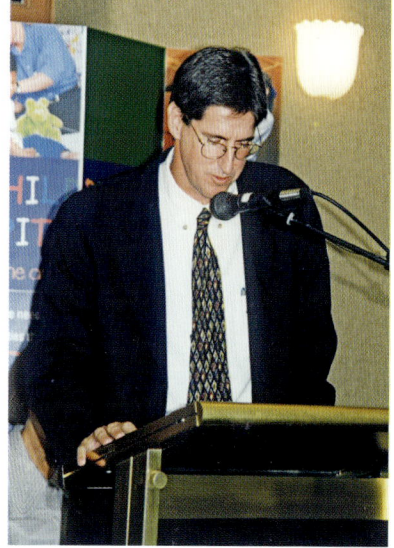

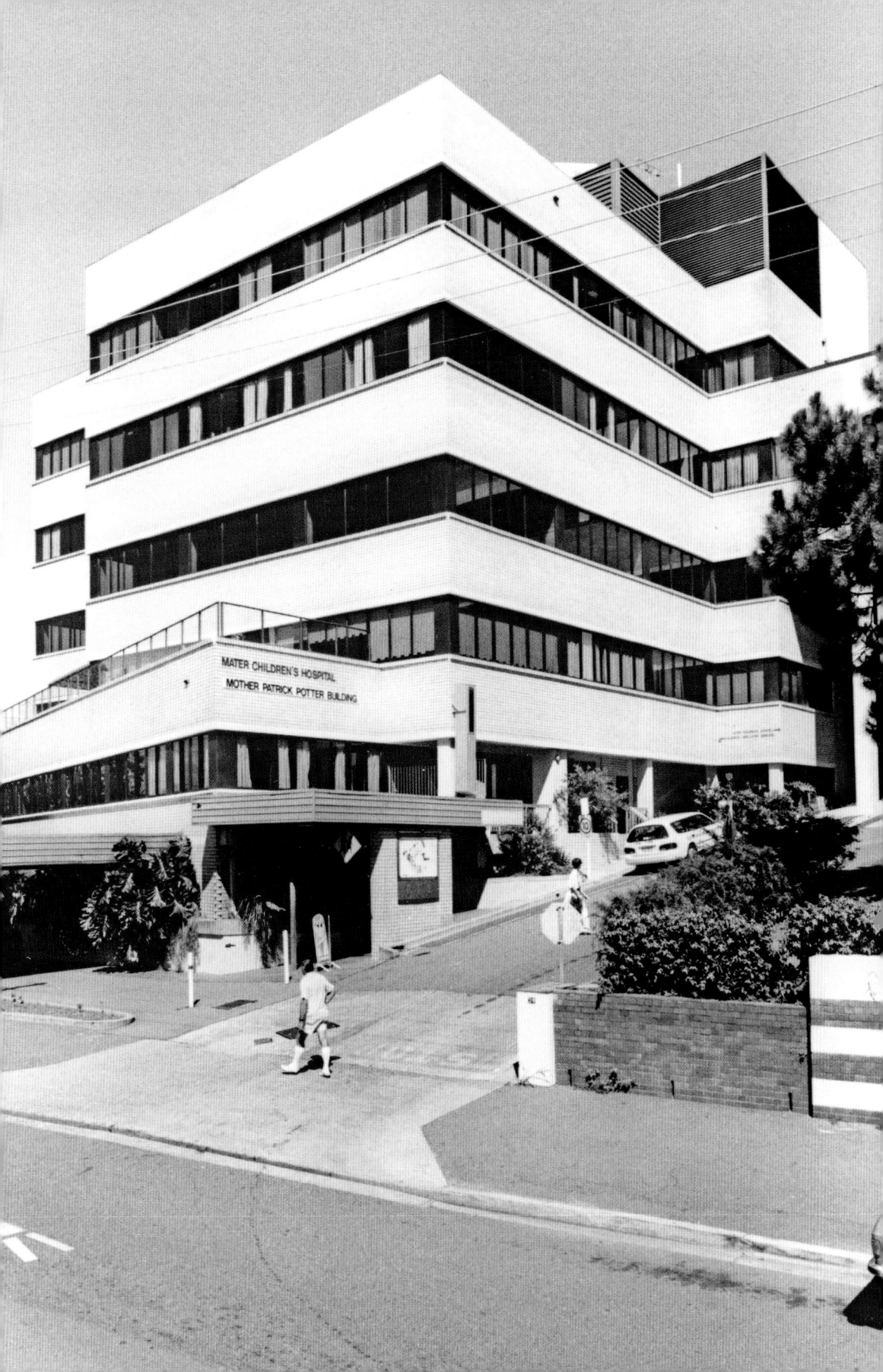

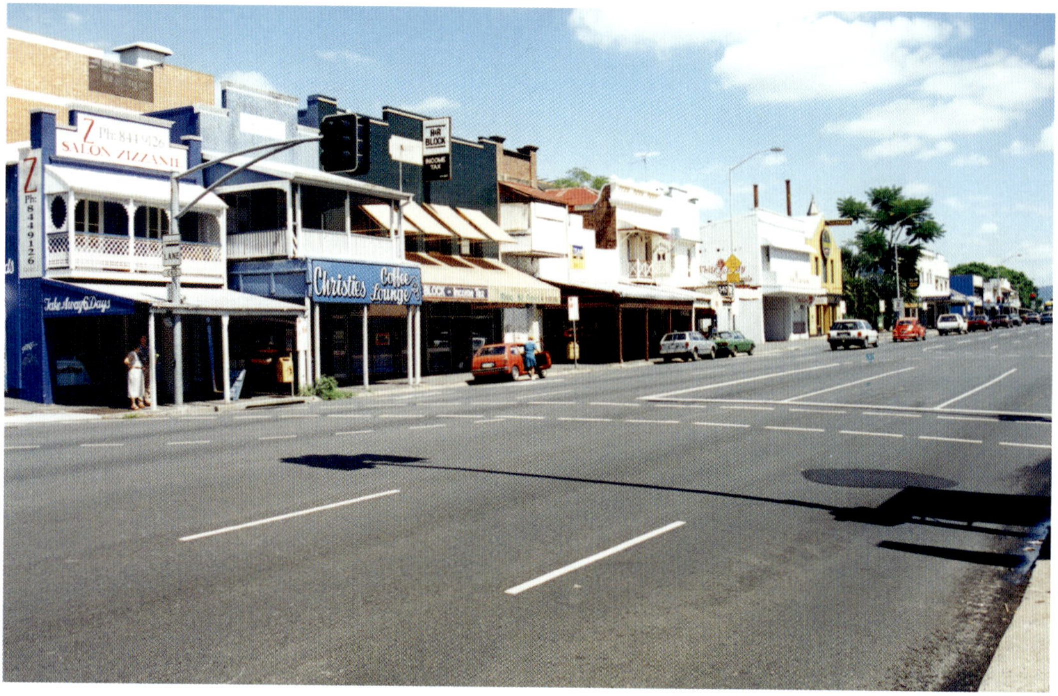

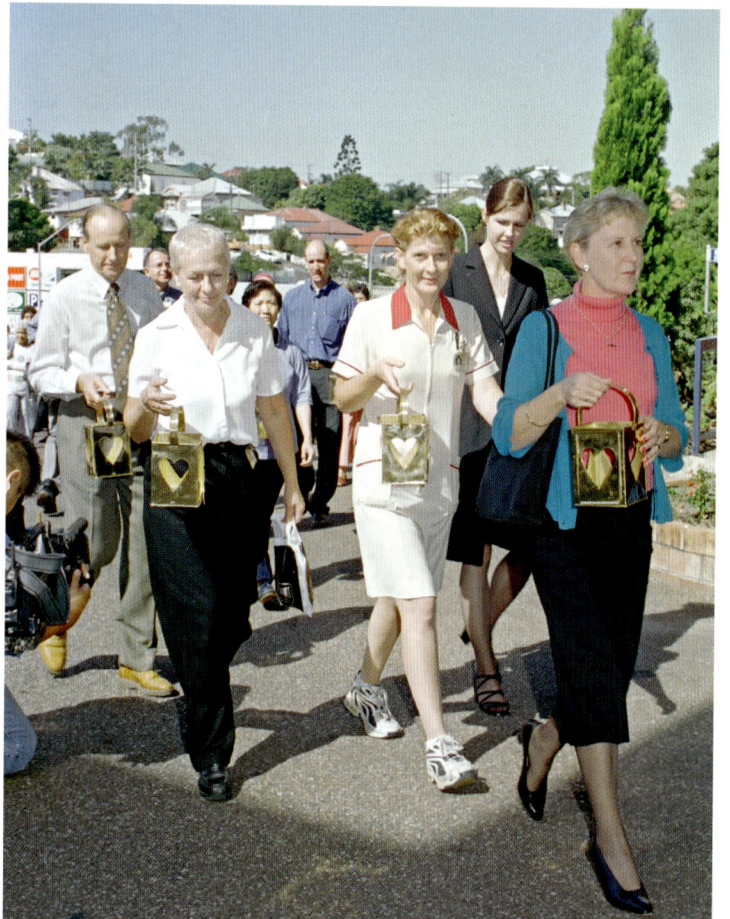

The shops in Stanley Street that made way for the new hospital.

LEFT: The lantern procession from the original Mater Children's Hospital to the splendid 2001 Mater Children's Hospital.

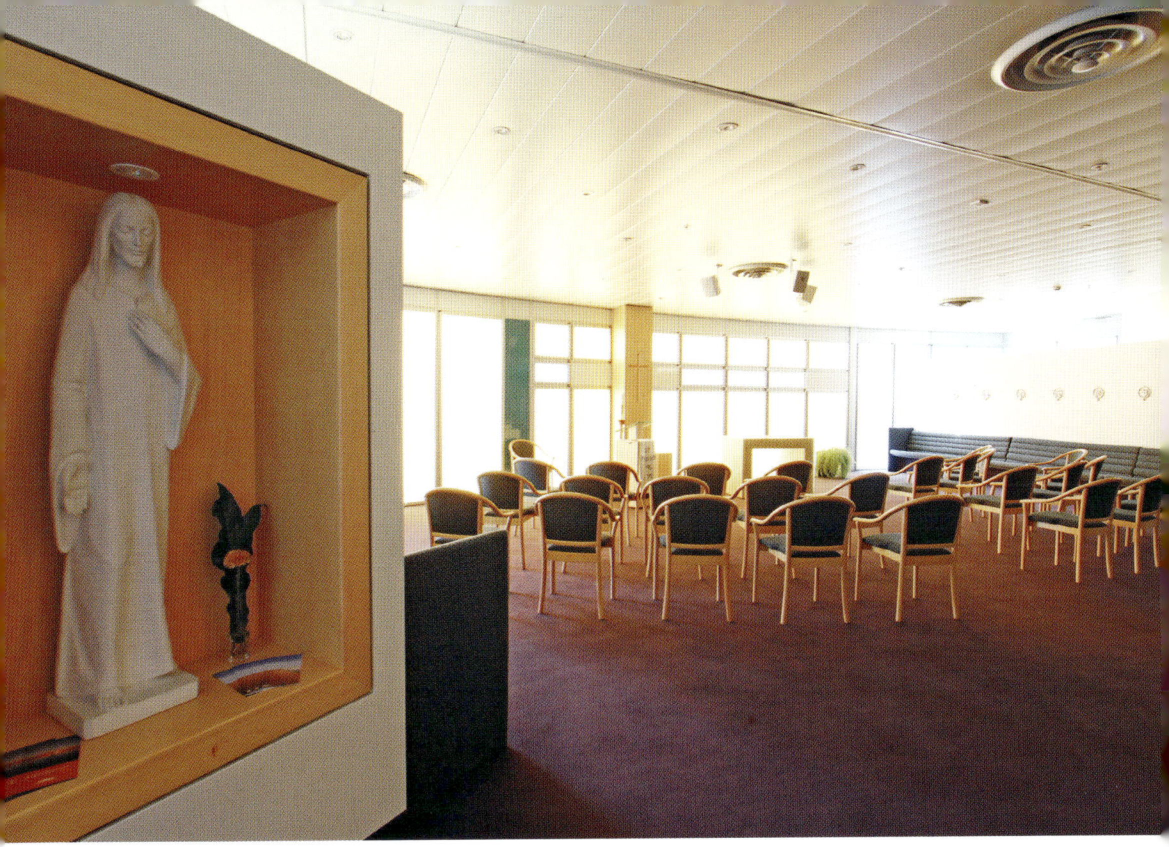

The light, airy chapel in the 2001 Mater Children's Hospital.

LEFT: A beautiful pet-therapy dog ready for work.

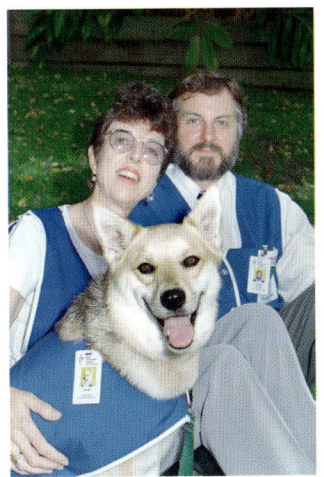

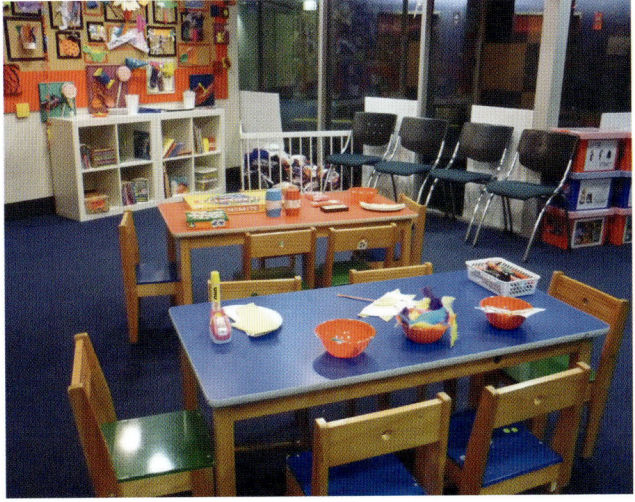

A cheerful play area in the 2001 Mater Children's Hospital.

FOLLOWING PAGES: Banks of tiles on the walls of level 8.

8

Children's Hospital Lift
Level 8

Children's Private → Hospital
Beds C801 - C831

Beds C832 - C864
8 South

← Parent's Lounge

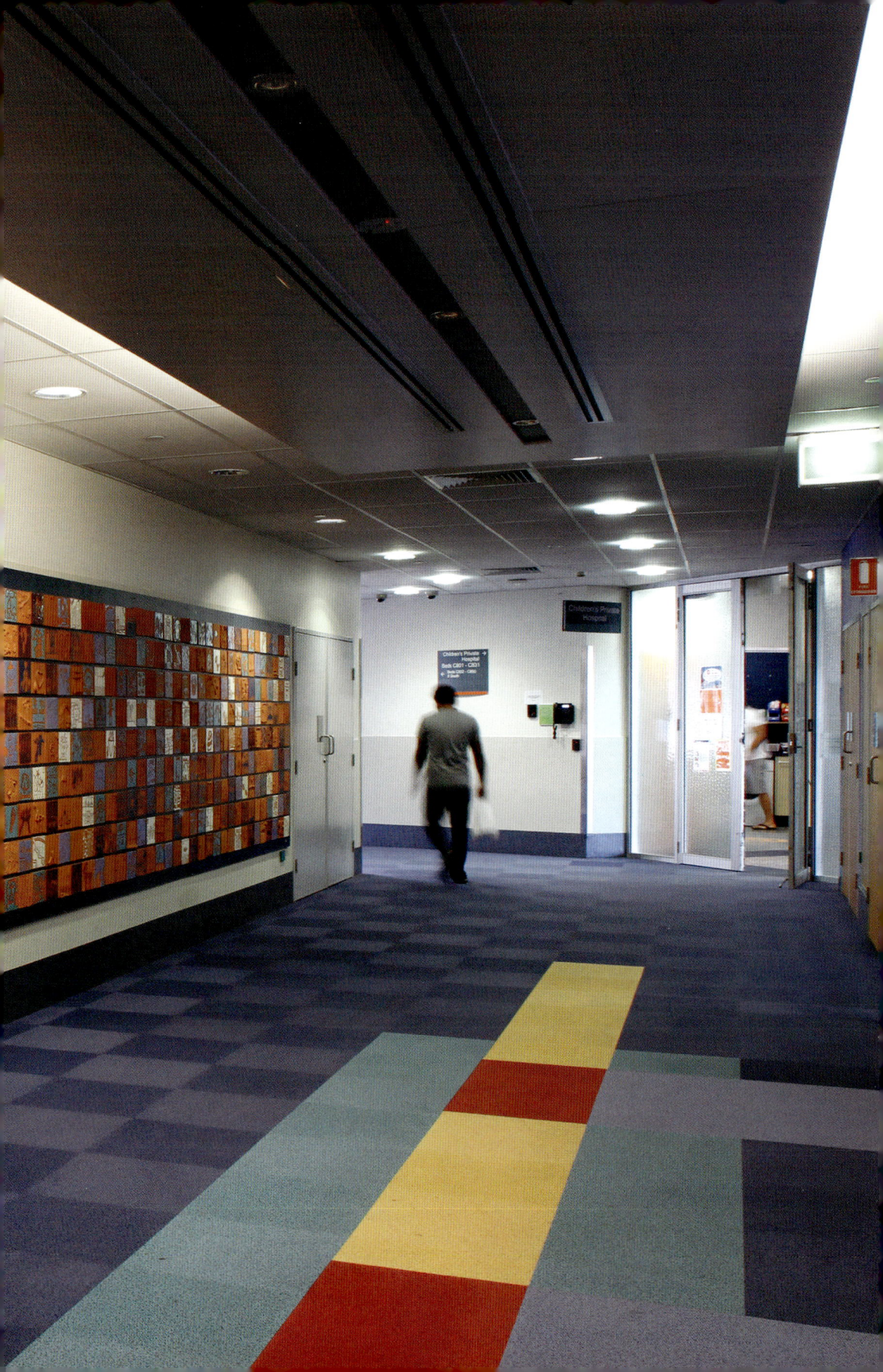

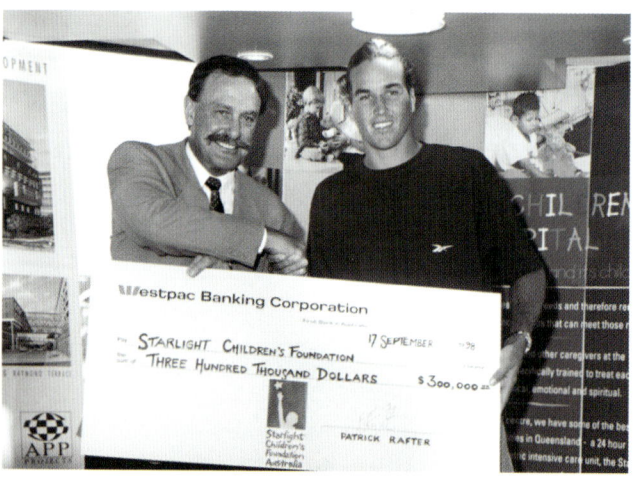

Benefactor of the Starlight Express Room Pat Rafter (right) with fellow tennis star and Starlight Room enthusiast John Newcombe (left).

RIGHT: The reception area at the Mater Children's Private Hospital in 2012.

OPPOSITE PAGE, BOTTOM: The magical Circus of Dreams play area, which brought great joy to patients at the 2001 Mater Children's Hospital.

BELOW: Crowds of people walking their '5Ks for Kids'.

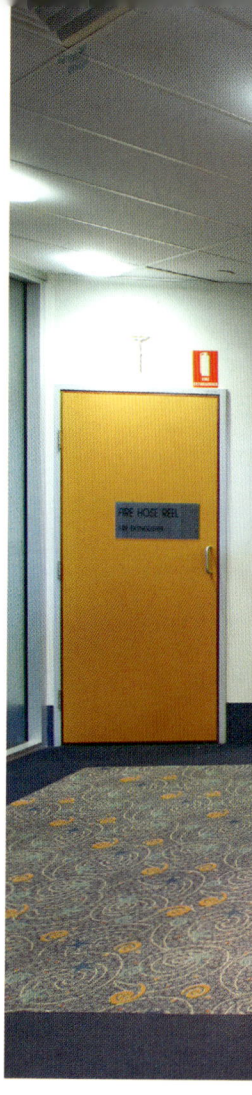

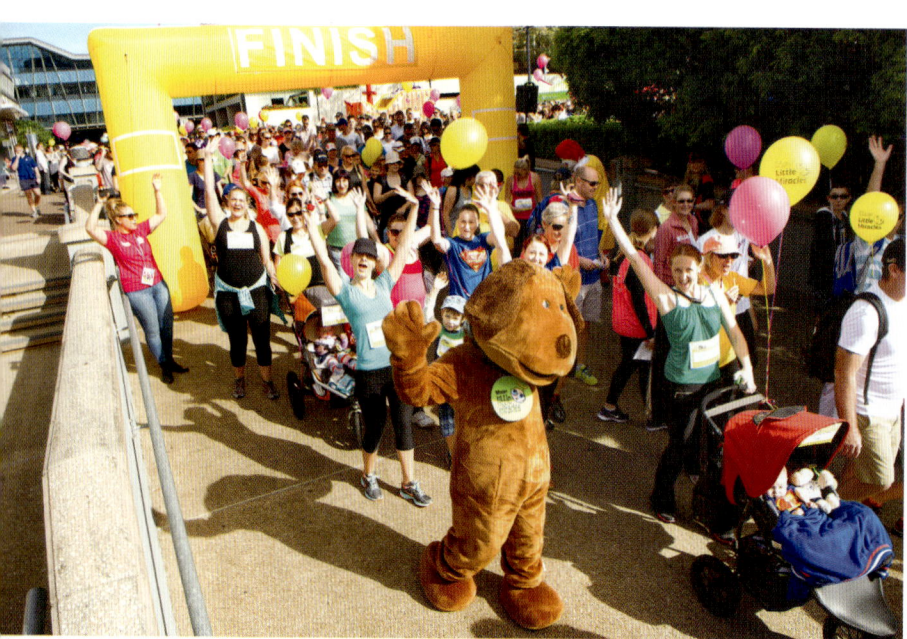

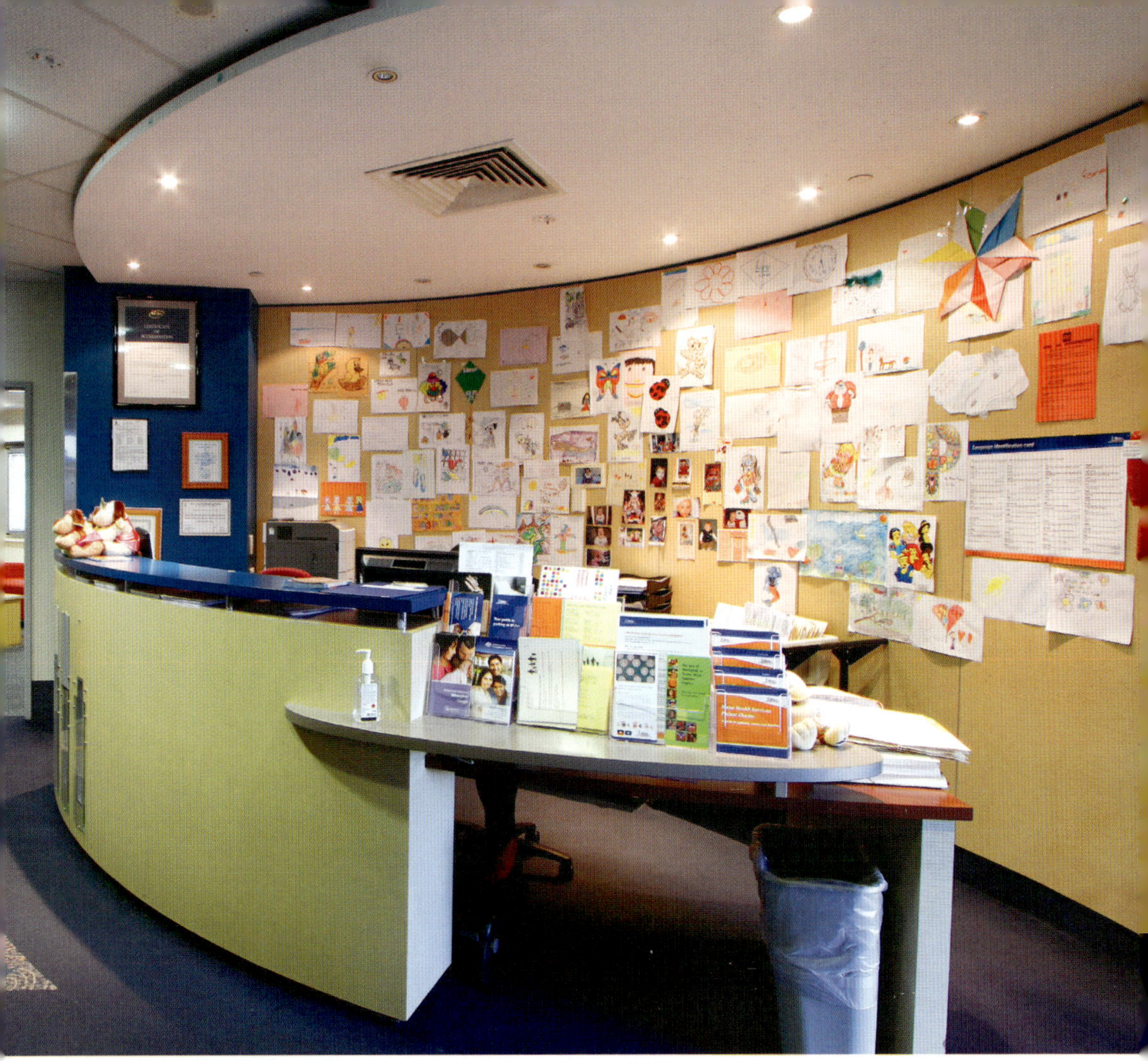

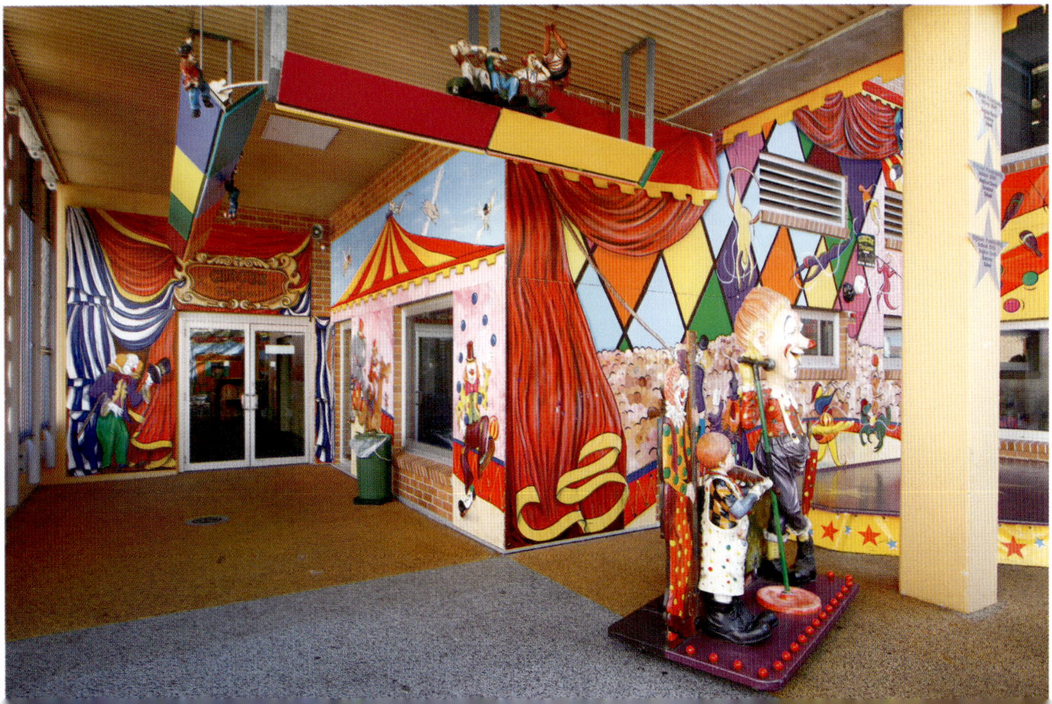

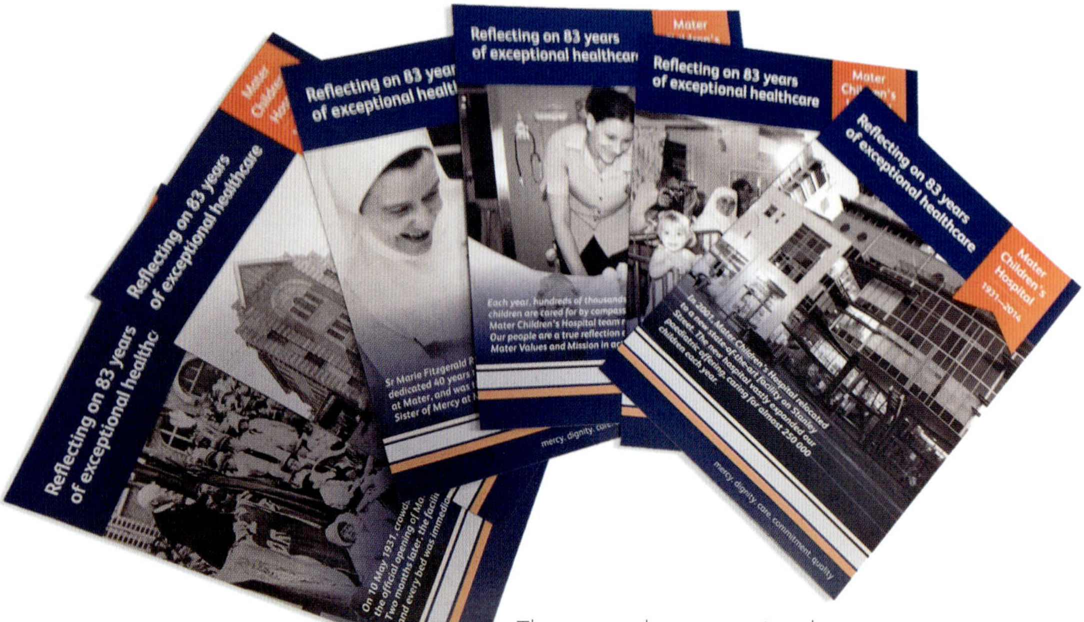

The postcards encouraging the recording of memories and thoughts about the Mater Children's Hospital.

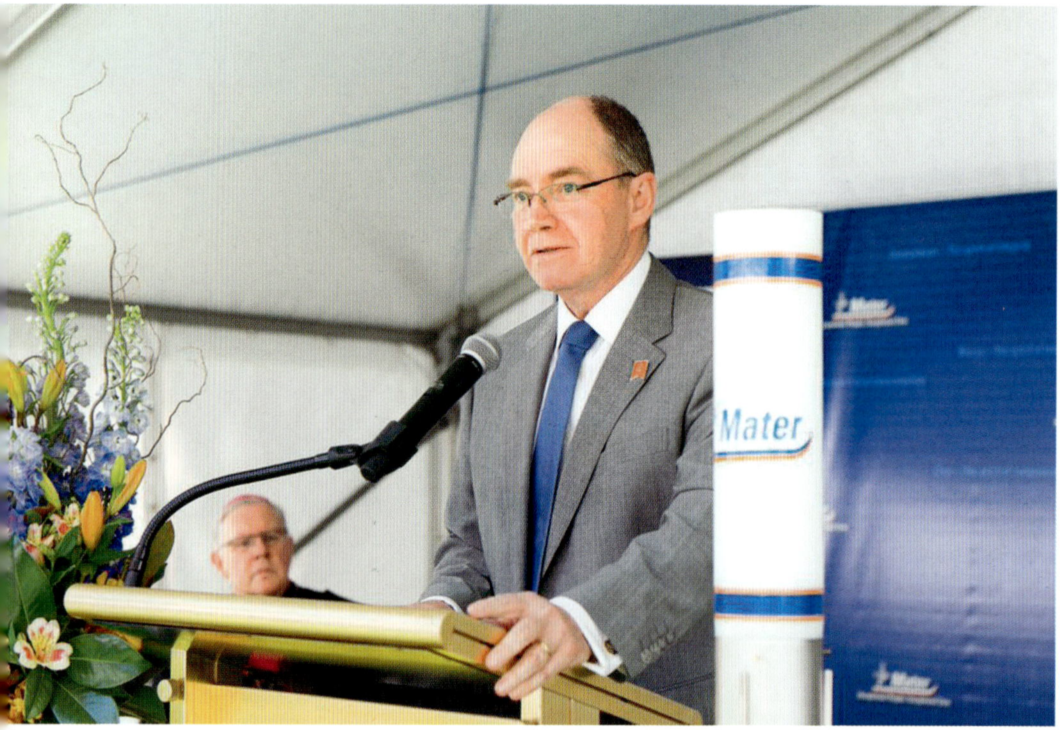

Dr John O'Donnell, chief executive officer, Mater Health Services, speaking at the special farewell ceremony for the Mater Children's Hospital on 1 November 2014.

There would also be greater community outreach and a stronger focus on working with other health-care providers. Projects in partnership with the University of Queensland Department of General Practice were directed towards creating the 'boundaryless hospital'. Continuity of care between the hospital and community clinics would be a very high priority. Child and adolescent mental health and development assessment teams were functioning as models of integrated service delivery across the region.

Ideas for the new hospital were drawn from the United States, Canada and England. On their visit to Hasbro Children's Hospital in Providence, Rhode Island, the Mater chief executive officer, Mark Avery, and the executive director of the Mater Children's Hospital, Peter Steer, had been impressed by its cooperative care centre and by the co-location of the children's and women's hospitals.[43] The resource centre at the much older Hospital for Sick Children in Toronto, founded in 1875, attracted the attention of Margaret Murphy, assistant director of nursing, clinical, at the Mater Children's Hospital, when she visited. The Great Ormond Street Hospital in London had been developed and redeveloped since its foundation in 1852 and its new Variety Club building, opened in 1994, was also a pertinent example of modern clinical buildings in children's hospitals. There was plenty to tell the architects, Bligh Voller Nield, appointed in 1997.[44]

Extensive experience of patients, families, nurses and doctors, not to mention the intricacies of dealing with the hospital administration, was invaluable in bringing a new hospital to reality. Rosalie Lewis, director of nursing at the Mater Children's Hospital since 1986 and acting executive director of nursing for the Mater group since Rex Ducat's retirement in 1996, was appointed as project coordinator for the redevelopment.[45] This was a demanding brief: coordinating information between project managers, architects, builders and Mater Children's Hospital staff from the earliest stage of design to completion and opening the new hospital. Wide consultation with parents and the local community became an integral part of planning, which was sufficiently detailed to consider the housekeeper's concern that the wider beds would mean new sheets – a considerable expense.[46]

There were several mandatory inclusions in addition to a vast range of clinical facilities. Radio Lollipop needed a studio as close as possible to the wards so that patients and their families could visit as often as possible.[47] There was also to be Queensland's first Starlight Express Room, supported generously by the Australian tennis star Pat Rafter. Fun and mayhem, the latest computer games, movies, crafts and activities have enlivened children's hospitals since the Starlight Children's Foundation was established in 1988. Children too ill to leave the wards could join in the fun through daily Captain Starlight shows broadcast to television sets at every bed.

Construction began in August 1999. A large, colourful building replaced the old shops and Raymond Court. The transformation of Stanley Street, which had begun with the new Mater Private Clinic and the Mater Hill stop on the southern busway, was accelerating.

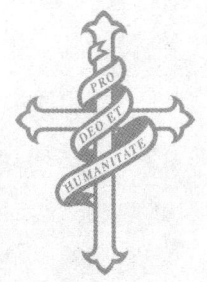

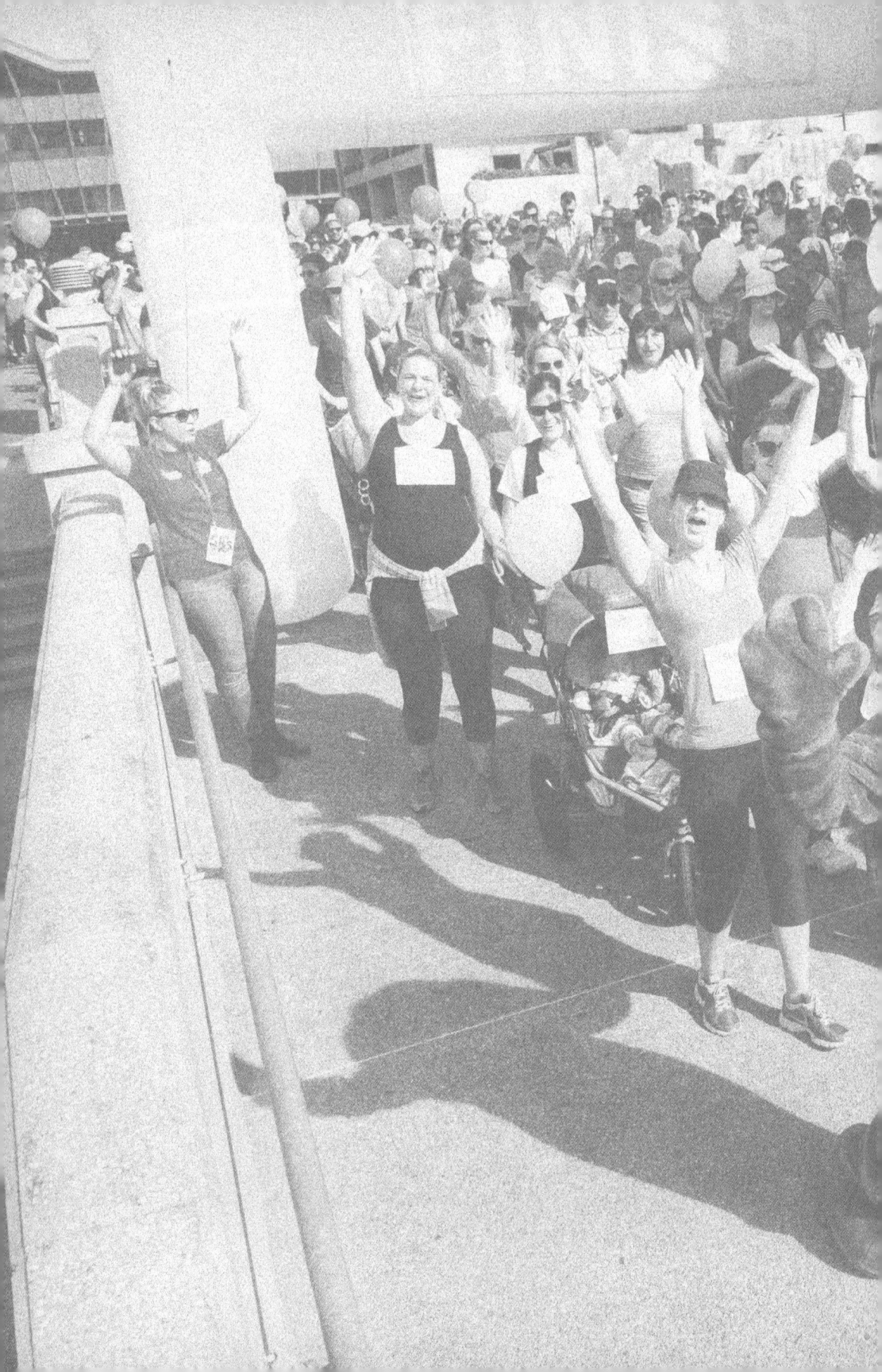

Part Four
The 2000s

Chapter 14

The Sparkling New Hospital in Stanley Street

Care and love, as symbolised by the lights and lanterns, were carried to the new hospital.

Margaret Murphy RN, 2001

Almost 70 years to the day that the original hospital received its first patients, ceremony and celebration on 16 May 2001 marked the opening of the long-awaited new hospital. But the original hospital was not forgotten – children made golden lanterns carried in a procession linking old and new. The rich symbolism of the lantern procession expressed the care and love carried to the new hospital and recalled the founder of the Sisters of Mercy, Catherine McAuley, who believed that the Christian symbol of light belonged to everybody.[1]

Celebrations and parties had always been part of life at the Mater Children's Hospital. The staff and children had made 6 July 2000 – the hospital's last birthday in the old buildings – a special celebration. All children, whether bed-bound or not, were included, as they had been in all Mater Children's Hospital's parties, a tradition continued at the party celebrating the new building. Some of the hospital's favourite people were also part of the celebratory opening of the new hospital, among them Sister Mary Colette Anderson RSM, who had been part of the hospital for 30 years, and Sister Marie Fitzgerald RSM, the gentle 'Sister Butterfly', who had moved swiftly, but lightly, through the wards and operating theatres for 40 years. The continuity from past to present was also recalled in the history section of a booklet specially prepared for the opening.[2]

The patients had to wait for almost a fortnight before they could move to the new wards and clinics. Moving day, 29 May 2001, was carefully organised to be both safe and enjoyable, with Captain Starlight and Miss Lollipop on duty to greet the patients. A large newspaper feature told the stories of some of the patients who made the transition, among them many children undergoing treatment for very serious and complex conditions.[3]

The model of care for the new Mater Children's Hospital, developed by Rosalie Lewis and the staff, was an obvious expression of continuity between the old and the new. The philosophy of the Sisters of Mercy – as expressed by the Mater's core values: mercy, dignity, care, commitment and quality – underpinned the model of care. Expert clinical care, health promotion, emotional development and spiritual support were all part of the Mater Children's Hospital's mission.

The model of care also had to respond to the Queensland government's metropolitan health-care plan. The Mater was required to provide tertiary-level support to regional hospitals and community services, as well as to children in its immediate neighbourhood. Skilled staff and active research programs were necessary to support the Mater Children's Hospital as a tertiary teaching hospital providing level 5–6 general paediatric medical and surgical services. Level 6 services for the entire state of Queensland included respiratory medicine, endocrinology, radiology, haematology–oncology, orthopaedics, plastic and craniomaxillary surgery, urology, developmental paediatrics and child and adolescent mental health services.

The Model of Care Document was no overnight creation. It was years in the making. Wide consultation with patients and families, the local community and hospital staff was essential from the earliest stages.[4] A family-centred approach was expressed in the belief that parents and carers were equal partners with clinicians in the care of their children. Parents could stay with children while anaesthetics were administered, and were supported during hours at bedsides by facilities such as parent lounges with tea- and coffee-making facilities; some of the lounges had beds and televisions, and all lounges were adjacent to bathrooms. Parents could also sleep on special beds beside their children. Nourishing meals at reasonable prices were available and an area on level 1 was designed to provide a pleasant break from the wards.

Any suggestion of dark, gloomy spaces, all too familiar in the original building, was eliminated in the new hospital. It was light, airy and colourful, designed to appeal to patients ranging from infancy to late adolescence. An old theme in health care, the benefits of contact with nature and the outside world, was re-emphasised in the 1990s in the design of children's hospitals.[5] At the Mater Children's Hospital, large windows in different shapes and colours had low windowsills, so that children could see the view from their beds. External sunshades allowed blinds to be open during the day. Curtains were avoided as much as possible, but privacy was maintained through internal venetian blinds and special finishes on the window glass.

Shaded balconies, designed as outdoor play spaces, were equipped with power points, oxygen and suction outlets to allow bed-bound children access to the open air. A playground and coffee shop, highly visible from Stanley Street, was to be an active and friendly entry to the hospital and also a diversionary area where families could retreat, and yet remain in contact with the hospital. Special attention to floor surfaces, wall and roof fittings and outdoor furniture design helped to ensure a safe outdoor environment.

Art has also become increasingly important in humanising hospitals. Major artworks at the Mater Children's Hospital included a large mosaic set into the floor of the entry foyer, emphasising the healing power of light and water through a pebble river, a globe of the world and the sun, along with Queensland themes represented through an Indigenous story and images of the Queensland outback, rainforests, sea and city. The mission and philosophy of the Sisters of Mercy and their Mater hospitals were represented in a collage.[6]

Inside the hospital, banks of decorated tiles were arranged on walls on each floor. All 5,500 tiles were designed and decorated by thousands of children to represent life in Queensland through their imaginations.[7] One designer, a little girl from Moranbah, had been a pupil in the Flying Arts program, itself an illustration of the vastness of Queensland and the sparsely spread population that the hospital's tertiary services had to reach; another was the daughter of a Mater staff member with more than 30 years' service.[8] Nothing in the design or decoration of any part of the hospital highlighted any specific age group: there were no Disney pictures or rock band posters. The colour scheme incorporated bright areas with more neutral areas.

No matter how beautifully decorated, a hospital must be focused on patient care. Day-patient areas were adjacent to the operating theatres with their own admission, discharge and parent facilities.[9] Many bed areas had ensuite bathrooms. Separate dining rooms were incorporated in the in-patient areas so that children could have their meals away from their beds. Children with disabilities, whether admitted as in-patients, day patients or out-patients, were considered. Bench heights were sufficiently low to be accessible by children in wheelchairs and they could use every bathroom. There was a special telephone for children and parents with severe hearing impairments; signage in braille helped blind children and their visitors.

Entertainment had been part of life at the Mater Children's Hospital since the 1930s, when personalities from radio and the stage regularly visited the hospital. Radio Lollipop – the hospital's own radio station – had been important in the old hospital and continued in the new with radio, television and a telephone at each bed. The Starlight Express Room was an exciting new feature, important in giving children and their families a break from the wards. The Pets As Therapy Scheme (PATS) continued to delight the children. PATS began in 1998 when the German shepherd Honey began to visit patients. Dr Wendy Moody, the PATS consultant, held the only Australian doctorate in animal–human behaviour.[10]

The Mater hospitals, located in South Brisbane since 1910, had always responded to the special needs of Brisbane's most ethnically and culturally diverse area. Brisbane – and Queensland generally – had become much more culturally diverse in the late twentieth century. It was, therefore, essential that the Mater Children's Hospital respected the many and varied religious and cultural needs of its community. It was a Roman Catholic hospital, but the chapel was designed to be ecumenical, and signs were printed so that people whose first language was not English could easily understand them.

The building's relationship to other Mater buildings and their facilities was one of the most important features of the new hospital. Links to the Mater Adult Hospital, the Mater Mothers' Hospital and the Radiation Oncology Mater Centre created essential efficiencies in sharing expensive services. The new helipad on the roof of the Mater Children's Hospital led to covered access to the Mater Mothers' and Adult hospitals through the links between the hospitals. The slogan 'a family of hospitals for all of the family' was increasingly expressed in the physical organisation of the campus, as well as in the philosophy of care.[11]

The staff had struggled with many of the crowded and inconvenient features of the old buildings. Better lighting, air-conditioning, more conference rooms and less congested staff rooms all helped, particularly as comforts such as tea- and coffee-making facilities were close to the various wards and departments.

Safety and security were important features. Family breakdown had become more common; it was important to ensure that only the parents with legal access to the children could reach them. Security systems were unobtrusive but sophisticated: closed-circuit television, mobile and static duress alarms, and key-pad access to certain areas. The basic design enhanced security. Public spaces were at the front of the building, ambulatory services were on the lower levels, with in-patient areas above.

Each level of the eight-storey building reflected the principles underpinning the model of care. Level 1, the main entry from Stanley Street, included a large plaza, as well as space for the school. Level 2 included a second entrance – this one from Raymond Terrace – and the entry to the walkway that linked the children's hospital to the adult hospital. The main reception area for the children's hospital and the pharmacy shared by the children's and adult hospitals were included on level 2 with a suite of offices.

On level 3, the chapel, with beautiful glass walls, was linked to the remainder of the floor by bridges that gave a view of the mosaic in the floor of level 1. An important innovation, the Australian Centre for Paediatric Pharmacokinetics, was designed for this level. The pharmacokinetics project, a partnership between the Mater Children's Hospital and the University of Queensland, studied the action of various drugs in children ranging from premature babies to older children.[12]

Several key clinics were also located on level 3, with others on level 4. These included the child protection unit, the nutrition and dietetics clinic, and the clinic specialising in the rehabilitation of brain-injured children and those with neuromuscular disorders (ROBIN). These services all required teamwork, particularly from the physiotherapy, occupational therapy, social work and psychology departments – all conveniently located on level 3.

Critical care units on level 4 included the emergency department, the cardiology department, medical imaging – as radiology had become known – and the respiratory and sleep studies units. Several specialist services, including the epilepsy clinic and the ear, nose and throat and eye clinics, were also on level 4. A plan suggested several times in earlier days – sharing ear, nose and throat services with the adult hospital – was implemented on level 4. Unlike practitioners in many other specialties, most ear, nose and throat specialists continued to treat children and adults. In many ways, level 4 was the centre of the hospital. It was certainly the centre for entertainment. The Starlight Express Room, Radio Lollipop and the Red Cross Play Scheme area were located directly above the chapel.

Level 5 accommodated the six operating theatres, the intensive care unit and the recovery unit. Pre-admission tours and orientation programs for children preparing for surgery, familiar in the old hospital, continued in the new. Both the public and private day-surgery units were located close to the operating theatres. Operating-theatre change rooms on level 6 serviced the adult and children's hospitals.[13]

The main medical and surgical wards, or 'care units' as they became known, were located on level 7, with day units for patients with diabetes and other endocrine disorders. The in-patient and out-patient services managed by the Child and Youth Mental Health Service (CYMHS) were located on this level. The babies' ward, the haematology and oncology unit and the larger Mater Children's Private Hospital occupied level 8.

As executive director of both Mater Children's hospitals, Fiona Brewin-Brown supervised the restructure of the nursing staff needed to manage this complex new hospital. In July 2001, Judy Perrin was appointed director of specialty services at the Mater Children's Hospital. Her responsibilities included endocrinology, cardiology, respiratory medicine, developmental medicine, rehabilitation, epilepsy, gastroenterology, haematology, oncology and child protection.[14] Dr Peter Steer, who had been executive director of the Mater Children's Hospital since 1995, left to work in Canada in 2001. Dr Peter Leslie acted as executive director of the Mater Mothers' and Mater Children's hospitals with Dr David Wood as director of paediatrics.[15]

There were other developments at the Mater in 2001. Mater Health Services became an incorporated company on 1 July 2001 and the brand new Mater Private Hospital Redland, co-located with Redland Hospital, joined the Mater family.[16] There was also a new chief executive officer. Mark Avery, who had held the post since 1993, left the Mater in 2001, and was succeeded by John O'Donnell.

When John O'Donnell arrived, the Mater was facing a serious financial situation: annual losses amounting to millions of dollars. Flatter administrative structures – fewer people between the chief executive officer and the

> JOHN O'DONNELL, MBBS, MHP (UNSW), FRACMA, FACHSM, FAIM, FAICD, graduated in medicine at the University of Adelaide. As well as several years in medical practice, John O'Donnell had a master's degree in health planning from the University of New South Wales and many years' experience in hospital management at the Royal Adelaide Hospital, the Royal Canberra and Woden Valley hospitals, the Port Macquarie Base Hospital, St George Private Hospital, Prince of Wales Private Hospital, and as national director of clinical services and quality at Mayne Health Care, which owned 62 private hospitals around Australia.[17]

patients – was one of the measures employed to address the situation.[18] The Mater Mothers' and Mater Children's hospitals had already been combined administratively under one executive director; the combination of these two with the adult hospital came next. The change from the original Mater Children's Hospital to the new building, swiftly followed by new management structures, was challenging for the staff. Doctors and nurses had not liked sharing directors with the Mater Mothers' Hospital; the idea that there would be one director for all three hospitals was even worse.[19]

Further complicating the situation, neither the nurses nor the medical staff were particularly impressed by the saving in costs that the integration of nursing administrations at the Mater Mothers' and Mater Children's hospitals had accrued.[20] Although the board and the chief executive officer were determined that the Mater hospitals would be identified as one organisation, there were administrative difficulties: the public hospitals were in one executive director's portfolio and the private hospitals in another.[21]

A survey of employees by Best Practice Australia, just before John O'Donnell's arrival, told a worrying tale: ratings for organisational culture, job satisfaction, leadership and performance were poor, a situation compounded by lack of communication between management and staff, adding to a perception of significant mistrust between management and employees. Doctors admitting patients to the Mater Adult and Children's Private hospitals in 2002 brought important issues to the board's attention: a call for better communication with visiting doctors and the need to establish clear directions and standards of care.[22]

The families of Mater Children's Hospital patients who responded to a statewide survey reported that they were generally unaware they could make a complaint – or how to do it – and thought that the staff did not encourage feedback. They also wanted more information on the hospital before a child was admitted and on managing a child's recovery at home after discharge. There were, however, bright spots. Parents liked the staff's caring attitude and the hospital's facilities and cleanliness.[23] Despite these ups-and-downs, the Mater Children's Hospital's intensive care unit was accredited by the Australian College of Emergency Medicine in 2001 and the hospital was surveyed by an American health-care measurement and improvement company and rated the No. 1 paediatric hospital for patient satisfaction in Australia and New Zealand.[24]

These were very busy times, complicated by a national shortage of nurses. Nurses from private agencies filled some gaps, particularly in the intensive care unit, but this was an expensive solution.[25] The paediatric intensive care unit introduced a new computerised clinical information system, the first of its kind in the world. The new system monitored the patient's condition in real time and ensured that drugs were administered correctly and, in the process, eliminated a great deal of paperwork that could consume hours of nursing time. The nurses were freed for their real jobs: patient care.

Life in the emergency department was also very hectic; it was rapidly cementing its place as the busiest paediatric emergency centre in Queensland.[26] The Mater Children's Private Hospital was also in great demand: unexpectedly high activity in its new quarters also strained the available staff; looking after acutely ill children in private rooms was labour-intensive. It seemed inevitable that private beds would have to be capped at 22 until additional staff could be found.[27] There was, however, time for the more joyous side of life. A Mad Hatter's Morning Tea, when 1,270 cupcakes were served, celebrated the first birthday of the new hospital on 16 May 2002.[28]

Some patients continued to travel great distances for treatment. Operation Smile brought children from Vietnam and the Philippines for surgery. Mater staff also travelled: to Vietnam to set up a craniofacial unit for South-East Asia and to Russia to continue Project Nadezhda. In 2002, the relationship with Russia was in its sixth year, with plans to continue the visits.[29]

Outreach included destinations closer to home. Children with diabetes continued to use their insulin pumps at home; the cochlear-implant outreach program, established in 2001, extended its reach further into rural and remote Queensland in partnership with the Royal Children's Hospital. Through connections with the Mater hospitals in Townsville and Rockhampton, specialist services were made available to children in those centres.[30] In Brisbane, the MOSHPIT – Mobile Outreach Support and Health Program by Integrated Teams – reached young Indigenous people in their own communities.[31] Children, as well as adults, were included in the refugee health service introduced in 2003.[32] The continuity of patient care between hospitals, general practitioners and community organisations was made easier when the original Mater Children's Hospital was refurbished to become the Mater Community Services Building.[33]

In 2003, a major health concern of the age – childhood obesity – expanded the range of outreach services. A new program examined eating patterns and exercise regimes in children's homes and schools and linked general practitioners, paediatricians, psychologists and allied health workers on Brisbane's south side. The National Health and Medical Research Council also focused on the obesity issue and Michael O'Callaghan from the Mater chaired a group that wrote a handbook for use in these types of programs.[34] Accidents continued to be a major concern. The Queensland Injury Surveillance Unit (QISU), as the Queensland Injury Surveillance and Prevention Program (QISPP) had become known, continued its nationally significant work, but without the level of funding that supported equivalent programs in the southern states.[35] QISU had at least one significant reward: swimming pool drownings had decreased by two-thirds since the late 1980s.[36]

Young people's mental health was also an increasingly prominent concern in the early twenty-first century. The Mater's Child and Youth Mental Health Service could accommodate 12 patients, and there were also clinics for day patients at the Mater and at four centres in the wider community. In 2003, technology expanded the program's reach with the launch of Kids in Mind on the internet. The website focused on removing the stigma of mental illness, especially important as one in every 10 to 15 young people was affected. Explaining what happens in mental health services, it was hoped, would encourage more young people to use them. The website was rewarded with 45,364 hits in one month, and there were plans to investigate the feasibility of online counselling.[37] The Adolescent Drug and Alcohol Withdrawal Service, ADAWS, went from strength to strength. The Health Minister,

Wendy Edmond, launched the Queensland-wide ADAWS, with provision for training state Health Department staff, on 16 September 2003. The original five-bed unit at South Brisbane could not cope with the demand and, in 2006, the Mater built a new house for ADAWS.[38]

ADAWS was one illustration of innovation – John O'Donnell's theme for 2003. Extraordinary surgery was another. Dr Geoff Askin pioneered endoscopic surgery to correct the common, but serious, spinal condition of scoliosis. The spinal research group was also working on new ways of working with magnetic resonance imaging to assess the degree of spinal curvature more accurately than had previously been possible.[39] Some children followed their parents into the operating theatres. A patient who had corrective surgery in the craniofacial unit in 1976 for Crouzon syndrome – a condition affecting the development of bones in the skull and face – spent many hours at the Mater in the early twenty-first century while her two children underwent numerous procedures for the same condition. Other children needed delicate surgery for unusual conditions. In 2005, surgeons removed a large mass between a little girl's eyes. This dermoid cyst became known as Xanthie's 'diamond cyst'.[40]

The Mater Hospital Special School was very important to children with serious illnesses who spent long periods in hospital, or who had frequent hospitalisations for chronic illnesses. The design of the new Mater Children's Hospital allocated space to relocate the school from Clarence Street, but two years of negotiation with the Department of Education was necessary. Eventually, the Department of Education decided that the school should continue, but with concentration on children who needed complex care and long stays in hospital.[41] In return for rent-free premises in the new hospital, the Department of Education gave the former school to the Mater to become a childcare centre. The bright and cheerful school, with its own entrance from Stanley Street, opened on 5 May 2003.

The school went from strength to strength in its new location. In 2004, it was one of ten schools selected as a case study for the National Safe School framework; in 2005 and 2007, it won the regional Showcase Education regional award for inclusive education. In 2006, it was selected as a national 'Kids Matter' pilot school. The Mater Special School became a national reference centre for best practice in hospital schooling, particularly recognised for including students at secondary-school level.[42]

Country families whose children were in hospital, or were receiving treatment as out-patients, continued to stay at Ronald McDonald House. The original house in Allen Street was too small; its nine units struggled to keep up with demand. Reg Leonard House, which accommodated families of very ill patients in the other Mater hospitals, was also busy and not able to relieve Ronald McDonald House. In any case, Reg Leonard House was not easy for children with disabilities to access. Ronald McDonald House in Allen Street was extended from 12 to 22 self-contained units on land donated by the Mater. Ronald McDonald House Charities provided $2,200,000 for the refurbishment.[43]

As well as the normal regime of clinical care, the two busy Mater Children's Hospitals supported research projects, including a project to investigate children's reactions to hospitalisation for tonsillectomy and adenotonsillectomy, surveying 85 patients aged between four and 18. On a broader scale, Prabha Ramritu, clinical nurse consultant, research, was deeply involved in the development of the international paediatric nursing research network. With Mary Mackinnon, clinical nurse consultant, rehabilitation and complex care services, Prabha Ramritu completed a study into services for children with multiple disabilities and their families.[44]

The Mater Children's Private Hospital was in such demand only a year after the new hospital opened that thoughts turned to using the small ward on level 8 East as a private hospital ward, which could also be used by oncology patients from the public hospital when necessary.[45] By the middle years of the new Mater Children's Hospital's first decade, demand seemed to be outgrowing the facilities. There were calls for additional psychology services, more funding for physiotherapy, speech pathology and occupational therapy and the parent aide program, and relief for overcrowding in the specialist out-patient clinics.[46] There was even discussion on acquiring more space for the children's hospital in the building vacated when the Mater Mothers' Hospital moved into its new building in 2008.[47] Funding for a statewide epilepsy service, managed by the Royal Children's and Mater Children's hospitals, was secured and there was hope that, at last, the Mater Children's Hospital would have its own nuclear medicine department. Imaging was updated when the Mater attracted 'Smart State' funding for magnetic resonance imaging.[48]

Many adolescent patients, like their younger counterparts, were treated at home whenever possible. The Mater Children's Hospital had steadily developed its home-care programs for many years, as had children's hospitals everywhere.[49] By 2007, home treatment for a wide range of conditions had become so common in Australia that the Hospital In The Home (HITH) Society amalgamated a number of earlier home-treatment associations to provide education, promote networking and lobby governments for improved funding. The HITH Society represented all ages, but there was a special paediatric interest group.[50]

In December 2009, the Mater Children's Hospital's home-care programs, which had developed over many years, were consolidated in two services: Hospital In The Home and the Post-Acute Care Program. These programs enabled many young patients to reduce their hospital stays and receive continuing care in their home environment, but it was a delicate balance to ensure that children were not discharged too soon.[51] There could be no denying the efficiency advantages of Hospital In The Home and the Post-Acute Care Program: these two programs saved a total of 1,000 bed days in 2009.[52] But such programs were not suitable for all patients. Patients with cystic fibrosis were treated at home as often as possible, but still required frequent admissions to hospital.[53]

Improved treatment had extended the life span of children with life-threatening, chronic conditions to the extent that many continued to be treated in their teenage and young adult years. Nor were adolescents spared the more routine acute illnesses and accidents that required hospital care. Appropriate care for adolescents had preoccupied clinicians and hospital administrators all over the world for many years. A study in England showed that, contrary to most assumptions, hospital bed use increased in adolescence.[54]

Dr Russell Viner, a consultant in adolescent medicine at University College London, researched the number of bed days taken by teenagers in hospitals in England, Wales and Scotland. Viner's study revealed that there were 17 in-patient bed days per 10,000 youngsters aged 12, rising to 24.6 per 10,000 for 19-year-olds. More boys than girls occupied hospital beds at the age of 12; by the age of 17, more teenage girls than boys were in-patients. Despite the fact that experts in the 1960s had advocated separate wards for teenagers, only a quarter of hospitals in England made some accommodation available for their adolescent patients. The situation had become more acute as the age of patients in children's wards decreased, but increased in adult wards.[55] Dedicating special adolescent wards was an obvious possibility, but Great

Ormond Street Hospital in London had developed a section of an ordinary ward for adolescents, with specially trained staff.[56]

Adolescent wards had been opened in several Australian hospitals.[57] A broader definition of 'young people' as a range between ten and 25 years was emerging. This span recognised different levels of maturity, a flexibility prohibited by rigid chronological age divisions.[58] Whether at the younger or older end of the spectrum, many young people found it difficult to access health-care programs, which often did not take into account the special problems of adolescence. Community programs such as ADAWS, Pregnancy Help and university health clinics had gone part of the way to filling the need, but could not accommodate the situation when acute hospital care was required. The review team found that teenagers chose different sites for different problems. They might, for instance, consult general practitioners for physical illnesses, but not for drug abuse or emotional problems.

Illnesses such as cystic fibrosis, asthma, diabetes and spina bifida fitted more easily into the usual acute hospital system than lifestyle problems. The Mater already had one possible model. Its adolescent diabetic centre had been functioning since the late 1990s, and was staffed by an adult endocrinologist, as well as a paediatric endocrinologist, nurse educators, a dietitian and a psychologist. Patients from the first year of high school were seen at the centre. Some patients wanted to move to adult care when they were 17, or even younger, but others preferred to continue with the centre until they were 21 or 22. The centre's work in supporting patients through the transition from parental control to autonomous management was critical in helping patients with diabetes to manage a lifelong condition.

The attitude and approach of the staff was found to be more important than the environment, but teenagers reported that they liked opportunities to discuss their situation with others in their own age group.[59] The Mater Adult Hospital treated patients over the age of 14, but had no specific adolescent programs. Most nurses thought there needed to be a formal mechanism for the handover from paediatric to adult care and more training for nursing staff. Paediatricians at the Mater Children's Hospital favoured a ward at the adult hospital where doctors at adult and children's hospitals had admitting rights. Out-patient clinics staffed by both hospitals were also suggested for patients with chronic illnesses.[60] Apart from the Child and Youth Mental Health Service, and special clinics for patients with cystic fibrosis and diabetes, not a great deal changed at the Mater. In 2006, there were calls for a coherent plan for adolescent care and a common age for transition from paediatric to adult care. Each unit had developed its own transition process, a situation which seemed to apply everywhere in Queensland.[61]

In the first five years of the new hospital, many of the original Mater Children's Hospital services had expanded, and new ones developed. At the same time, however, an old idea was re-emerging: a single Queensland children's hospital, a concept that most clinicians at both hospitals favoured, but one which would bring down the curtain on Brisbane's two independent children's hospitals.[62] The Mater Children's Private Hospital could continue, but the Mater Children's Hospital could not.

Chapter 15

Transition: The Queensland Children's Hospital

... Queensland needs to construct a single, integrated, purpose built, new Queensland Children's Hospital (QCH) in metropolitan Brisbane.

Mellis Review, 2006

In November 1970, Queensland's first Professor of Child Health, John Rendle-Short, advocated the replacement of Brisbane's two children's hospitals with one well-resourced Institute of Child Health.[1] In ensuing decades, a single children's hospital was the subject of frequent discussions and repeated arguments. The Royal Children's and the Mater's Children's hospitals continued as separate entities, but discussions about the rationalisation of health services in the 1980s and 1990s reprised the single children's hospital concept.

In 1993, the South East Hospital Planning Project options paper identified a single tertiary hospital as one of three options for future paediatric services.[2] In 1996, the Mater Children's Hospital Paediatric Staff Society discussed the possibility of merging the two children's hospitals but, after an acrimonious meeting between the staff societies of the two children's hospitals in October that year, reported that 'any proposed amalgamation of services seems very unlikely'.[3] In 1997, however, clinicians at both hospitals agreed that a single tertiary hospital would be the best solution for Brisbane. Disagreement on an appropriate location, first aired in the 1970s, persisted: neither hospital would willingly cede its identity or its location.[4]

In the late 1990s, the relationship between the two hospitals was competitive, rather than collaborative, and there was little action at the political level, perhaps because governments were reluctant to offend voters on either side of the river. The debate resurfaced in the early twenty-first century. In 2002, the strategic plan for super-specialist paediatric services in Queensland recognised that the Mater Children's Hospital should be part of statewide planning. As well as providing renal transplantation, craniofacial and sleep study services, the Mater Children's Hospital would retain its own paediatric intensive care unit and be an equal partner with the Royal Children's Hospital in services such as metabolic medicine, cochlear implantation, oncology, medical imaging, respiratory medicine, neurosurgery, neurology, endocrinology, orthopaedics, developmental medicine and behavioural paediatrics.[5]

Children needing treatment for more than one condition faced a difficult situation. Crossing the city from a specialist unit at one hospital to another specialist unit at the other was trying for patients and wearing for their parents. A three-year-old child with complex medical problems exemplified this situation. This child was born at the Mater Mothers' Hospital in 2008 and spent three months in the neonatal intensive care and high-dependency units. Subsequently a patient at the Mater Children's Hospital, the child received regular care from five medical teams, as well as intermittent care from a further eight, spending eight months in intensive care units, undergoing six operations, 11 general anaesthetics, and multiple invasive tests and procedures. Then followed a series of transfers: in April 2009, to the Royal Children's Hospital for a form of nutrition available for long-term home use only through its gastroenterology department and, between 2009 and early 2011, to the Mater Children's Hospital for overnight hospital admissions necessary to monitor respiratory support available for home use only through the Mater.[6]

The 2005 Queensland health systems review – the Forster Review – found that Queensland's population was not sufficiently large to support two tertiary children's hospitals.[7] The Forster Review team met the Mater Board and praised the Mater's strong positive culture, particularly discernible in its patient-centred staff.[8] The Forster Review was replete with advocacy for health networks, such as the 'bub-hubs' recommended in the March 2005 report on Queensland's maternity services and endorsed enthusiastically by the Health Minister.[9] 'Bub-hubs' would provide seamless transition from maternity services to paediatric care. The physical connection between the Mater Children's and Mater Mothers' hospitals, and the organisational structure bringing both hospitals under one executive director, was a ready-made 'bub-hub'.[10] The Forster Review criticised the duplication of expensive tertiary subspecialty services at the two children's hospitals.[11]

The Forster Review became the spark that lit a powerful fire. Paediatric cardiac services were reviewed by a team chaired by Professor Craig Mellis in 2006.[12] Several factors prompted the review: a series of deaths following paediatric cardiac surgery at The Prince Charles Hospital, the coroner's findings in an inquest into a cardiac death at the Royal Children's Hospital and comments in the Forster Review on the need for rationalisation.[13]

The Mellis Review found that two competing tertiary children's hospitals was 'far from ideal for clinical care, training, resource allocation, and research'.[14] In 2004, the Cardiac Society of Australia and New Zealand criticised the Queensland situation and recommended that a cardiac unit be installed in a single, child-friendly environment.[15] Paediatric cardiac surgery by surgeons who treated all age groups ignored the proposition – accepted for decades – that children should always be treated separately from adults. In many instances, a child's heart problem was only one of several health issues, best managed in a tertiary paediatric hospital, where appropriate support was available.

Philosophy was one element; cost was another. The existing situation had created three expensive paediatric intensive care units in one city, an unsustainable situation, as it was impossible to ensure that all were adequately staffed with appropriate expertise; paediatric intensivists could not receive comprehensive training at any one of the three small units.[16] This situation had been anticipated at the Mater years earlier. In 2002, the Mater Board indicated that, perhaps, cardiology should be integrated at the Royal Children's Hospital, and that the two paediatric intensive care units should be amalgamated.[17] By 2006, when the Mellis Review was underway, the Mater's view was different. The review team visited the Mater, which proposed that it should host paediatric cardiac surgery, a position supported by the patient advocacy group HeartKids Queensland.[18]

The Mellis Review highlighted the shortage of paediatric cardiologists and cardiac surgeons. The review report continued:

... Queensland needs to construct a single, integrated, purpose built, new Queensland Children's Hospital (QCH) in metropolitan Brisbane. Once commissioned, the existing children's hospitals would close and ... their resources would be consolidated into the new, well-resourced QCH ... To achieve this goal within five years, a strong commitment from the Government is required ...[19]

The government needed a change of mind. In March 2006, the Health Minister, Stephen Robertson, asserted that a new hospital would be too costly, and unnecessary because staff had already been increased at The Prince Charles Hospital.[20] A few months later, however, the government needed a 'good news' health story. The Queensland public hospital system seemed to be unravelling in the wake of allegations that patients had died at Bundaberg Hospital after surgery by Dr Jayant Patel.[21] A taskforce, chaired by the Director-General of Health, was appointed immediately to examine how the Mellis Review's recommendations could be implemented. The taskforce – a large gathering of clinicians, parents and the chief executive officers of Mater Health Services and the Royal Children's Hospital – endorsed the Mellis Review's recommendation that a new, single children's hospital should be created.[22] In coming to its recommendations, the taskforce examined the sites of both children's hospitals and assessed their strengths and weaknesses.

The taskforce noted that the Royal Children's Hospital was already recognised as a centre of excellence with proven capacity to attract and train specialist staff. The University of Queensland medical school, close to the hospital, helped in this regard, as did research at the nearby Queensland Institute of Medical Research (now QIMR Berghofer Medical Research Institute). The Mater Medical Research Institute was smaller, but was more focused on the translation of research findings to clinical care.[23]

The Mater Children's Private Hospital, a key difference from the Royal Children's Hospital, enhanced the Mater Children's Hospital's already good reputation for attracting and retaining clinical expertise. Procedural specialists with part-time public appointments liked the private practice option. It was an important factor in the international competition for talented specialists. About 26 per cent of the children treated at the Mater in 2004–05 were private patients. There was evidence that 36 per cent of children under the age of ten had private health insurance, as did 38 per cent of children in the

10–14 years age group.[24] Admitting children to private hospitals enhanced the capacity of public hospitals to treat more patients, a position reflected in Mater discussions with Queensland Health.[25]

Outreach to the wider Queensland community was another factor. Historically, the Royal Children's Hospital had been the main provider of statewide tertiary services through a network of outreach clinics. The Royal Children's Hospital was also recognised as the centre of statewide telemedicine – even though the Mater Children's Hospital had begun telemedicine broadcasts of grand rounds in 1996[26] – and coordinated a number of medical rotations to regional hospitals. The Mater Children's Hospital had not led as many statewide services, but provided tertiary services in renal transplantation, craniofacial surgery, sleep studies, epilepsy management, child and adolescent mental health, and alcohol and drug rehabilitation.[27]

The development of adolescent services and the appropriate management of the transition to adult care were also regarded as important in any new tertiary paediatric hospital. In a submission to the taskforce, the Faculty of Health Sciences at the University of Queensland pointed out that 'Brisbane seems to be the only major capital city without specific arrangements for older adolescents', even though the evidence indicated that properly planned transition programs resulted in better disease control and improved patient satisfaction.[28]

After all the services had been examined and the options considered, the taskforce reported that:

> The Royal campus provides the best option when it comes to a new children's hospital being linked with other specialities and services. The Mater Children's Hospital does have established links with the Mater Adult and Mater Mothers' hospitals and, significantly, a good working relationship with the Princess Alexandra Hospital's cardiac unit with which it currently shares expertise.[29]

The taskforce left the touchy decision on a site for the new hospital to the government, apart from recommending that it be located adjacent to the Mater Mothers' Hospital or the Royal Brisbane and Women's Hospital. The Sisters of Mercy, the Mater Board and its Executive supported the single tertiary hospital – wherever it was located – in the interests of excellence in paediatric care,[30] a brave decision only 14 years after the fight to avoid moving the Mater Children's Hospital to Mt Gravatt.[31] Neonatology was a significant factor. The Mater Mothers' Hospital unit was by far the largest in Australia with the highest patient acuity, likely to increase in the new Mater Mothers' Hospital, under construction when the taskforce reported.[32]

The taskforce spotlighted the most difficult challenge:

> A priority for the planning process should be the creation of a new, single, child-centred culture that overcomes current barriers to achieving a unified service. These barriers result from the physical distance between the existing hospitals and from long-standing cultural and relationship issues.[33]

Unity would not come easily, but the taskforce had high hopes:

> One of the key advantages of building a new tertiary hospital would be the establishment of a new joint culture. Considerable effort would need to be made in the planning phase to work with clinicians, parents and patients on the development of this new culture for the new facility.

The Premier, Peter Beattie, had already ruled out the closure of the Mater Children's Hospital in favour of one children's hospital, presumably on the Royal Children's Hospital site. In a fiery debate in Parliament in March 2006, the Premier proclaimed that the Mater Children's Hospital would close 'over my dead body'.[34] Although other factors seemed to favour the Royal Children's Hospital site, the taskforce had noted that the Mater was more easily accessible by public transport and, unlike the Royal Children's Hospital, had a prominent, accessible street frontage. The advocacy group HeartKids Queensland – and other parents – emphasised that the proximity of the South Bank Parklands, a stimulating and pleasant place to take children on breaks from hospital, was an important advantage at South Brisbane. A number of options on the Mater site would provide more than adequate space for a 350–400-bed hospital. The Mater nominated land it owned adjacent to the current Mater Children's and new Mater Mothers' hospitals. This area – between 16,000 and 18,000 square metres in size – already had Brisbane City Council approval for a ten-storey building.

Queensland Health did not conduct its own analysis of the South Brisbane and Herston sites, relying instead on the government's capital works agency, which reported that the Mater site had good access for construction. There were also cost and efficiency advantages. Existing hospital operations would not be disrupted during construction at South Brisbane and there were convenient linkages to necessary services at the other hospitals on the campus. Even better, a new hospital could be built and operational on the Mater site within five years, if the Mater Children's Hospital building was extended onto the adjoining site.[35]

On the other hand, the older Royal Children's Hospital buildings would have to be replaced completely by new buildings on land occupied by the heritage-listed north and south towers of the old Lady Lamington Nurses' Home. This site was smaller – between 12,000 and 16,000 square metres – and was some distance from the Royal Brisbane and Women's Hospital. Nor was it an easy site. Blasting hard, high-level rock would be required to create a basement car park, a 'prohibitively' expensive exercise. Traffic access was difficult, public transport was poor, and the site would not have the street presence demanded by a world-class hospital. The tight site was not sufficiently large for an outdoor playground or a garden. Construction access was poor. Building a new hospital and associated facilities would take more than five years.[36]

Celebrations marking 100 years since the first Mater hospital was established in 1906 and 75 years since the Mater Children's Hospital opened in 1931 made 2006 a momentous year. In August 2006, mere days after the taskforce reported – but in time for the 2006 Queensland state election campaign – the government announced that a new Queensland Children's Hospital would be built adjacent to the Mater campus at South Brisbane and that Mater Health Services would share in its management.[37] The time for prevaricating over a single children's hospital was over.[38] The imminent election had left little time for investment planning and analysis, health service planning or comprehensive construction and implementation planning processes. The absence of plans and analyses set the scene for costs to escalate.[39]

Immediate and vociferous opposition ensued.[40] The powerful Queensland branch of the Australian Medical Association (AMA) opposed the decision on the site and the manner in which it was made.[41] There were complaints that the site selection was rushed and not based on the best available evidence, ignoring a recommendation in the Forster Review that Queensland Health base decisions on locating health facilities on advice from technical experts and wide community and stakeholder consultation.[42] Criticism was exacerbated by the imminent election and the government's decision not to release the taskforce report.

Medical opposition persisted for years. In July 2008, for instance, doctors opposed to the South Brisbane site wrote to the government claiming that cost estimates had blown out to $2,500,000,000 from the original $770,000,000. The lower figure was, however, based on re-using and extending the 2001 Mater Children's Hospital building, and sharing existing clinical and support infrastructure, an option the Bligh government rejected.[43]

The government was unwilling to pay in cash the full value of the Mater Children's Hospital and adjacent Mater land.[44] Tense negotiations followed.

Eventually, an agreement based on 'exchange of value' was forged. Though the contract between Queensland Health and the Mater Board stipulated that the operation of the Mater Children's Hospital would be government funded until 2022, the Mater Board agreed to forgo this right. The offer to re-use the Mater Children's Hospital building – with the exception of the Mater Children's Private Hospital – for accommodation and some clinical services was included in the agreement. Additional Mater land in Stanley Street and Hancock Street would also be transferred to the government for $1.

In return, the Mater received the right to operate the new hospital's car park, equivalent in value to the land. Unlike the health department in Victoria, Queensland Health did not own or operate car parks.[45] New car parks were essential; the Mater's car park in Raymond Terrace was resumed as part of the new hospital's site. The Mater secured an agreement with a neighbour, St Laurence's College, for a 105-year lease of part of its land to construct a car park for both the new hospital and the Mater, and, in return, to construct an auditorium for the school with a playing field on the car park roof.[46] This ingenious $100,000,000 project delivered an enormous car park in South Brisbane, where no other land was available. Despite this contribution, and ceding its contractual rights for funding to operate the Mater Children's Hospital, the Queensland Auditor-General's 2014 report surprised the Mater in estimating that the Mater would benefit considerably at the state's expense.[47]

The Queensland branch of the AMA maintained its opposition and recommended a total reconsideration of the project, citing concern that patient care and research would suffer, as well as fear that there would be 'religious interference', even though the government had supported the Mater public hospital services financially for decades.[48] The Mater reassured the government that Catholic teaching did not impose any restriction on any practice that might occur in a tertiary children's hospital, a position later affirmed by the Health Minister.[49] As if this were not enough, the proposed governing board – three representatives from the Mater, three from the Royal Children's Hospital, with a chairman chosen by Queensland Health, but who was also acceptable to Mater – was somehow construed to be 'too Mater-focused'.[50]

The furore over the site for the new hospital highlighted the strength of the culture and institutional loyalty that had developed at the Royal Children's Hospital. In 2007, 98 per cent of paediatric clinicians had been in favour of a single children's hospital but, when the site was announced, only 50 per cent of the clinical community supported the South Brisbane location.[51] The Mellis Review had warned that there would be resistance to change. Previous experience elsewhere had indicated that there would be 'reluctance ranging from inertia and foot dragging' to 'active vocal and political resistance' often 'disguised as altruistic regard for history and tradition'.[52] Two members of the review panel had experienced personally this form of resistance and grieving when the Royal Alexandra Hospital for Children moved to the Westmead site in Sydney.[53]

The Mellis Review recommended that the planning process engage as many stakeholders as possible to increase understanding of the decision. In September 2008, the Health Minister described consultation on the proposed hospital:

> We have been engaged in a progressive consultation to design the new hospital. That has involved an extensive range of clinicians, doctors, nurses, allied health professionals, parent groups and children's groups ...[54]

The Mellis Review had highlighted an intransigent Brisbane factor: the sociological and psychological division between the north and south sides of the river. Nevertheless, staff at all levels, in all disciplines, and from all three hospitals (Mater Children's Hospital, Royal Children's Hospital and The Prince Charles Hospital), had recognised that existing arrangements were inconvenient, inefficient, hazardous and unsustainable. Strong leadership, the

Mellis Review continued, would be necessary to harness the professionalism of the best elements of all three institutions to build a new world-class Queensland children's hospital.[55] Dr Leigh Atkinson, a former Mater neurosurgeon, wrote to Brisbane's main daily newspaper of his anger that the 'north–south neurosis', which had 'ruined Brisbane' for decades, was affecting the badly needed Queensland children's hospital.[56] Some clinicians felt so strongly that they threatened to leave Queensland if the new hospital did not proceed.[57]

The 'great divide' was, however, about to shrink, physically at least. Two new cross-river road links, the Go Between Bridge and the Clem Jones Tunnel beneath the river, opened while the new hospital was still in its planning and early construction stages. The northern and southern 'busways' – roads used by buses exclusively – further tightened the link. The South Bank railway station was close by, as was a ferry terminal.[58]

In 2006, the state Opposition offered a measure of comfort to those distressed by the government's decision. It planned a new stand-alone tertiary paediatric hospital, with the original two children's hospitals remaining to offer secondary-level services. The government, however, pressed on. The design for the Queensland Children's Hospital by architects Conrad Gargett Riddel in conjunction with Lyons Architecture was accepted, the master plan was approved in June 2008, the health services plan was announced in July 2008 and the project definition plan was approved in October 2008.[59]

There had, however, been some tense times. A staunch advocate for the South Brisbane site, the Premier, Peter Beattie, retired in September 2007 and was succeeded by the member for South Brisbane, Anna Bligh. The global financial crisis constrained government finances and Queensland Treasury warned that the new hospital might be unaffordable.[60] The Mater was concerned that the new hospital might not survive the change of premier, a change of government, or the global financial crisis, and insisted that the Mater's land gift be conditional on the hospital proceeding, reflecting concern that if the Royal Children's Hospital raised sufficient issues, the government might abandon the project.[61] As late as August 2008, discussions about using part of the Mater Children's Hospital building were continuing.[62]

The Bligh government's decision that the new hospital would not share facilities with the Mater reduced the potential for cost saving through sharing expensive diagnostic services and utilities with the Mater. Co-locating the Mater Children's with the Mater Mothers' and Mater Adult hospitals had demonstrated the benefits of shared services. The 'stand-alone' decision meant, for example, two back-up power plants, two information and communication technology systems, duplicated oxygen reticulation, and two paediatric pathology laboratories in adjacent buildings. The Bligh government was much less enthusiastic about access to beds at the Mater Children's Private Hospital.[63] The cost of the new hospital more than doubled.[64] Cabinet capped the cost of at $1.1 billion, but this proved to be an underestimate of the final cost: $1.75 billion.[65]

Governance was also affected. The new hospital had originally been planned as a joint venture between the government and the Mater, with Mater representation on the governing board. However, the Bligh government changed the board's status to an advisory board, indicating that there was little point in the Mater participating in the governance of the new free-standing hospital.[66]

The Memorandum of Understanding between the Mater and the government, signed late in 2008,[67] stated that if the Queensland Children's Hospital did not proceed, the land reverted to the Mater, including any additional land acquired by the state for the hospital. If the hospital was built, but not operated as a tertiary children's hospital, the land and improvements would revert to the Mater.[68] After 60 years – far longer than the usual life of modern hospitals – the land and buildings would revert to the Mater. If, however, the government wished to retain the hospital as a tertiary children's hospital for more than 60 years, it would pay land rent to the Mater until 90 years had passed. The land and buildings would then revert to the Mater unconditionally, a precaution to provide for the Mater's twenty-second-century expansion, as the site of the new children's hospital would be the only land available in the area.[69]

This confidential agreement effectively 'gagged' the Mater. Public discontent continued. The chief executive officer of the Queensland Children's Hospital, Professor Alan Isles, attempted to defuse allegations that the hospital would have insufficient beds by pointing out that the combined hospital would have more beds than the total available in the two existing original hospitals: 359 public beds compared with 288 public beds in the Royal Children's and Mater Children's hospitals. In September 2008, the Health Minister, Stephen Robertson, stated that the government was committed to a 400-bed hospital. In addition, the Mater Children's Private Hospital was expected to expand.[70] A few months later, however, the project plan was leaked to the press, indicating that the new hospital would have only 200 overnight beds; the remainder of the 359 beds would be day beds.[71]

A forum convened by Queensland Health and the AMA in September 2008 was attended by 150 clinicians, achieving, in the Health Minister's words, 'remarkable consensus'.[72] Nevertheless, the furore raged again during the 2009 election campaign. The Leader of the Opposition, Lawrence Springborg, promised to abandon the new hospital project and to expand the two existing children's hospitals.[73] The Premier, Anna Bligh, attempted to alleviate community concern that children – particularly on the north side – would be left without sufficient emergency services. Children's emergency departments would be upgraded at The Prince Charles, Redcliffe and Caboolture hospitals in Brisbane's north, at Redland Hospital in the east, at Ipswich Hospital in the west and at Logan Hospital in the south.

Despite these assurances, a few Royal Children's Hospital doctors continued to claim that it would be less expensive to abandon the South Brisbane project and return to Herston.[74] The situation for newborns particularly troubled them. Overlooking the reality that there were almost twice the number of births at the Mater Mothers' Hospital, which contained 30 level-3 neonatal intensive care beds compared with seven at the Royal Brisbane and Women's Hospital, they feared that the separation of the new hospital from the Grantley Stable Neonatal Unit at the Royal Brisbane and Women's Hospital might decrease its patient numbers.[75]

Dr Peter Steer, formerly medical director of the Mater Children's Hospital, returned from Canada early in 2009 to succeed Alan Isles, who, it was later claimed, warned the Premier that the project was flawed.[76] Steer tried to address doctors' concerns. He recognised that even those who supported the Queensland Children's Hospital moved into stages of grief and loss at the prospect of the closure of the two hospitals.[77] Dr Steer pointed out that the Hospital for Sick Children in Toronto had only 330 beds for a population of 4 million and that services in Queensland would not merely be combined, but also expanded.[78]

A senior Mater paediatrician, Dr David Wood, and colleagues Professor Ross Pinkerton, Dr Cameron Ward, Dr Rosslyn Walker and Professor Kim Oates in Sydney addressed their concerns in a letter to the editor of the *Courier-Mail*.[79] They emphasised that one children's hospital was essential for highly complex treatment by people who saw enough patients to maintain their skills and train their successors. Rotation of specialist staff to regional hospitals – as already existed between the emergency departments at the Mater and Logan hospitals – would be an additional advantage. They pleaded for a change of attitude to put children first.

Even before construction began with the turning of the first sod on 9 March 2010, senior clinical appointments to the Queensland Children's Hospital were announced.[80] Dr David McCrossin, director of paediatric health services at the Mater Children's Hospital, was appointed to lead the medical staff, but ill health later forced his resignation. Fiona Brewin-Brown, who had worked in the planning and coordination branch of Queensland's Health Department after she left the Mater for further study, continued in senior roles.[81] In contrast, hundreds of staff members of the two hospitals remained uncertain about their future prospects. There was to be no transfer of staff from either hospital: all had to apply for jobs, with the likelihood that there would not be room for everyone.

The longevity of complaint and resistance to the project did nothing to settle apprehension on either side of the river. Research was the focus of later protests. Despite the Premier's assurance that research would be included in a new building close to the hospital, there were fears that its funding would be diverted to a childcare centre, shops and car parks.[82] In 2012, earthworks began for a building to house the Queensland Children's Medical Research Institute, as well as pathology, translational research and university researchers.[83]

Country families feared that they would have nowhere to stay close to their children, but there would also be a new building for them: a Ronald McDonald House on land donated by the government.[84] Fundraising was also part of the project. The old Bank of New South Wales building on the corner of Stanley and Vulture streets was earmarked as the future home of the Children's Health Foundation Queensland.

In preparation for the new hospital, significant changes at both children's hospitals created the first fully integrated services. Rather than be couched in language of gains and losses, the new arrangements were portrayed as improvements. The Mater Children's Hospital's oncology unit moved to the Royal Children's Hospital to create the Queensland Children's Cancer Centre, providing a comprehensive statewide cancer service.[85] In the wake of the Mellis Review, which had initiated the controversy, cardiac surgery and cardiology were transferred from The Prince Charles Hospital to the Mater Children's Hospital.

Extensive renovations began at the Mater in May 2007 to house the Queensland Paediatric Cardiac Service. Three paediatric cardiac surgeons were appointed; the paediatric intensive care unit was expanded; a new cardiac catheter laboratory, a dedicated operating theatre and perfusion area were added; and facilities for parents, physiotherapists, social workers and clinical leaders were enlarged. Dozens of new staff transferred with the unit.[86] Cardiac surgery began at the Mater on 20 May 2008. The paediatric intensive care unit became Australia's second largest.[87]

The first few months were not without controversy.[88] A nurse who had moved to the Mater with the cardiac unit claimed that some of the equipment was 'archaic', that the workload at the hospital was too heavy, and that some practices were unsafe. In the unit's defence, the director pointed out that the equipment was new and that twice as many operations were being performed.[89] Queensland's first three specialist paediatric cardiac surgeons had been appointed, exemplifying the benefits of a single tertiary children's hospital; surgeons at The Prince Charles Hospital also operated on adults. In May 2009, one year after the Mater unit opened, the fatality rate – less than 2 per cent – compared very favourably with other Australian cardiac units and internationally. There were no infections and a six-month waiting list had been slashed to zero.[90]

In October 2009, the Queensland Paediatric Cardiac Service registered the nation's first paediatric cardiac patient to use a remote monitoring system. The technology enabled patients like a seven-year-old boy from Katherine in the Northern Territory, some 3,000 kilometres from Brisbane, to transmit data electronically from implanted cardiac devices – pacemakers, cardiac defibrillators and electrocardiography monitoring devices – directly to the hospital, saving a great deal of travel for regular hospital assessments.[91]

Only a couple of years later, the cardiac unit recorded a world first when Professor Tom Karl began to use a new patch, which mimicked human tissue, to repair congenital heart defects – a condition affecting about eight children in every 1,000 births. The CardioCel® patches were expected to allow patients to live a normal life, free of implanted tissue-related complications.[92] Technology was becoming increasingly important in cardiac care, as it was in most medical and surgical practice. The Extracorporeal Membrane Oxygenation (ECMO) machine, which the Mater introduced to Queensland, provided cardiac and respiratory support to patients whose hearts and, often, lungs, were so severely diseased, or damaged, that they no longer functioned.[93] Children who needed heart transplants were sent to Melbourne, with an ECMO machine supporting them on the journey.

New heights were also being reached in orthopaedic surgery at the Mater Children's Hospital. Dr Geoffrey Askin and a group of specialists operated on an eight-year-old girl who had a congenital deformity of the neck and thoracic spine. Without surgery, her spine would have continued to deform and eventually compromise vital organs. The spinal team developed a plan to correct her spine in a single operation, followed by traction to improve the curve. This procedure replaced the series of operations that children with severe curvatures had undergone in earlier times.[94]

The orthotist Gary Bateman designed many mechanical aids to support orthopaedic treatment, including a traction apparatus that didn't confine children to bed when their spines needed to be stretched before operations for scoliosis.[95] Technological innovations and the products of research permeating many specialties was a reminder of the essential work of 'behind the scenes' teams. When the sleep studies unit needed a new impedance meter, a device used to check that electrodes placed on a patient's body were within an acceptable range for a sleep study, the Mater's biomedical engineers found a solution.[96] In July 2009, the paediatric urologist Dr David Winkle hosted the first Asia–Pacific seminar on cutting-edge computer game technology to treat incontinence in children. The Mater's Mars Clinic, a partnership between Dr Winkle and rehabilitation physiotherapists, had been established in 2008 for specialist treatment of children's incontinence.[97]

Ideas also came from other places. Dr Caroline Grant, a Mater engineer, was awarded a Queensland International Fellowship to spend 13 weeks at the University Children's Hospital in Bern, Switzerland, working with the respiratory research group, which was at the forefront of research on mechanical ventilation and electrical impedance tomography, a non-invasive medical imaging technique. The aim was better understanding of lung physiology in order to improve mechanical ventilation and reduce the risk of ventilator-induced lung injuries.[98] In 2007, an AxiliM navigator was introduced to support brain surgery at the Mater Children's Hospital. Like a global positioning system for the brain, the new device helped to accurately identify the position and extent of brain lesions.[99] In 2011, after completing demanding requirements, Mater speech pathologist Inge Kaltenbrunn qualified as a Listening and Spoken Language Specialist Certified Auditory-Verbal Therapist at the Alexander Graham Bell Academy in the United States. The ability to provide Auditory-Verbal Therapy helped to expand the range of intervention services available to patients and their families at the Mater Cochlear Implant Clinic.[100]

Patients helped others to overcome fear of hospitals and the procedures that might come their way. In 2010, the Mater developed a video designed to introduce children to magnetic resonance imaging (MRI). Annabel, aged eight, was the narrator in the video, which took children through the entire MRI experience. It was thought that if children felt more comfortable, they would keep still for their MRI scans, reducing the need for general anaesthesia. In the first few months after the video's introduction, 53 fewer children, including some as young as four years old, had general anaesthetics.[101]

Despite kidney problems from birth, Jordan Fothergill was able to lead a relatively normal life for nine years until his health began to deteriorate. His treatment involved daily dialysis and he was placed on a transplant waiting list. While waiting for his transplant, Jordan required regular blood tests, which he did not enjoy. He wrote a book, *Be Brave*, published by Mater Pathology, encouraging children to tolerate needles and injections. After his kidney transplant in August 2010, Jordan was able to resume an active life.[102]

Bringing new ideas to clinical reality and supporting established services could be expensive. As always, fundraising was essential. In 2011, the Mater's fundraising arm, the Mater Foundation, helped to fund a library of specialised equipment and resources for the domiciliary and acute care rehabilitation team (DART), as home-care services had become known, and which had grown to assist more than 700 families.[103]

The Mater Little Miracles Easter Appeal became an important initiative of the Mater Foundation. The first Easter Appeal in 2004 set a pattern of engaging the community in the work of the Mater Children's and Mater Mothers' hospitals. The '5Ks for Kids' walk became a highly visible feature. The visibility of the entire Easter appeal was enhanced in 2007 by the presence of Miracle Max, a huge dog mascot.[104] Many stories of families coping with difficult problems lay behind the people striding out for their '5Ks for Kids'. In 2011, for instance, Lilly Munn's family and friends took part in the five-kilometre walk. Lilly was diagnosed with congenital adrenal hyperplasia (CAH), an inherited condition that affected the ability of her adrenal glands to produce hormones essential for growth and metabolism. Lilly needed many procedures and frequent visits to the Mater Children's Hospital.

On Good Friday 2010, babies and children at the Mater Mothers' and Mater Children's hospitals touched the hearts of people all over Australia when Channel Nine broadcast the Mater Little Miracles Telethon live from the Aubigny Place forecourt. A team of Mater volunteers joined Channel Nine celebrities and former Olympians Grant Hackett and Giaan Rooney to take calls from generous donors around the country. Almost $1,200,000 was raised in the 2010 Easter Appeal.[105] Great sadness could also inspire fundraisers. The Mater Foundation's Preston James Fund commemorated a little boy who died in 2003 from an overwhelming infection. The fund in Preston's memory, organised by his mother and a special committee, was dedicated to research funding for the intensive care unit where Jordan had been treated.[106]

Fundraising for the Mater Children's Hospital had engaged legions of volunteers ever since the hospital was a mere twinkle in the Sisters of Mercy's eyes. Volunteers also worked in many other roles in the hospital itself. In 2009, a joint initiative between Mater Volunteer Services and the paediatric intensive care unit (PICU) brought a supportive presence to the sickest children. In September 2009, two Mater volunteers, Vandra Neylan and Jenny Lord, became specially trained 'cuddle mums' in the intensive care unit. Their first task was to cuddle and comfort three-month-old Joseph and, in doing so, support Joseph's mother as she faced the daunting task of caring for Joseph in hospital and another child at home. The 'cuddle mum' concept had already been in successful operation in general wards at the Mater Children's Hospital and at the Mater Mothers' Hospital's special care nursery since 1992. Gwen Grant was a long-term volunteer, supporting families waiting while their children were in the operating theatre.[107] There was also a reminder of Mater Children's Hospital nurses who volunteered for foreign-aid work in Cambodia in the 1970s: Alison Pickering volunteered to work as a nurse in one of Africa's largest slums, Kibera, in Nairobi, as part of the African Inland Mission volunteer scheme.

Although the Mater Children's Hospital was in the shadow of its closure, the Mater Children's Private Hospital was anticipating its future with an encouraging plaudit. The Mater Children's and Mater Mothers' private hospitals were jointly awarded the national silver award and the Queensland silver award in a nationwide survey of 140 private hospitals conducted by the health fund Medibank Private. The survey covered every stage of the hospital experience from pre-admission to discharge and follow-up, the standard of medical treatment, privacy, cleanliness and food quality. The newest member of the Mater family, Mater Private Hospital Redland, put its senior siblings slightly in the shade by winning the gold award.[108] A parent's submission to a government inquiry explained some of the benefits: 'the Mater Children's Private Hospital has been our home away from home' and a 'mostly kind, welcoming and safe place for our child and family'. She continued: 'I believe that had we been in a shared public room on … very regular and long hospital stays, it would have added an enormous amount of additional, unnecessary pressure'.[109]

In the early years of the twenty-first century's second decade, staff at the Mater Children's Hospital had an ever-present reminder that their worlds would change. One of its immediate neighbours, the enormous new Queensland Children's Hospital, was steadily moving towards its opening date on 29 November 2014. Niggles remained, however, including the likelihood that only 288 beds – the same number in the two children's hospitals and not the 359 that were promised – would be available when the new hospital opened.[110]

Chapter 16
Changing Childhoods Forever

I like how the nurses play with me ... and look after me.

Jacob, aged eight, Mater Children's Hospital patient, 2014[1]

Hospitals, no matter how new and grand, are so much more than buildings, much more than institutions where issues of governance and finance – important as they may be – influence outcomes. Hospitals are lively human organisations, created to improve human health and to serve human needs.

Humanity is at the heart of the best clinical practice. In Mater hospitals, humanity is nourished by a unique blend: the Sisters of Mercy's philosophy of care bonded securely to their very practical approach to life and its challenges. Achieving the best health care possible was always the Sisters' goal for their Mater Children's Hospital, as it was for all their Mater hospitals. Tangible realities had to be created from vision and inspiration, sometimes by taking nerve-tingling risks. Money was merely a tool to be found somewhere, somehow. 'Mater' in a hospital title is a great deal more than a name: it identifies an entire philosophy of health care, with as much emphasis on 'care' as on 'health'.

Children mean families. The Mater Children's Hospital is a member of a family of hospitals: the Mater Adult Hospital, re-named Mater Hospital Brisbane in 2014; the Mater Private Hospital; the Mater Mothers' Hospital; the Mater Mothers' Private Hospital; the Mater Children's Private Hospital; the Mater Private Hospital Redland; and the twinkle in the family eye, the Mater Private Hospital Springfield, scheduled to open at the end of 2015. At the Mater Children's Hospital, family has many meanings: contemporary patients and their families; patients from earlier times who bring their children and grandchildren to the hospital; patients who grow up to join the Mater staff; children born at the Mater Mothers' Hospital who become parents of patients of the Mater Children's Hospital ... and so it goes on.

Relationships with the Mater Children's Hospital have crossed lifetimes and generations. Denise Martin began her association with the Mater's many dimensions when she was ten, assisting Sister Madeline Fishbourne on the handkerchief and plants stall at Mater fetes. At various times, her parents were patients in the Mater Adult and Mater Private hospitals. Denise's children were Mater Mothers' Hospital babies, and, in 1968, Sister Mary Mechtilde nursed her son in the Mater Children's Hospital. Years later, Denise's granddaughter was born at the Mater Mothers' Hospital.[2] In the 1970s, a small girl, seriously ill with osteomyelitis, was a frequent patient at the Mater Children's Hospital for four years; as an adult, she spent 23 years as a scientist in Mater Pathology and as a parent of children who needed Mater Children's Hospital care.[3] Dr Geoff Wallace, a patient in the 1960s, returned to the Mater for his first medical job and, in 2014, was director of neurosciences at the Mater Children's Hospital.[4]

The story of the Mater Children's Hospital encompasses much more than a saga of development from one small building in 1931 to the enormous building opened in 2001, of facing challenges as formidable as sacrificing the Mater Children's Hospital to achieve even higher standards of care for Queensland children in a merger with the Royal Children's Hospital to create a single tertiary hospital. This new state-of-the art facility was named the Lady Cilento Children's Hospital in December 2013, recalling Phyllis Cilento, a doctor whose extensive – and sometimes controversial – practice included many mothers and children.[5] But some promises await fulfilment. Early in 2015, only 288 beds had been commissioned; the remainder of the 359 beds were in 'shell' form.

Statistics can tell part of the story – from 1,266 in-patients, 2,872 out-patients, 1,153 emergencies and 1,445 surgical procedures in the Mater Children's Hospital's first full year (1931–32) to 18,304 in-patients, 86,062 out-patients, 46,729 emergencies and 6,451 surgical procedures in 2013, the last full year of the Mater Children's Hospital's life.[6]

Changes have, however, been far more significant than mere numbers. The early, simple division into medicine and surgery expanded to numerous subspecialties; patient treatment directed by doctors and carried out by nurses developed into care by multidisciplinary teams. Patients arrived on foot, in trains, buses, ambulances and cars and, in more recent decades, by plane from remote parts of Queensland and overseas and, when the need was urgent, by helicopter.

However they arrived – and whether they came as emergencies, as in-patients or to an out-patient clinic – children passing through the doors of the Mater Children's Hospital met the staff. For more than half a century, Sisters of Mercy matrons, from Sister Mary Marcelline Kehoe in 1931 to Sister Mary Dorothea Sheehan, the last 'Sister Matron' in the 1980s, managed the nursing staff. Sisters of Mercy were once in charge of every ward and every department, with eagle eyes on the junior staff, usually nurses from the Mater's own nurse training school. In later decades, secular directors of nursing managed highly qualified staff with university degrees and additional training in a variety of disciplines.

Decades of change expanded the medical staff from Dr Percy Alan Earnshaw, the revered 'PA', in charge of the medical wards and Dr Harry 'Daddy' Windsor in charge of surgery in the 1930s – assisted by one resident medical officer – to clinicians in charge of disciplines ranging from mental health to critical care, teaching groups of resident medical officers and registrars. Legendary orthopaedic surgeons, assisted by physiotherapists in the 1940s, were succeeded by specialists in several disciplines, supported by speech pathologists, audiologists, physiotherapists, occupational therapists, psychologists, nutritionists and social workers. As well as looking after in-patients and out-patients, visiting specialists attended numerous meetings and gave their time and expertise to writing plans and submissions to improve the hospital and worked with colleagues at the Royal Children's Hospital to prepare new models of care for the Lady Cilento Children's Hospital.

Patterns of illness have also changed: poliomyelitis has disappeared and lead poisoning and osteomyelitis are much less common. Their prominence has given way to conditions that once could be treated effectively only rarely, or not at all. Cardiac surgery and kidney transplants, neurology and plastic surgery, care for patients with diabetes, cystic fibrosis and brain injuries all became part of life at the Mater Children's Hospital. Innovations continued to the end. In 2014, for instance, a gaming 'app', Pepster, was trialled to encourage cystic fibrosis patients to be diligent with breathing exercises. Pepster uses a young patient's breath as the controller of computer games.[7]

As in all human creations, development has not been uniformly smooth. There have been periods of rapid change interspersed with quieter spells, disappointments and lost opportunities, along with exciting breakthroughs, times of friction and clashes of opinion, as well as warm camaraderie. Always, however, there has been the primacy of the patient.

Weeks in hospital, enlivened by visiting entertainers and lessons in the hospital school, have given way to care at home wherever possible. Entertainment and education remained and grew, but parents, once consigned to a weekly visit on Sunday afternoons, became essential partners in care teams at home, or at the hospital bedside.

But some things don't change: the kindness of volunteers, from parent aides to cuddle-mums, and the generosity of donors, from members of the public who deposited coins into Mater Children's Hospital collection boxes in the 1930s and 1940s, to hard-working auxiliary committees, to enthusiastic participants in the Mater's Little Miracles events in the twenty-first century. Finance was always a worry: necessity mothered invention many times in fostering innovation and supporting everyday care.

There have been many 'firsts' at the Mater Children's Hospital: craniofacial surgery; appointing Queensland's only specialist in growth and development; the pet therapy scheme; orthopaedic treatment for children in Russia; and Australia's first children's private hospital. But there have to be 'lasts': the last surgery in the operating theatres, the final clinic in out-patients, the end of nursing at the Mater's Children's Hospital and the last patient to leave the hospital. They will walk through a new door to the Lady Cilento Children's Hospital, but that door is very close to the familiar door to the Mater Children's Hospital in Stanley Street.

Tangible evidence of the Mater Children's Hospital will remain in its original 1931 building, full of life as the Mother Patrick Potter Building, housing community services, and in the 2001 building living on, re-named as the Salmon Building, in honour of a distinguished Sister of Mercy, Mother Alban Salmon. It will be a centre for neurosciences and adult intensive care, and a long-held goal – adolescent care – will be realised. The Queensland Centre for Adolescent and Young Adult Care will receive patients from the Lady Cilento Children's Hospital; many will progress to the adult hospital, Mater Hospital Brisbane.

Dr David Wood is a member of the Lady Cilento Children's Hospital board. The new hospital will include almost 1,000 staff members from the Mater Children's Hospital, among them Cathy Keyte, director of critical care nursing, formerly director of nursing at the Mater Children's Hospital, and Sue McKee, general manager, who was Cathy Keyte's predecessor at the Mater Children's Hospital.

Ends of significant eras prompt reflections. The great 'cupcake' party for the Mater Children's Hospital final birthday in July 2014 prompted memories of the balloons, music and laughter of more than 80 birthday celebrations before it. Postcards dotted throughout the hospital tempted patients, parents and staff to record memories. And there were conversations and tears, many tears, well before the moving ceremony farewelling the Mater Children's Hospital on 1 November 2014.

Vale Mater Children's Hospital

I have immense respect for those who made this decision, based not on what was best for the Mater, but on what was best for the community of Queensland.

Dr John O'Donnell, 1 November 2014

Celebrations, ceremonies and commemorations mark rites of passage in human society. Numerous celebrations have marked the opening of whole hospitals and many new buildings on the Mater campus. On 1 November 2014, there was a very different ceremony – a farewell.

The lawn between the original Mater Private Hospital, the first building on Mater Hill, and the original Mater Adult Hospital, the second building, is the centre of the Mater campus, featuring in numerous Mater photographs. The markers of the decades since 1910 and 1911, when the first Mater hospitals opened, are visible from the lawn: the enormous weeping figs edging the space, the smart 2008 Mater Mothers' Hospital immediately below, the 1980s Mater Adult Hospital beside the 1911 building a little further on, the 1961 Mater Mothers' Hospital building to the west, the 1931 Mater Children's Hospital building below to the east and, between upper and lower levels, the beautiful sculpture, 'Embrace', commemorating every one of the 263 Sisters of Mercy who served wards, laboratories and offices so faithfully.

The brightly coloured 2001 building housing the Mater Children's and Mater Children's Private hospitals, linked securely to the Mater Mothers' and the Mater Adult hospitals, is also visible from the lawn, and to its west are the upper storeys of the immense Lady Cilento Children's Hospital.

On 1 November 2014 – All Saints' Day – white chairs in neat rows faced the lawn. On each chair, a typical Mater touch: a bottle of cool water, as this was a very warm spring afternoon in subtropical Brisbane. Birds chirped and flew from fig to fig and a cooling breeze fluttered the profusion of blossoms on the mauve jacaranda. Every chair was occupied: Mater Children's Hospital patients and parents, past and present; rows of Sisters of Mercy; previous and current Mater Children's Hospital doctors, nurses, therapists, volunteers, administrators, caterers and maintenance staff.

They all faced a small, neat, white marquee, where valedictorians would take the stage. First, Uncle Des Sandy welcomed the gathering to his traditional country with grace, humour and his own reflections on the meaning of the Mater Children's Hospital to Aboriginal and Torres Strait Islander people, and to the whole Queensland community. The Roman Catholic Archbishop of Brisbane, the Most Reverend Mark Coleridge, encouraged reflections on beginnings and endings and the service of the Sisters of Mercy. The Congregational Leader of the Brisbane Sisters of Mercy, Sister Catherine Reuter's expression of the 'intertwining of life's joys and sorrows' echoed the feelings of many in the audience. The Director-General of Queensland Health, Ian Maynard, spoke of past and future partnerships between the Mater and Queensland Health. Susan Johnston, the first person to chair the new Children's Health Queensland Hospital and Health Board, looked firmly to the future of the Lady Cilento Children's Hospital, where the very best would be combined when 'two magnificent heritages' were joined. The host of the gathering, the Chief Executive Officer of Mater Health Services, Dr John O'Donnell, placed the painful decision to close the Mater Children's Hospital in its context:

> I am very proud of the decision taken by the Mater Board, the executive team and the Sisters of Mercy, to support a single children's hospital no matter where it was to be located. I have immense respect for those who made this decision, based not on what was best for the Mater, but on what was best for the community of Queensland. This adherence to the Mission of the Sisters of Mercy, above all else, was certainly a test of courage and conviction, and I believe we passed the test with the same degree of optimism and decisiveness shown by Catherine McAuley, who closed ministries when the circumstances demanded it.[1]

Catherine McAuley also opened new ministries when circumstances demanded it. And there is a bright future for the 2001 Mater Children's

Hospital building. The Mater Children's Private Hospital will grow to care for many more children, neurosciences will expand and Mater, in partnership with Queensland Health, will fulfil a long-felt need: a new Queensland-wide adolescent and young adult health service to include mental health. This new initiative will, in the Mater tradition, be linked – to two hospitals: the Mater Hospital Brisbane (the Mater Adult Hospital, re-named to incorporate this new direction) and the Lady Cilento Children's Hospital.

Modern tertiary-level care at its most complex and innovative will be available at the Lady Cilento Children's Hospital. The Mater Children's and Royal Children's hospitals had each to face a painful reality: neither hospital was 'capable of the level of excellence in clinical service, teaching and research to which we must all aspire, and which we must demand on behalf of the community we aim to serve'.[2]

The anguish of the loss of two vibrant children's hospitals, each with their own traditions and culture, will eventually fade as new traditions and a new culture emerge at the Lady Cilento Children's Hospital. Archbishop Duhig's remarks are as relevant in 2014 as they were in 1926, when the decision to establish the Mater Children's Hospital was announced:

> Children ... are Queensland's greatest asset ... more precious than gold or silver mines and more to be treasured than wealth or pastoral lands, and as brilliant as the sun ...[3]

There was grief when the patients left the Mater Children's Hospital on 29 November 2014, but their hospital's caring culture, character, warm 'personality' and achievements will remain in the memories and stories of patients and families and in the training countless doctors, nurses and therapists use at the new hospital – and all over the world – every day. All of these will continue to exert a special Mater Children's Hospital influence on the future.

Acknowledgments

I was very privileged to be asked to research and write the history of a well-loved Brisbane institution: the Mater Children's Hospital. In many ways, this was a different task from writing the history of all seven Mater hospitals, *Expressions of Mercy*, published in 2006 to celebrate the centenary of the first Mater hospital. The history of the Mater Children's Hospital was written, not to foreshadow future development, but to mark its closure. In its 83-year history, the Mater Children's Hospital etched a warm place in the hearts of many thousands of Queenslanders, a place that the continuing Mater Children's Private Hospital will perpetuate.

It should come as no surprise, therefore, that Mater people – both past and present – would willingly contribute their insights and opinions. The views of people with lived experience enliven the documentary record and contribute valuable perspective. I recognise that this listing of those whose generosity has contributed greatly to this history is inadequate, but, nevertheless, my gratitude to them is profound for answering numerous questions, reading sections and finding time in busy clinical lives for meetings: Sister Michaeleen Mary Ahern RSM, Dr Leigh Atkinson, Cathy Bagley, Dr Robyn Brady, Fiona Brewin-Brown RN, Dr Rob Campbell, Linda Ewing RN, John Gilmour, Cathy Keyte RN, Erica Lee, Kathryn McCarthy RN, Mary McCarthy RN, Professor Brett McDermott, Dr Terry McGuire, Dr Michael O'Callaghan, Judy Perrin RN, Dr Ian Robertson, Dr Sadasivam Suresh, Dr John Thearle, Elizabeth Trickett RN and Dr Geoff Wallace.

A committee of experts to review drafts of chapters adds greatly to any history project. The reviewers of this project – Sister Angela Mary Doyle RSM, Marie Hand RN, Nigel Harris, Rosalie Lewis RN OAM and David Wood – tackled drafts and, often, re-drafts, conscientiously and with warm spirit. Their assistance, and their willingness to chase up elusive details, was essential and greatly appreciated. In any history that reaches to the present day, legal issues can arise. The Mater's solicitor, Laurie Rogencamp, unerringly applied his skills to areas where doubts arose.

Jackie Chamberlin, the Mater archivist, made the years of documentary research not only extremely productive, but very enjoyable. Her meticulously organised collection of documents and photographs, and her intrepid ventures into the hospital cellar to retrieve boxes of material unexplored for decades, ensured that opportunities for research were as comprehensive as possible. Images do tell their own stories and, in addition to the collection in the Mater Archives and Heritage Centre, the doyenne of Mater photography, Vicki Adams, willingly researched her extensive collection for essential items. Veena Herron, Marketing and Communication Officer, was unstinting in her assistance in arranging permissions to use images and locating photographs in the Marketing collection.

It is always a pleasure to work with Greg Bain and his staff at the University of Queensland Press. Their attention to ensuring that every outcome is the best that it can be is challenging to any writer, but is always enjoyable and stimulating. Janet Parker edited the manuscript with great care and sensitivity and made dozens of helpful suggestions, Stan Lamond created a lovely design that is both interesting and accessible and, in managing the project through its production stages, Jacqueline Blanchard somehow kept all the balls in the air tactfully and carefully.

Most thanks of all, however, must go to the retiring Chief Executive Officer of Mater Health Services, Dr John O'Donnell. He inspired this project, kept it on track and, in the midst of tremendous demands on his time, read many drafts, identified errors, answered questions promptly and offered ideas and suggestions that added immeasurably to the finished product.

Helen Gregory
May 2015

Endnotes

Introduction

1. Anna Price statement, MCH presentation, Mercy Day 2014, Mater Archives and Heritage Centre (MAHC).

Chapter 1

1. The *Brisbane Courier*, 14 November 1925, p. 6.
2. JR Laverty, *The making of a metropolis: Brisbane 1823–1925*, Brisbane History Group, Brisbane, 2009, p. 42.
3. JR Laverty, *The making of a metropolis*, p. 45.
4. The tramline opened to Dutton Park in 1908 and Annerley in 1915. The train line on the south side was extended to Greenslopes and Coorparoo during the First World War.
5. For an account of the foundation of the Mater Public Hospital, see H Gregory, *Expressions of Mercy: Brisbane's Mater Hospitals 1906–2006*, UQP, Brisbane, 2006 and HJ Summers, *They crossed the river: The founding of the Mater Misericordiae Hospital, Brisbane*, UQP, Brisbane, 1979.
6. Centre for the Government of Queensland, http://queenslandplaces.com.au/moreton-district, accessed 1 December 2011. The combined population was about 250,000 in 1925: the *Brisbane Courier*, 31 May 1923, p. 6; P Hall, *Royal Children's Hospital Brisbane, 1878–1978: A century of care*, Royal Children's Hospital, Brisbane [Herston], 1978, pp. 49–50.
7. Minutes of Honorary Board, 8 September 1925, Meetings of Honorary Board, 16 May 1912–22 August 1930, Mater Archives and Heritage Centre (MAHC).
8. The *Daily Mail*, 12 June 1924, Press clippings, MAHC.
9. P Hall, *A century of care*, pp. 2–12. The hospital began in small rented quarters in inner Brisbane suburbs, first at Spring Hill and then in Fortitude Valley before moving to Herston.
10. *Queensland Past and Present: 100 Years of Statistics, 1896–1996*, Government Statisticians Office, Brisbane, c. 1998, p. 264. The infant mortality rate had fallen to 6.4 in 1995.
11. MJ Thearle, 'Turner, Alfred Jefferis (1861–1947)', *Australian Dictionary of Biography*, National Centre of Biography, Australian National University, http://adb.anu.edu.au/biography/turner-alfred-jefferis-8883/text15601, accessed 9 January 2012. The service expanded and infant mortality in Queensland dropped from 50.7 to 35.6 per thousand births, the second lowest rate of all the Australian States.
12. For more information on childhood illnesses, see H Gregory and MJ Thearle, 'Casualties of Brisbane's growth: Infant and child mortality in the 1860s', *Brisbane: Housing, health, the river and the arts*, Brisbane History Group Papers No. 3, Brisbane History Group, Brisbane, 1985; H Gregory and MJ Thearle, 'Saving the children: Brisbane and medical triumphs of the 1890s', *Brisbane: Housing, health, the river and the arts*.
13. For further information on AJ Turner, see MJ Thearle, *Dr Alfred Jefferis Turner, 1861–1947: His contribution to medicine in Queensland*, MD thesis, University of Queensland, 1987.
14. R Patrick, *A history of health and medicine in Queensland 1824–1960*, UQP, Brisbane, 1987, p. 237.
15. Heine did not recognise the contagious nature of the disease. Even during relatively large outbreaks of polio in Europe during the second half of the nineteenth century,

teething, stomach upset, and trauma were usually described as the cause of the illness. It was finally recognised as an infectious disease after epidemics in Europe in the 1880. See e.g. JR Paul, *A history of poliomyelitis*, Yale University Press, New Haven, 1971.

16 R Patrick, *A history of health and medicine in Queensland*, p. 238.
17 Philip Drinker and Louis Shaw developed the iron lung in 1928. It was a large metal tank equipped with a pump to assist respiration. The iron lung went into commercial production in 1931. An epidemic in New York in 1916 affected thousands of children and some adults; widespread panic ensued.
18 R Patrick, *A history of health and medicine in Queensland*, p. 237; the *Brisbane Courier*, 25 January 1932, p. 12.
19 JH Pearn, *To Teach the Sick*, Amphion Press, Brisbane [Herston], 2009, p. 55.
20 H Gregory and MJ Thearle, 'Child abuse in nineteenth century Queensland', paper presented at 6th International Congress on Child Abuse and Neglect, Sydney, 1986, Pergamon Press, Sydney, 1988.
21 For background on Ireland in this period, see A Jackson, *Ireland 1798–1998*, Blackwell, Oxford, 1999; R Dudley Edwards, *Daniel O'Connell and his world*, Thames and Hudson, London, 1975; RB McDowell, *Public opinion and government policy in Ireland, 1801–1846*, Studies in Irish History, vol. 5, Faber and Faber, London, 1952; N Davis, *The Isles: A history*, Macmillan, London, 1999.
22 For more information on the early Sisters of Mercy, see MB Degnan, *Mercy unto thousands*, Browne and Nolan, Dublin, 1958, pp. 20, 25–7.
23 Committees of women in Brisbane also established the Women's Refuge, which sheltered destitute and abused women, and the Brisbane Servant's Home to care for young women immigrants 'of good character' to train them for work as servants in affluent households.
24 Degnan, *Mercy unto thousands* p. 54; R Longhurst, *In the footsteps of the Mercies: A History of Nursing at the Mater Misericordiae Public Hospitals, Brisbane*, Mater Misericordiae Hospitals, Brisbane, 1992, pp. 15–17; B Abel Smith, *The Hospitals 1800–1948*, Heinemann, London, 1964.
25 Untrained male orderlies cared for patients in British military hospitals; they were described as 'worn out pensioners' in a scathing report in the London *Times*. William Howard Russell in the *Times*, quoted in E Bolster, *The Sisters of Mercy in the Crimean War*, Mercier, Cork, 1964, p. 11.
26 After her term as Superior at Baggot Street, Mother Vincent regularly sought permission to join a Mercy venture overseas. It was, she said, 'the real desire of my heart', which she had held for 20 years. Mother Vincent to Reverend Mother, 14 July 1860, 15 November 1860, Sisters of Mercy, *Mercy women making history: From the pen of Mother Vincent Whitty*, Congregation of the Sisters of Mercy, Brisbane, 2001, p. 1.
27 CK Killerby, *Ursula Frayne: A biography*, University of Notre Dame, Perth, 1996, pp. 172, 239.
28 The Mater Misericordiae Hospital in Dublin opened in 1861.
29 The Sisters took charge of St Stephen's school in the city.
30 Mother Vincent constantly worried about the debt on Adderton. The debt was a great problem in a poor society without, as Mother Vincent expressed it, 'government aid for anything'. Mother Vincent to Reverend Mother, 19 October 1863, in *Mercy women making history*, p. 72.
31 Even the modest rental of £5 per week for Aubigny worried Mother Patrick. Mother Patrick to Dottie, 27 February 1906, Letters from Mother Patrick Potter to GW Gray, Mother Patrick Potter collection, Sisters of Mercy Congregational Archives (SOMCA).
32 C Maggs, *The origins of general nursing*, Croom Helm, London, 1983, p. 63.
33 The Dublin Mater, for instance, earned valuable income by hiring out many of its nurses to private patients. E Nolan, *One hundred years: A history of the School of Nursing and of developments at Mater Misericordiae Hospital 1891–1991*, Sisters of Mercy, Dublin, 1991, p. 16.
34 Mother Mary de Chantal RSM, 'The Mater Private Hospital story', unpublished manuscript, MAHC; *History of the Movement for the establishment of the Mater Misericordiae Hospital from 1 January 1906–31 October 1911*, Sapsford & Co., Brisbane, n.d., MAHC; *The Mater Misericordiae Hospital's Illustrated Publication*, Innes Millbank,

Brisbane, 1934, p. 3; H Summers, *They crossed the river*, pp. 4–14; R Longhurst, *In the footsteps of the Mercies*, p. 26.

35 An early patient, Sister Mary Consilio's mother, insisted on the new Mater. Dr Lilian Cooper was her doctor. Initially very reluctant, as she feared that the Mater staff was not adequately trained, Dr Cooper overcame her concerns and became one of the early Mater's strongest supporters. L Williams, *No easy path: The life and times of Lilian Violet Cooper, MD, FRACS (1861–1947), Australia's first woman surgeon*, Amphion Press, Brisbane [Herston], 1991, p. 41.

36 The *Brisbane Courier*, 4 January 1906, p. 2, 5 January 1906, p. 2.

37 H Gregory and C Brazil, *Bearers of the tradition: Nurses of the Royal Brisbane Hospital, 1888–1993*, Boolarong, Brisbane [Bowen Hills], 1993, p. 3. The year of the award of Sister Mary Antonia Brosnan's certificate was taken from the official records of the Royal Brisbane Hospital.

38 Mother Mary de Chantal RSM, 'The Mater Hospital story', unpublished manuscript, MAHC.

Chapter 2

1 The *Brisbane Courier*, 24 May 1926, p. 7.

2 For more information on Gray, see B Crouchley, 'George Wilkie Gray', *Australian Dictionary of Biography*, Vol. 9, MUP, Melbourne, 1983, pp. 84–5. The family firm, Quinlan Gray & Co. amalgamated with the Victorian Fitzgerald family business. Castlemaine Brewery and Quinlan Gray & Co established a brewery at Milton in Brisbane. Gray was an entrepreneur with investments ranging from schooners in the 1860s Brisbane–Ipswich river trade, the Bendigo pottery, land in Melbourne and the Queensland sugar industry. He became a director of leading Queensland companies, such as the Queensland National Bank and the *Daily Mail* newspaper and persuaded the government to extend scholarship benefits to Catholic schoolchildren so they could enjoy the same subsidy for secondary education as state school children.

3 Mater Public Hospital Annual Report, 1924, Mater Archives and Heritage Centre (MAHC); Thynne and Macartney to Reverend Mother Patrick, 26 June 1918, Mater Children's Hospital files, MAHC.

4 The *Brisbane Courier*, 15 May 1926, p. 17. The Mater Children's Hospital was to be connected to the Mater Adult Hospital, but to have its own kitchen and other essential services.

5 The *Brisbane Courier*, 24 May 1926, p. 11.

6 The *Brisbane Courier*, 24 May 1926, p. 7.

7 Estimate published in article on 1926 Mater Ball, the *Brisbane Courier*, 5 June 1926, p. 20.

8 The *Brisbane Courier*, 20 May 1925, p. 20.

9 The *Brisbane Courier*, 26 September 1925, cutting file, Mater Children's Hospital, 1926–1970, MAHC.

10 Convenors included the Lady Mayoress, Lillie Jolly; the widow of a former Premier, Mrs TJ Ryan; the President of the All Hallows' Past Pupils Association, Mrs McKenna; and Mrs HJ Windsor, wife of a senior surgeon at the Mater Adult Hospital, The *Brisbane Courier*, 21 November 1926, p. 17.

11 The *Brisbane Courier*, 20 November 1925, p. 10; *Catholic Advocate*, 26 November 1926, p. 21, cutting file, Mater Children's Hospital, 1926–1970, MAHC.

12 Ticket enclosed in letter, CF Bagley to Mother Patrick, 16 October 1926, Art Unions file, MAHC.

13 P Hall, *Royal Children's Hospital Brisbane, 1878–1978: A century of care*, Royal Children's Hospital, Brisbane [Herston], 1978, p. 46.

14 The *Brisbane Courier*, 28 June 1926, p. 13, 27 November 1926; p. 19, *Daily Standard*, 15 May 1926, cutting file, Mater Children's Hospital, 1926–1970, MAHC.

15 The *Brisbane Courier*, 5 June 1926, p. 20.

16 The *Queenslander*, 7 July 1927, pp. 26–27; the *Brisbane Courier*, 30 June 1927, p. 18.

17 The *Brisbane Courier*, 1 July 1927, pp. 18, 19. There was a large photograph of the debutantes in the *Brisbane Courier* on 7 July 1927, p. 27.

Endnotes

18 J Hogan, 'Hall, Thomas Ramsay (1879–1950)', *Australian Dictionary of Biography*, National Centre of Biography, Australian National University, http://adb.anu.edu.au/biography/hall-thomas-ramsay-7055/text11205, accessed 30 December 2011.
19 Sister Mary St Pierre McCormack, 'Mater Misericordiae Children's Hospital', typescript, Mater Sisters of Mercy L–M, MAHC.
20 Mater Annual Report, 1926–27, MAHC, refers to excavations for the foundations.
21 Report of 1928 Annual General Meeting, the *Brisbane Courier*, 31 October 1928, p. 23.
22 R Evans, *A History of Queensland*, Cambridge University Press, Cambridge, 2007, pp. 180–2. At 19 per cent, Queensland's unemployment rate during the Depression was 10 per cent below the Australian average.
23 Mater Annual Report, 1928, MAHC.
24 The *Brisbane Courier*, 8 May 1931, p. 6.
25 Mater Annual Report, 1931, MAHC.
26 Sister Mary St Pierre McCormack, 'Mater Misericordiae Children's Hospital', typescript, MAHC.
27 F Hagelthorn, the *Catholic Leader*, 14 May 1931, p. 19.
28 Mater Children's Hospital, first Annual Report, 1932–33, MAHC.
29 The centenary of the foundation of the Sisters of Mercy was 10 December 1931; the *Brisbane Courier*, 25 April 1931, p. 3.
30 Sir John was seen frequently at the Mater during his years in office and, in 1928, the year after his arrival in Queensland, had opened Queensland's first cancer clinic at the Mater Adult Hospital. For further information on Sir John, see P & S Forrest, *All for Queensland: The Governors and the people*, Shady Tree, Darwin, 2009, pp. 193–200.
31 The *Brisbane Courier*, 11 May 1931, p. 10.
32 The *Brisbane Courier*, 8 May 1931, p. 6.
33 P Hall, *A century of care*, pp. 54–5.
34 F Hagelthorn, the *Catholic Leader*, 14 May 1931, p. 19.
35 ibid.
36 ibid.
37 The *Brisbane Courier*, 8 May 1931, p. 6.
38 ibid.
39 HJ Windsor, 'The Australian memoirs of Dr HJ Windsor, 1914–1976', manuscript, MAHC.
40 From data on Mater Sisters, MAHC.
41 Mater Children's Hospital, first Annual Report, 1932–33, MAHC.
42 Sister Mary St Pierre McCormack, 'Mater Misericordiae Children's Hospital', MAHC.
43 ibid.
44 J Pearn, *Focus and innovation: A history of paediatric education in Queensland*, Amphion Press, Brisbane [Herston], 1986, pp. 209–301.
45 MJ Thearle, 'Meehan, Arthur Vincent (1890–1955)', *Australian Dictionary of Biography*, National Centre of Biography, Australian National University, http://adb.anu.edu.au/biography/meehan-arthur-vincent-11103/text19767, accessed 10 January 2012; M Gallagher, *A history of orthopaedics at the Mater Misericordiae Hospitals*, Boolarong, Brisbane, 2004, pp. 2–11. During World War II, AV Meehan was consultant to the Australian Military Forces and the Royal Australian Air Force and orthopaedic surgeon at the 112th Base Hospital, Greenslopes.
46 Obituary, JRS Lahz, *Med J Aust*, 26 March 1960; Mater Public Hospital Annual Report, 1959–1960, p. 15, MAHC.
47 Mater Children's Hospital, first Annual Report, 1932–33, MAHC.
48 ibid.
49 ibid.
50 Dr ES Jackson, cited in BLW Clarke, 'Foundation of cancer treatment in Queensland', *Med J Aust*, 20 December 1969, pp. 1271–4.
51 Sister Kenny opened her first clinic in Townsville in 1932. R Patrick, *A history of health and medicine in Queensland 1824–1960*, UQP, Brisbane, 1987, pp. 238–9; the *Brisbane Courier*, 12 January 1932, p. 9.
52 M Gallagher, *A history of orthopaedics at the Mater Misericordiae hospitals*, pp. 7–8; Sister Gertrude Mary Lyons, Sisters of Mercy L–M file, MAHC.

53 Sister Marie Fitzgerald, speech at the Mater Children's Hospital Golden Jubilee celebrations, Sisters of Mercy staff writings, MAHC.
54 Mater Children's Hospital, first Annual Report, 1932–33, MAHC.
55 For more information on Montrose Home, which admitted its first patients in December 1933, see H Gregory, *MontroseAccess: A history*, MontroseAccess, Brisbane, 2011.
56 Sister Mary St Pierre McCormack, 'Mater Misericordiae Children's Hospital', MAHC.
57 ibid.
58 Sister Marie Fitzgerald's speech at the 69th birthday celebrations of the Mater Children's Hospital, Sisters of Mercy file, MAHC; Stories by Sister Germaine Greathead and 'Justine', http://www.mater.org.au/Home/Hospitals/Mater-Children-s-Hospital/Farewell-Mater-Children-s-Hospital/MCH-Reflections, accessed 10 October 2013.
59 The Sisters believed that aligning the terms of honorary medical officer appointments at the Mater Children's and Adult hospitals was the best way to manage their complex public health-care responsibilities in the trying economic climate of the 1930s when the two hospitals shared many doctors, including the radiologist, Dr BLW Clarke; the urologist, Dr Stanley Roe; and the pathologist, Dr George Taylor. A letter from Mother Alban informed the doctors that appointments of all honorary staff terminated on 30 June 1934, but all honoraries would be reappointed until further notice 'to enable the appointment and the Mater Public [Adult] and Mater Children's hospital to be brought into line at a future date'. Draft letter, Mother Alban to Medical Board, 3 June 1933, Correspondence re establishment of Advisory Board, 0030/001, MAHC; Mater Public Hospital Annual Report, 1935, MAHC.
60 Mother Alban to Medical Board, 1 September 1933, cited in Minutes, Meetings of Honorary Board, 12 September 1930–5 November 1936. MAHC.
61 The Act established hospital districts throughout Queensland, each of which would be controlled by a district hospital board. However, the district to be controlled by the Brisbane and South Coast Hospitals Board was the only district proclaimed initially.
62 Dr Ellis Murphy, chairman of the medical board, wrote that 'I consider that the Advisory Board will be most representative and if they meet with your approval I am sure that a new era of progress and peace will ensue'. Murphy to Mother Alban, 20 May 1933, Correspondence re establishment of Advisory Board, 0030/001, MAHC.
63 Minutes of Honorary Board, 25 August 1936, Meetings of Honorary Board, 16 May 1912–22 August 1930, MAHC. All board terms were to be one year.
64 Dr English to Dr Ralph Weaver, 12 July 1937, Correspondence re establishment of Advisory Board, 20 May 1933–23 June 1937, 0030/001, MAHC.
65 Mother Alban's letter to all staff laying down policy, 17 June 1937, Correspondence re establishment of Advisory Board, 20 May 1933, 0030/001, MAHC.
66 Dr Hemsley, first resident medical officer to be appointed at the Mater Public Hospital, to Mother Alban, 9 March 1938, MAHC.
67 Circular to staff, 9 March 1938, in reply to Hemsley to Mother Alban, 25 February 1938, Correspondence re establishment of Advisory Board, 0030/001, MAHC. Mother Alban wrote to JC Hemsley 'the planned position is that the Administration has checked an attempt by the Honorary Staff to proceed from co-operation to control of the Mater Misericordiae Public [Adult] Hospital'. This, she was aware, would not be tolerated in any public hospital.
68 At a meeting at BMA House on 11 March, Drs Hoare, Ahern, Roe, Foxton, Macartney, Reye, Macdonald, Betchel, Geaney, Foote, Taylor, Maclean, Kelley and Hemsley thanked the Sisters for appreciation of their services and said 'it has at all times been an honour and a pleasure to them to co-operate with the Sisters of Mercy in the relief of suffering', but continued that they couldn't continue their services under a conjoint board. JC Hemsley to Salmon, 12 March 1938; Horace Johnson, Hon Sec BMA Qld, to 'Administration', 9 April 1938, offering BMA's assistance in mediating the dispute. Sisters of Mercy to BMA, 11 April 1938, 'I regret to inform you the matter in dispute, within the ambit of which were principles from which the Sisters of Mercy will not deviate, is not one which admits of arbitration or mediation', Correspondence re establishment of Advisory Board 0030/001, MAHC.
69 The *Courier-Mail*, 4 April 1938, p. 3, 5 April 1938, p. 3, 15 September 1938, p. 2; the *Telegraph*, 2 April 1938, p. 1.

70 Sister Mercia Mary Higgins, 'Mater Public [Adult] Hospital', typescript, 1962, Sisters of Mercy staff writings, MAHC.
71 Minutes of Honorary Board, 1 November 1935, Meetings of Honorary Board, 12 September 1930–5 November 1936, MAHC. The subcommittee recommended an alternative to the public service contribution scheme.
72 Recommendations of subcommittee, Minutes, Medical Board, 1 November 1935, MAHC; Meetings of Honorary Board, 16 May 1912–22 August 1930, MAHC. The doctors also suggested that the Mater adopt the Victorian Charities Board Schedule for assessing public hospital patients.
73 Minutes of Honorary Board, 15 November 1935, Meetings of Honorary Board, 12 September 1930–5 November 1936, MAHC. It was suggested that 10 per cent of the professional fees collected from intermediate patients be set aside in a separate fund to defray operating theatre expenses and to purchase scientific equipment.
74 The *Courier-Mail*, 2 November 1933, p. 12, 9 November 1933, p. 9. The Public Service Assistance Fund, which had caused such angst, raised £1,200 for the hospitals, Mater Annual Report, 1935, MAHC.
75 See, for example, articles about the Mater Ball and the debutantes, the *Courier-Mail*, 20 June 1933, pp. 18–19; a bridge benefit for Mater Children's Hospital, the *Courier-Mail*, 9 November 1933, p. 16; three hostesses having a party for the Mater Children's Hospital, the *Courier-Mail*, 14 November 1933, p. 17. The Sisters at All Hallows' raised £391/7/4, of which £300 came from street collections, Mater Children's Hospital, first Annual Report, 1932–33, MAHC.
76 Sister Mary St Pierre McCormack, 'Mater Misericordiae Children's Hospital', MAHC.
77 The *Courier-Mail*, 6 August 1936, p. 13.
78 The altar was donated by Mrs Martin Crane, the chalice by relatives of Sister Mary Marcelline, a ciborium in memory of Mary Kidner, altar linens, vestments, set of Stations of the Cross from the Smith family and a Communion tray from Monsignor Molony.

Chapter 3

1 PA Earnshaw, letter of condolence, 8 January 1972, Mater Sisters of Mercy file L–M, Mater Archives and Heritage Centre (MAHC).
2 Mater Sisters of Mercy file L–M, MAHC.
3 PA Earnshaw wrote of Sister Mary St Aidan, 'Her work was exemplary whether it was in her management of the ward, her attention, and concern of individual patients, and her instruction of the Nursing Staff ... I knew of none better'; Sister Mary St Pierre McCormack, Mater Misericordiae Children's Hospital, typescript, Sisters of Mercy L–M file, MAHC.
4 The *Courier-Mail*, 3 January 1941, p. 11.
5 Mater Children's 1926–1986 file, Box 146: Mater Public Hospital, Sisters of Mercy Congregational Archives (SOMCA).
6 Minutes of Advisory Board, 27 October 1944, Minutes Mater Public Hospitals Advisory Board 1938–1956, MAHC.
7 J Pearn, *Focus and Innovation. A history of paediatric education in Queensland*, Amphion Press, Brisbane [Herston], 1986, pp. 303–4.
8 Sister Mary Dorothea Sheehan, Eulogy for Sister Mary St Pierre, MAHC. In her retirement, Sister Mary St Pierre assisted the Superior at the Mater Convent and helped to maintain the medical records at the Mater Adult Hospital.
9 McCormack file, Mater Sisters of Mercy file L–M, MAHC. Her sister, Lily, Sister Mary Mathias, had entered earlier.
10 Minutes of Advisory Board, 27 October 1944, Minutes Mater Public Hospitals Advisory Board 1938–1956, MAHC.
11 ibid.
12 ibid.
13 Minutes of Advisory Board, 27 October 1944, Minutes Mater Public Hospitals Advisory Board 1938–1956, MAHC; M Gallagher, *A history of orthopaedics at the Mater Misericordiae Hospitals*, Boolarong, Brisbane, 2004, pp. 24–25.

14 *Hospital Benefits Act (Commonwealth) 1945*.
15 Minutes of Advisory Board, 27 October 1944, Minutes Mater Public Hospitals Advisory Board 1938–1956, MAHC.
16 The *Courier-Mail*, 1 January 1946, p. 3
17 Mater Doctors file A–D, MAHC.
18 Minutes of Advisory Board, 7 March 1949, 6 November 1950, Minutes Mater Public Hospitals Advisory Board 1938–1956, MAHC.
19 Minutes of Advisory Board, 22 June 1946, Minutes Mater Public Hospitals Advisory Board 1938–1956, MAHC.
20 David Jackson began tertiary study at the University of Queensland and, in 1932, enrolled in Medicine at the University of Melbourne. He lived at Trinity College, entering fully into the life of that college in rowing and as editor of its journal and later established a bequest to allow other 'Churchie' students to study in Melbourne and live at Trinity College.
21 *Worcester* blocked the path of the German battleships *Scharnhorst, Gneisenau* and the *Prinz Eugen*, a heavy cruiser, which were trying to leave Brest harbour.
22 R Eastgate, College Roll, David Clements Jackson, https://www.racp.edu.au/page/library/college-roll/college-roll-detail&id=546, accessed 10 January 2012. Jackson's publications included *The discovery of childhood: A paediatric triad; One ship, one company: The story of H.M.S. "Worcester" 1650–1950; The six horseshoes: Memoirs of a personal and professional life*.
23 DC Jackson to Matron, Minutes of Advisory Board, 22 April 1949, Minutes Mater Public Hospitals Advisory Board 1938–1956, MAHC.
24 ibid.
25 Board secretary to Jackson, Minutes of Advisory Board, 4 October 1949, Minutes Mater Public Hospitals Advisory Board 1938–1956, MAHC. Many ear, nose and throat patients requiring surgery were usually seen first by PA Earnshaw.
26 Lahz to administration, Minutes of Advisory Board, 29 June 1949, Minutes Mater Public Hospitals Advisory Board 1938–1956, MAHC.
27 Minutes of Advisory Board, 2 October 1950, Minutes Mater Public Hospitals Advisory Board 1938–1956, MAHC.
28 DC Jackson's letter to Matron, Minutes of Advisory Board, 22 April 1949, Minutes Mater Public Hospitals Advisory Board 1938–1956, Minutes of Advisory Board, 4 August 1952, MAHC.
29 The *Brisbane Courier*, 11 May 1931, p. 10.
30 Minutes of Advisory Board, 1 August 1949, Minutes Mater Public Hospitals Advisory Board 1938–1956, MAHC. The Sisters did not agree that the university should veto the appointment of staff members it believed would be unsuited to teaching students.
31 Correspondence re establishment of Advisory Board, 20 May 1933, 0030/001, MAHC.
32 The Mater was also completing its application for approval to train surgical registrars for admission to the Royal Australasian College of Surgeons.
33 The *Courier-Mail*, 2 September 1947, p. 3.
34 The *Courier-Mail*, 11 December 1951, p. 2, 1 October 1953, p. 3. The problem persisted and, in 1953, the Queensland Medical Research Council warned in its Annual Report that vigilance to ensure that healthy milk was distributed and properly stored was essential.
35 The *Courier-Mail*, 5 January 1952, p. 1; *Maryborough Herald*, 26 July 2006, p. 15.
36 The *Courier-Mail*, 22 October 1954, p. 3.
37 The *Courier-Mail*, 27 November 1950, p. 3, 1 September 1954, p. 1.
38 The *Courier-Mail*, 1 June 1954, p. 1.
39 The *Courier-Mail*, 15 June 1954, p. 1.
40 The *Courier-Mail*, 7 July 1951, p. 4.
41 Letter to editor from BMA Member, the *Courier-Mail*, 17 July 1953, p. 2.
42 The 1943 amendments created a power to declare certain hospitals as medical schools.
43 The *Courier-Mail*, 18 February 1936, p. 13. At the same time, there were plans to extend the Mater Private Hospital with advice from the specialist hospital architects, Stephenson, Meldrum, and Turner, of Sydney.
44 R Patrick, *A history of health and medicine in Queensland 1824-1960*, UQP, Brisbane, 1987, pp. 378–9.

45 HJ Summers, 'The hospitals on Mater Hill', the *Courier-Mail*, 13 May 1952, p. 2.
46 In 1950, for instance, the Mater Ball at Cloudland, richly decorated with jonquils and roses from the Darling Downs, added considerably to the Mater Mothers' Hospital appeal funds: the *Courier-Mail*, 25 May 1950, p. 8.
47 Minutes of Advisory Board, 17 March 1947, Minutes Mater Public Hospitals Advisory Board 1938–1956, MAHC.
48 Minutes of Advisory Board, 3 April 1950, 11 December 1950, Minutes Mater Public Hospitals Advisory Board 1938–1956, MAHC.
49 Sister Mary Colette Anderson, Sisters of Mercy file A–D, MAHC.
50 Minutes of Advisory Board, 23 June 1951, 21 April 1952, Minutes Mater Public Hospitals Advisory Board 1938–1956, MAHC.
51 Minutes of Advisory Board, 2 March 1953, Minutes Mater Public Hospitals Advisory Board 1938–1956, MAHC.
52 Lahz to Sister Mary St Gabriel, Administrator, Mater Public Hospitals, 1 October 1954, MAHC.
53 Orthopaedic Department (Lahz, McSweeny and Gallagher) to Board, 10 September 1956, MAHC.
54 Minutes of Advisory Board, 21 February 1955, Minutes Mater Public Hospitals Advisory Board 1938–1956, MAHC.
55 Mater Misericordiae Public Hospitals Annual Report, 1958–59, MAHC.
56 ibid.

Chapter 4

1 Mater Annual Report, 1967–68, Mater Archives and Heritage Centre (MAHC).
2 Australian Bureau of Statistics, Australian historical population statistics, cat. no. 3105.0.65001, Table 18, Population capital cities and balance of states and territories, 30 June 1901 onwards, www.abs.gov.au, accessed 18 February 2014.
3 JP Kelly, Chairman's Report, Mater Advisory Board Annual Report, 1959–60, MAHC. In its first five months, 425 babies were born at the Mater Mothers' Hospital.
4 JP Kelly, Chairman's Report, Mater Advisory Board Annual Report, 1959–60, MAHC.
5 ibid.
6 JP Kelly, Chairman's Report, Mater Advisory Board Annual Report, 1963–64, MAHC.
7 JP Kelly, Chairman's Report, Mater Advisory Board Annual Report, 1965–66, MAHC.
8 Sister Mary St Pierre McCormack, Report of the ICN Conference, 1961, MAHC.
9 JP Kelly, Chairman's Report, Mater Advisory Board Annual Report, 1963–64, MAHC.
10 Both boards were chaired by JP Kelly. The Medical Board included representatives of the University of Queensland.
11 After two years at St Bartholomew's Hospital and as house surgeon to TG Illtyd James, M Chir, FRCS, senior surgeon and director of the neurosurgical unit at the Central Middlesex Hospital, Brian Purssey worked as senior casualty officer at St Mary Abbot's Hospital in London for six months in 1955, where he had considerable experience in emergency surgery, as well as general surgery. During his time in England, he also worked as a surgical registrar at Queen Alexandra Hospital, Portsmouth; Solihull Hospital; and Little Bromwich Hospital; and in orthopaedics at the Rowley Bristow Orthopaedic Hospital in Surrey. HA Hegerty to Registrar, University of Queensland, 15 December 1958, Mother General to Purssey, 4 December 1958, Purssey to Mother Damian, 7 December 1961, Doctors file L–R, MAHC.
12 ED O'Callaghan, application for Director of Medical Services, 25 January 1962, Doctors file N–R, MAHC.
13 In 1958, the paediatrician Dr Geoffrey Bourke had recommended a separate committee for the Mater Children's Hospital, so that it had direct access to the administration. Discussion on the future of Mater Children's Hospital as a paediatric centre, March 1958, Dr Geoffrey Bourke's files, MAHC.
14 Doctors file A–D, MAHC; the *Telegraph*, 23 March 1971, Press clippings, MAHC.

15 Discussion on the future of Mater Children's Hospital as a paediatric centre, March 1958, Dr Geoffrey Bourke's files, MAHC.
16 JP Kelly, Chairman's Report, Mater Advisory Board Annual Report, 1960–61, MAHC.
17 B Purssey, Director of Medical Services Report, Mater Advisory Board Annual Report, 1960–61, MAHC.
18 Minutes of Medical Advisory Board, 6 March 1961 and 8 May 1961, Box 150, Sisters of Mercy Congregational Archives (SOMCA).
19 J Pearn, *Focus and innovation: A history of paediatric education in Queensland*, Amphion Press, Brisbane [Herston], 1986, pp. 165–72.
20 Professor Rendle-Short recommended that a space near out-patients would be the best location for the medical records section, which might also need to make provision for microfilm.
21 Sister Mary St Pierre McCormack's journal and press clippings, Mater Chronicles, 1962–68, MAHC.
22 H Gregory, *MontroseAccess: A History*, MontroseAccess, Brisbane, 2011; J Pearn, *To Teach the Sick: The hospital schools of Queensland*, Amphion Press, Brisbane [Herston], 2009. The 1950–53 polio epidemic was the most severe. 1,200 cases were reported by 1952, with an 8 per cent fatality rate. A special polio school opened at the Wattlebrae Infectious Diseases Hospital with the teacher Rowland Griffiths, who had contracted the disease in 1951.
23 J Pearn, *To Teach the Sick*, pp. 38, 51, 59.
24 J Pearn, *To Teach the Sick*, pp. xix, xx.
25 Director-General of Education to JJ O'Brien, 10 October 1962, File 9, MCH – staff, Box 143, SOMCA.
26 Sister Mary St Pierre's journal and press clippings, Mater Chronicles, 1962–68, MAHC.
27 Entry, 14 December 1967, Sister Mary St Pierre's journal and press clippings, Mater Chronicles, 1962–68, MAHC. Joy Engwicht, the teacher in 1967, organised a grand break-up celebration. The Matron, Sister Mary St Pierre admired the teachers and the 'special vocation' they demonstrated.
28 Rendle-Short to JJ O'Brien, Secretary, Mater Advisory Board, 11 October 1962, MCH 1926–86 file, Box 146, SOMCA; 'The Blessing of our new Mater Children's Hospitals, 16 May 2001', commemorative booklet, 2001, MAHC.
29 Sister Mary St Gabriel to Mother General, File 9, MCH staff, Box 143, SOMCA.
30 Sister Marie Fitzgerald, 'An overview of paediatric nursing practice', MAHC.
31 The other projects on the books were an extension of the adult hospital to provide 105 additional beds, a new operating theatre block and new X-ray and pathology departments, a new wing at the Mater Private Hospital and a convalescent and terminal care hospital to provide 100 beds, Mater Advisory Board Annual Report, 1964–65, MAHC.
32 JP Kelly to Editor, the *Courier-Mail*, 16 May 1962, Press clippings, MAHC.
33 Mater Advisory Board Annual Report, 1961–62, MAHC.
34 Mater Advisory Board Annual Report, 1960–61, MAHC.
35 Mater Advisory Board Annual Report, 1965–66, MAHC.
36 Sister Mary St Pierre McCormack's journal and press clippings, Mater Chronicles, 1962–68, MAHC.
37 Mater Advisory Board Annual Report, 1964–65, MAHC.
38 Mater Advisory Board Annual Report, 1965–66. MAHC. The total cost was $97,708 and the state subsidy was $48,854.
39 Sister Mary St Pierre approved of the Chapel changes, particularly the refurbishment of the St Joseph statue who 'came back wearing an attractive mauve gown and cream cloak. He looks a youthful figure'. Sister Mary St Pierre McCormack's journal and press clippings, Mater Chronicles, 1962–68, MAHC.
40 Director of Medical Services Report, Mater Advisory Board Annual Report, 1966–67, MAHC.
41 Mater Advisory Board annual reports, 1965–66, 1966–67, MAHC.
42 DC Jackson, Mater Children's Hospital Honorary Medical Staff Society Report, Mater Advisory Board Annual Report, 1966–67, MAHC.
43 Sister Mary St Pierre's journal and press clippings, Mater Chronicles, 1962–68, MAHC.

44 Entry, 27 June 1965, Sister Mary St Pierre's journal and press clippings, Mater Chronicles, 1962–68, MAHC.
45 Mater Misericordiae Public Hospitals, Study of Community attitudes and analysis of financial resources, Confidential Report, Compton Associates, 1969, p. 1, Box 145, SOMCA.

Chapter 5

1 Sister Angela Mary Doyle, *Mercy, Mater & me: Sister Angela Mary (a memoir)*, UQP, Brisbane, 2010, p. 78.
2 The division between old and new nurseries was removed on 30 June 1967, and the move into the new nursery was completed on 3 July 1967, leaving the old babies' ward available for reconstruction.
3 Mater Sisters E–K, Mater Archives and Heritage Centre (MAHC).
4 Patricia Mexted (nee Mahony), 14 October 1991, Interviews and documents collected for *In the footsteps of the Mercies*, MAHC.
5 PA Earnshaw to Sister Mary Mechtilde, 29 December 1961, Medical E–I, MAHC. Dr Earnshaw enclosed a cheque for 'some small item in your ward that you would like to replace'.
6 Instructions for nurses kept by Sister Mary St Pierre, Mater Children's Hospital Records, Box 2, MAHC.
7 Mater Past Nurses Association (MPNA) Newsletter, Vol. 1, No. 1, May 1965. In 1964, there were 9 Sisters of Mercy, 10 full-time lay trained sisters, 8 part-time lay trained sisters, 61 student nurses and 14 nursing aides. The lay staff included Sister Joan Geyer, Sister Tephting Arkfun, Sister Janet Orr, Sister Sheila Carroll, Sister Nancy Nolan, Sister Nanette Flynn, Sister Bettie Kennedy, Sister Jan Thynne, Sister Carmel McCormack and Sister Diane Rigby.
8 Sister Mary St Pierre's journal and press clippings, Mater Chronicles, 1962–68, MAHC.
9 R Longhurst, *In the footsteps of the Mercies: A history of nursing at the Mater Misericordiae hospitals*, Brisbane, 1992, p. 95.
10 Sister Administrator's Report, Mater Advisory Board Annual Report, 1963–64, MAHC; R Longhurst, *In the footsteps of the Mercies*, p. 95.
11 Sister Administrator's Report, Mater Advisory Board Annual Report, 1963–64, MAHC.
12 Patricia Mexted (nee Mahony), 14 October 1991, Interviews and documents collected for *In the footsteps of the Mercies*, MAHC.
13 Chairman's Report, Mater Advisory Board Annual Report, 1961–62, MAHC.
14 Sister Mary St Pierre's journal and press clippings, Mater Chronicles, 1962–68, MAHC. The pool and squash court cost £50,000, paid by the Sisters of Mercy, Mater Advisory Board Annual Report, 1966–67.
15 Sister Mary St Pierre's journal and press clippings, Mater Chronicles, 1962–68, MAHC.
16 Director of Medical Services Report, Mater Advisory Board Annual Report, 1959–60, MAHC.
17 Sister Mary St Pierre's journal and press clippings, Mater Chronicles, 1962–68, MAHC.
18 Director of Medical Services Report, Mater Advisory Board Annual Report, 1964–65, MAHC.
19 Entry, 24 February 1969, Sister Mary St Pierre's journal 1968–79, MAHC.
20 Minutes of Advisory Board, 2 May 1962, Mater Public Hospitals Advisory Board, Box 150, Sisters of Mercy Congregational Archives (SOMCA).
21 Minutes of Advisory Board, 7 October 1963, Mater Public Hospitals Advisory Board, Box 150, SOMCA.
22 K Wilkinson, J Craig, J Bourke, Anaesthetic Registrars, to ED O'Callaghan, Director of Medical Services, 27 April 1962, Box 146, SOMCA.
23 ibid.
24 Sister Mary St Pierre's journal and press clippings, Mater Chronicles, 1962–68, MAHC. Dr Tess Brophy, one of the honorary anaesthetists, was appointed to the Faculty of the College of Anaesthetists, the first Queensland anaesthetist to achieve this distinction.

25 Minutes of Children's Hospital Committee, 23 September 1964, Mater Public Hospitals miscellaneous file, 1911–86, Box 146, SOMCA.
26 Alexander Inglis, Director of Medical Services, 30 September 1964, Mater Public Hospitals miscellaneous file, 1911–86, Box 146, SOMCA.
27 Toakley to Director of Medical Services, 28 September 1964, Box 146, SOMCA.
28 Stephen Suggit to ED O'Callaghan, Director of Medical Services, 25 September 1964, Mater Children's 1926–1986 file, Box 146, SOMCA.
29 Stephen Suggit to ED O'Callaghan, Director of Medical Services, 25 September 1964, Dr EF McGuinness to Director of Medical Services on 23 September 1964, Mater Public Hospitals miscellaneous files, 1911–86, Box 146, SOMCA.
30 Toakley to Director of Medical Services, 24 September 1964, JG Hynes to Director of Medical Services, 25 September 1964, A Inglis to Director of Medical Services, 18 September 1964, Mater Public Hospitals miscellaneous files, 1911–86, Box 146, SOMCA. The specialists also reminded the administration that teaching duties used material from both hospitals in most specialties.
31 University of Queensland Registrar to Mater administration, 31 December 1964, Mater Public Hospitals Advisory Board, Box 150, SOMCA.
32 Minutes of Advisory Board, 7 October 1963, Mater Public Hospitals Advisory Board, Box 150, SOMCA.
33 L Swiss Davies, plastic surgeon, to Reverend Mother, 3 September 1966. Medical A–D, MAHC.
34 Statistics Mater Children's Hospital, Director of Medical Services, Mater Advisory Board Annual Report, 1964–65, MAHC.
35 Statistics Mater Children's Hospital, Director of Medical Services, Mater Advisory Board annual reports 1963–64, 1964–65, MAHC.
36 Entry, 19 May 1967, Sister Mary St Pierre's journal and press clippings, MAHC.
37 Entries, 11 August 1965 and 10 August 1970, Sister Mary St Pierre's journal and press clippings, MAHC.
38 Entry, 19 February 1968, Sister Mary St Pierre's journal and press clippings, MAHC.
39 Entries in 1965, Sister Mary St Pierre's journal and press clippings, MAHC.
40 Entries, 2 and 6 September 1967, Sister Mary St Pierre's journal and press clippings, MAHC.
41 Entries, 20 July 1967 and 17 July 1968, Sister Mary St Pierre's journal and press clippings, MAHC.
42 Entry, 16 January 1968, Sister Mary St Pierre's journal and press clippings, MAHC.
43 Entries, 5 June, 31 July 1967, Sister Mary St Pierre's journal and press clippings, MAHC.
44 Entry, 15 August 1969, Sister Mary St Pierre's journal and press clippings, MAHC.
45 Peggy Flenady to Sister Mary Dympna Hoare, 15 June 1966, Sister Mary St Pierre's journal and press clippings, MAHC.
46 Entry, 22 December 1970, Sister Mary St James Slattery's journal and press clippings, MAHC.
47 The *Courier-Mail*, 8 September 1969, Press clippings, MAHC.
48 Entries, 12 August and 6 October 1969, Sister Mary St James Slattery's journal and press clippings, MAHC.

Chapter 6

1 J Rendle-Short, short paper dated 26 November 1970, Blue file, 'Future of Mater Children's Hospital', Mater Archives and Heritage Centre (MAHC).
2 Quoted in P Hall, *Royal Children's Hospital Brisbane 1878–1978: A century of care*, Royal Children's Hospital, Brisbane [Herston], 1978, pp. 69–70.
3 J Rendle-Short, short paper, 'Future of Mater Children's Hospital', MAHC.
4 Dr Alan Dugdale returned to Brisbane in 1972 as senior lecturer in the Mater Children's Hospital unit of the Department of Child Health. For more information on Alan Dugdale, see J Pearn, *Focus and innovation: A history of paediatric education in Queensland*, Amphion Press, Brisbane [Herston], 1986, pp. 211–2, 273–6. The meeting on 27 November 1970 was attended by the Sister Administrator, Sister Angela Mary Doyle; the Mater

Children's Hospital Matron, Sister Mary St Pierre McCormack; the Paediatric Supervisor, Dr John Eckert; the Director of Medical Services, Dr ED O'Callaghan; Board Secretary, JJ O'Brien; Assistant Administrator, P Maguire; and the Mater architect, Harry Chapman, Alan Dugdale presentation, November 1970: Sister Angela Mary Doyle collection, MAHC.

5   S Clark Ryan, 'Thoughts and attitudes of members of honorary medical staff, Mater Children's Hospital', c.1969, Sister Angela Mary Doyle collection, MAHC.
6   Dr J Eckert, 'Mater Children's Hospital, present deficiencies and future needs', 17 November 1970, Sister Angela Mary Doyle collection, MAHC.
7   JR Tiernan to ED O'Callaghan, 26 November 1970, 'Future of Mater Children's Hospital', MAHC.
8   DC Jackson and N Anderson, 22 January 1970, 'Future of Mater Children's Hospital', MAHC; Dr Neville Anderson, 'The Mater Children's Hospital', c.1969, Sister Angela Mary Doyle collection, MAHC.
9   Sister Mary St Pierre, 27 November 1970, 'Future of Mater Children's Hospital', MAHC. A theatre nurse, Sister Geraldine (Mary Tarcissius) Doyle RSM, suggested both a new operating theatre and a second lift.
10 Sister Marie Fitzgerald, 30 November 1970, 'Future of Mater Children's Hospital', MAHC.
11 Dr Tess Brophy to Dr Peter O'Regan, 7 October 1986, Sister of Mercy files, A–D, MAHC.
12 Information on Sister Mary Dorothea from Sister Madonna Josey's eulogy, Sisters' obituaries file, MAHC; L Shields, 'Celebrating nursing achievement: Sister Mary Dorothea Sheehan RSM, 1916–1999'. *Neonatal, Paediatric & Child Health Nursing*, 1999, vol. 2, no. 4, pp. 5–7; the *Catholic Leader*, 15 September 1986, Press clippings, MAHC.
13 Sisters of Mercy files, A–D, MAHC; Mater Health Services Annual Report, 2006, MAHC.
14 Sister Mary Dorothea Sheehan, 27 November 1970, 'Future of Mater Children's Hospital', MAHC.
15 Chapman file, Box 4, Record Store, Mater Health Services.
16 Mater Advisory Board Annual Report, 1970–71, MAHC.
17 Sister Angela Mary to Tooth, 4 March 1971, Department of Health correspondence 1944–75, Box 152, Catholic Health Care file, Sisters of Mercy Congregational Archives (SOMCA).
18 Tooth to Sister Angela Mary, 27 September 1968, Department of Health correspondence 1944–75, Box 152, Catholic Health Care file, SOMCA. The $9,000,000 was made up of $4,000,000 for the Stanley Street block, containing new out-patient department and casualty section, pathology laboratories, a pharmacy, X-ray facilities, a central sterilising department, operating theatres and intensive care unit; $2,500,000 for a Stanley Street ward block containing 160 new in-patient beds; and $2,500,000 on a new nurses home to provide accommodation for 400 trainees.
19 ANZ Bank to O'Brien, Mater executive officer, 2 July 1970, notifying him that the Mater's overdraft had exceeded the $250,000 limit; ANZ Bank to O'Brien, 22 January 1971, the overdraft had reached $500,000, Catholic Health Care file, SOMCA.
20 Sister Angela Mary to Tooth, 18 March 1971, citing a report in the *Telegraph*, 3 February 1971, Catholic Health Care file, SOMCA.
21 Sister Angela Mary to Tooth, 4 March 1971, Department of Health correspondence 1944–75, Box 152, Catholic Health Care file, SOMCA.
22 The *Telegraph*, 12 May 1971, Press clippings, MAHC.
23 The *Australian*, 13 May 1971, Press clippings, MAHC.
24 The *Telegraph*, 13 May 1971, the *Courier-Mail*, 13 May 1971, Press clippings, MAHC.
25 The *Courier-Mail*, 13 May 1971, Press clippings, MAHC.
26 Examples of the press coverage outside Queensland include the *Sydney Morning Herald*, the *Australian*, and the *Age* and *Herald* in Melbourne. For offers of equipment and food see the *Courier-Mail*, 13 May 1971.
27 Tooth to Sister Angela Mary, 29 July 1971, Box 152, SOMCA.
28 Sister Angela Mary, Report to General Council, 31 July 1971, Box 151, Mater Public Hospitals reports to General Council, SOMCA. The government was determined to try to avoid duplication of services with the nearby Princess Alexandra Hospital.
29 Sister Angela Mary, Report to General Council, 31 July 1971, Box 151, Mater Public Hospitals reports to General Council, SOMCA.

30 Tooth to Sister Angela Mary, 21 August 1971, Catholic Health Care file, SOMCA.
31 The *Courier-Mail*, 21 October 1971, Press clippings, MAHC; Dr J Eckert file, Medical E–I, MAHC.
32 The *Courier-Mail*, 18 October 1971, the *Telegraph*, 18 October 1971, Press clippings, MAHC.
33 The *Telegraph*, 12 May 1971, the *Courier-Mail*, 13 May 1971, Press clippings, MAHC.
34 Editorial, the *Courier-Mail*, 21 October 1971, Press clippings, MAHC.
35 The *Courier-Mail*, 22 October 1971, the *Telegraph*, 22 October 1971, Press clippings, MAHC.
36 The *Courier-Mail*, 1 February 1972, Press clippings, MAHC.
37 ibid.
38 The *Courier-Mail*, 1 January 1972, 1 and 3 February 1972, 5 and 10 March 1972, 23 August 1972, 6 October 1972, Press clippings, MAHC.
39 Mater Advisory Board Annual Report, 1970–71, MAHC; the *Courier-Mail*, 3 September 1971, Press clippings, MAHC.
40 Chapman file, Box 4, Record Stores Boxes, Mater Children's Hospital series; Mater Advisory Board Annual Report, 1977, MAHC.
41 Mater Past Nurses Association (MPNA), *Newsletter*, April 1976.
42 Sister Angela Mary to Sister Mary Duchesne, 9 September 1974; Sister Mary Duchesne to Sister Angela Mary, 22 October 1974 and 11 June 1975, Box 4, MCH extensions, Record Store, Mater Health Services.
43 The *Courier-Mail*, 28 October 1974, Press clippings, MAHC.
44 The *Courier-Mail*, 29 August 1975, Press clippings, MAHC.
45 Report to General Council, 30 November 1972, Reports to General Council 1970–1974, Box 147, SOMCA; the *Courier-Mail*, 19 February 1972, Press clippings, MAHC. The microbiologist Sister Regis Mary Dunne RSM was highly qualified for this work. She had first joined the Mater laboratory in 1949 and had established Queensland's first cytogenetics laboratory in 1963. She became a Fellow of the Australasian Institute of Medical Laboratory Technology and was the founding director the Queensland Bioethics Centre in 1981. A new fluorescent microscope, costing $5,000, was an essential acquisition for her work. The microscope could be linked to a screen and showed chromosomes magnified 8,000 times.

Chapter 7

1 Sandra M Schneiders, 'Religious Life (Perfectae Caritatis)' in A Hastings, *Modern Catholicism: Vatican II and after*, SPCK, London, 1991, pp. 157. The decree was based on a 1960 draft called 'The States that aim at perfection'.
2 Information supplied by Rosalie Lewis.
3 The *Courier-Mail*, 16 January 1971, Press clippings, Mater Archives and Heritage Centre, (MAHC).
4 In 1971, Sister Pat Golik RN, a nurse educator, Sister Ailsa Curran RN and Sister Michaeleen Mary Ahern RSM studied at the College of Nursing.
5 Director of Nursing Report, Mater Advisory Board Annual Report, 1969–70, MAHC.
6 Director of Nursing Report, Mater Advisory Board annual reports, 1970–71, 1971–72, 1974–75, MAHC.
7 Director of Nursing Report, Mater Advisory Board Annual Report, 1970–71, MAHC. The Mater nursing school celebrated when Claire Walsh topped the state in her final examinations.
8 Director of Nursing Report, Mater Advisory Board Annual Report, 1969–70, MAHC. The nurse's aide course was available to applicants aged between 16 and 45, provided they had at least the 'junior' level of education, a standard acquired two years before matriculation.
9 Minutes of Paediatric Advisory Committee, 22 September 1978, Correspondence and minutes files, Record Store, Mater Health Services (MHS). Queensland had the lowest number of registered post-basic training courses in the nation.
10 Minutes of Paediatric Advisory Committee, 9 March 1979, MHS.
11 Sister Marie Fitzgerald, An overview of paediatric nursing practice 1971–81, Sisters of Mercy files, MAHC.

12 Minutes of Paediatric Advisory Committee, 9 March 1979, MHS.
13 Minutes of Paediatric Advisory Committee, 4 July 1979, MHS.
14 Edwards to Dr Grantley Stable, Minutes of Paediatric Advisory Committee, 30 October 1975, MHS.
15 The other members of the committee, chaired by Dr Ross Patrick, Director-General of Health, were Drs DP Bowler, H Connell, H Forbes, RN O'Reilly, G Stable, JF McFarlane.
16 Minutes of Paediatric Advisory Committee, 24 September 1976, MHS.
17 Dugdale Report, 21 July 1975, Blue file, Future of Mater Children's Hospital, MAHC.
18 To be successful, Dugdale thought that Mater staff would need to study McMaster University's methods and there would also be a need to attract senior paediatricians from overseas.
19 Report of meeting, 17 November 1975, Dr Geoffrey Bourke's files, MAHC.
20 Sister Angela Mary to McSweeny, 8 August 1977, Dr Geoffrey Bourke's files, MAHC. The Advisory Board established the committee on 1 August 1977.
21 Mater Children's Hospital, A study of the total function of physical facilities, File 143/05, Box 143, SOMCA.
22 Minutes of Paediatric Advisory Committee, 24 September 1976, MAHC.
23 Information supplied by Rosalie Lewis.
24 Mater Children's Hospital, 'A study of the total function of physical facilities', p. 15, Health Minister's speech, opening neonatal nursery, 21 December 1976, Dr Geoffrey Bourke's files, Cabinet 8, Box 4, MAHC.
25 The Montrose, Xavier and Cerebral Palsy League homes, which cared for children with physical disabilities, and Basil Stafford Centre at Wacol, which cared for children with intellectual disabilities, were particularly mentioned. An improved definition of the catchment areas from which country patients were drawn was also recommended.
26 Mater Advisory Board Annual Report, 1970–71, MAHC.
27 Doctors files, MAHC.
28 Mater Advisory Board Annual Report, 1976–77, MAHC; Dr Geoffrey Bourke's files, MAHC.
29 The *Catholic Leader*, 27 November 1977, Fundraising file, MAHC.
30 J Pearn, *Focus and innovation: A history of paediatric education in Queensland*, Amphion Press, Brisbane [Herston], 1986, p. 394. Professor Thong's previous appointment was at The University of Adelaide.
31 Y Thong to Sister Angela Mary, 15 July 1981, filed with Minutes, Mater Advisory Board, 15 July 1981, MAHC. All papers would be issued 'From the Centre for Paediatric Research, Mater Public Hospitals'; *Sunday Sun*, 6 December 1981, Press clippings, MAHC.
32 Mater Advisory Board Annual Report, 1979–80, MAHC. It was envisaged that many specialist appointments in these fields would be made jointly with the Royal Children's Hospital.
33 Mater Advisory Board Annual Report, 1977–78, MAHC; the *Telegraph*, 18 September 1981.
34 The registrars were Geoffrey Cleghorn, Carol Cox, Ross Diplock, Susan Dyer, Peter Ebeling, Anthony Leslie, Brent Masters, Patrick McCormack, Simone Peacock and Margaret Smyth.
35 Mater Advisory Board Annual Report, 1979–80, MAHC.
36 Report of the March 1975 study, MCH extensions loose bundle, Box 4, Record Store, MHS. On weekdays, the hours between 8.00am and 11.00am were the busiest, but on Saturdays, patients were spread more evenly across the day.
37 S Lovell, J Kibble, P Tennant, K Zabell, AE Dugdale, 'The functioning of a children's hospital casualty department', *Med J Aust*, 1975, Feb 1; 1(5): 135–138.
38 Casualty survey MCH, 1–7 March 1975, loose bundle, File 4, MCH extensions, MAHC.
39 Sister Angela Mary, Notes on Sister Assumpta Mary's letter of 19 December 1970, Sister Assumpta Mary to Sister Angela Mary, 6 January 1971, Sister Angela Mary Doyle collection, MAHC.
40 Submission 14445, Purchase of land for hospital purposes, Inala, Decision 16245, 13 September 1971, Z6868, Queensland State Archives (QSA).
41 Mother Marcella McCormick was particularly keen to explore this opportunity. Sister Claire Irving, oral history, MAHC.

42 Minutes of Medical Advisory Board, 3 February 1975, MAHC; Questionnaire signed by Sister Angela Mary, 30 November 1974; Building projects Public Hospital file, 1962–71, Box 147, SOMCA.
43 *Sunday Mail*, 24 October 1971, Press clippings, MAHC. A flight in bad weather brought a 2½-day-old baby with a blocked oesophagus from Rockhampton for a six-hour operation by Dr McGuckin, the *Courier-Mail*, 26 January 1974, Press clippings, MAHC; A two-year-old girl from Townsville with spina bifida had been in hospital for most of her first year, the *Courier-Mail*, 26 October 1971, Press clippings, MAHC.
44 The *Courier-Mail*, 31 October 1971, Press clippings, MAHC.
45 The baby, Chim, was rescued by Mrs Dumo, the *Courier-Mail*, 27 October 1971, Press clippings, MAHC.
46 Minutes of Paediatric Advisory Committee, 22 September 1978, Correspondence and minutes files, Record Store, MHS.
47 Entry for Michael O'Callaghan, Doctors file, MAHC.

Chapter 8

1 Golden Jubilee, calendar of events, Mater Archives and Heritage Centre (MAHC).
2 The *Telegraph*, Southside edition, 16 June 1981, Press clippings, MAHC.
3 Mater Advisory Board Annual Report, 1982, MAHC.
4 Mother Teresa to Sister Angela Mary Doyle, 25 May 1981, thanking her for the invitation to visit the Mater, Golden Jubilee file, Mater Children's Hospital files, Record Store, Mater Health Services (MHS).
5 The *Catholic Leader*, 22 March 1981, Press clippings, MAHC. Sister Marie Fitzgerald RSM presented a paper on paediatric nursing, later published in the *Australian Nurses' Journal*.
6 A Golden Jubilee seminar on 21 May 1981 featured Dr Brian Feery, medical consultant at Australia's Commonwealth Serum Laboratories.
7 Golden Jubilee file, Mater Health Services; File 9, staff, Mater Children's Hospital, Box 143, Sisters of Mercy Congregational Archives (SOMCA).
8 The *Courier-Mail*, 1 and 3 September 1981, Press clippings, MAHC.
9 Golden Jubilee, calendar of events, MAHC.
10 *Sunday-Mail*, 23 March 1980, Press clippings, MAHC. The architects, Peddle Thorp, prepared plans in 1980.
11 Peddle Thorpe Partnerships, *Quarterly Review*, September 1981. Peddle Thorp (G Fletcher) to Maguire, 23 January 1980; town planning approval, 9 June 1980; Sister Mary Dorothea to Maguire, 16 May 1980, 14 November 1980, requesting changes, Fletcher to Maguire, announcing that all tenders estimated the cost to be $1.2–$1.3 million, Mater Children's Hospital extensions, Mater Children's Hospital files, Box 5, Record Store, MHS; the *Courier-Mail*, 10 October 1981, Press clippings, MAHC.
12 Professor John Pearn to John McNee, 27 February 1984, requesting permission to name a room for David Jackson, Pat Maguire, Assistant Administrator, to Pearn, 12 September 1985, announcing the Mater's approval, MCH extensions, MCH files Box 5, MHS.
13 Sister Administrator's Report, 10 August 1983, Capital Works Report, 10 August 1983, Mater reports to Council file, Box 147, SOMCA.
14 Report on Mater Children's Hospital art unions for year ending 30 June 1983, Mater reports to Council file, Box 147, SOMCA.
15 Minutes of Advisory Board, 11 May 1983, MAHC. Report to meeting, 7 November 1985, Mater Hospital Council meetings 1985, Box 151, SOMCA. Mr and Mrs Burton Peterson, land developers, who had supplied much of the land for the Mater Prize Homes Art Union, donated $50,000 for equipment for the intensive care unit and new emergency department, Report 18 November 1986, Mater Hospital General Council meetings 1986, Box 151, SOMCA.
16 Mater Advisory Board Annual Report, 1987–88, MAHC. Intensive care patients had previously been nursed in a small end section of Ward One.
17 J Pearn, *To Teach the Sick: The hospital schools of Queensland*, Amphion Press, Brisbane [Herston], 2009, p. 155; the *Catholic Leader*, 1 November 1981, Press clippings, MAHC; Notes supporting budget projects 1982–83, Mater Hospital general file, Box 147, SOMCA.

Endnotes

18 *Sunday Sun*, 13 September 1981, Press clippings, MAHC.
19 *Sunday Mail*, 13 March 1977, the *Courier-Mail*, 2 October 1980, Press clippings, MAHC; Minutes of Mater Hospital Council, 6 and 14 June, 11 Oct 1978, MAHC; the *Catholic Leader*, 1 November 1981, Press clippings, MAHC.
20 J Pearn, *To Teach the Sick*, pp. 112, 119; Australian Schools Commission, Interim Committee, *Schools in Australia: Report of the Interim Committee for the Australian Schools Commission*, May, 1973, Australian Government Publishing Service, Canberra, 1973.
21 The *Catholic Leader*, 12 June 1983, Press clippings, MAHC.
22 Carmen Smith, 'A case study from the Mater Hospital School', Queensland Special Education Bulletin, 1984, cited in J Pearn, *To Teach the Sick*, p. 213.
23 Preceding principals included Mr Alwyn Thomas, 1977–79, and Mr Ron Kohler, 1980–81.
24 Vicki Sykes to John McNee, 21 October 1987, File 9, Mater Children's Hospital staff, Box 143, SOMCA; JL McNee to Pat Maguire, Chief Executive Officer, 26 October 1987, File 9, Mater Children's Hospital staff, Box 143, SOMCA.
25 The *Telegraph*, 5 September 1980, Children's Hospital 1980–84 files, MAHC.
26 The *Telegraph*, 2 October 1978, 3 September 1979, Press clippings, MAHC; Mater Advisory Board Annual Report, 1982, MAHC; the *Courier-Mail*, 22 September 1981, Press clippings, MAHC. Sir Reginald retired from Queensland Newspapers in 1982. In 1981, further facilities for parents were added when an empty shop opposite the hospital became a rest room for parents of children with respiratory diseases, *Sunday Mail*, 12 July 1981, Press clippings, MAHC.
27 The *Catholic Leader*, 18 and 26 February 1985, Press clippings, MAHC; Mater Advisory Board annual reports 1983, 1984, 1985, MAHC.
28 John McNee report, 26 February 1985, MCH future development Record Store file, Box 2, MCH various files, Record Store, MHS.
29 ibid.
30 The *Courier-Mail*, 18 February 1985, Press clippings, MAHC; Demographic Study, 1981, MCH future development file, Box 2, MCH various files, MHS.
31 *Sunday Sun*, 27 September 1987, Mater Children's Hospital file 1985–89, MAHC.
32 Report to Hospital Council, 24 February 1986, Mater Hospital Council meetings, Box 147, SOMCA.
33 Health Minister to Leonard, 31 May 1984, Minutes of Advisory Board, 17 March 1985. The sum of $1,300,000 was contributed by government, with $425,000 from Children's Hospitals' Appeal and $600,000 from art union, Mater Children's Hospital establishment and ceremonies, File 2, Box 143, SOMCA; the *Courier-Mail*, 8 May 1984, 18 February 1985, Press clippings, MAHC. The Children's Hospitals' Appeal raised $2,600,000 in its first ten years. The *Courier-Mail*, 4 July 1981; Mater Children's Hospital Redevelopment Plan, Mater Children's Hospital various files, Record Store, Box 2, MHS.
34 Report of the Golden Jubilee seminar, the *Catholic Leader*, 22 March 1981, Press clippings, MAHC.
35 Sister Mary Dorothea to Sister Catharine Courtney, 11 June 1980, Mater Children's 1926–1986, Box 146, SOMCA.
36 The *Catholic Leader*, 31 January 1988, Press clippings, MAHC.
37 Mary McCarthy to Sister Angela Mary Doyle, 30 December 1979, David Taylor to Sister Angela Mary, 31 May 1980, Kampuchea file, MCH extensions, Record Store, Box 4, MHS.
38 The *Catholic Leader*, 26 February 1985, *Sunday Sun* 30 August 1981, 8 July 1984, Press clippings, MAHC.
39 This genetic disorder was first recognised in the 1930s and, in those days, was often fatal in the first year of life. More than one child in a family could be affected. In June 1965, Sister Mary St Pierre recorded the death of the third child in one family from cystic fibrosis. There was one healthy child remaining in that family. Sticky mucus is secreted from many glands in the body. The pancreas is usually affected before birth and the lungs are affected soon after birth. The development of enzyme treatments helped children with cystic fibrosis to digest their food. Modern treatments greatly extended the life expectancy of children with cystic fibrosis. Australian Lung Foundation, 'Cystic fibrosis', www.nevdgp.org.au/info/lungf/cystic-fibrosis; the *Courier-Mail*, 21 December 1987, Press clippings, MAHC; information from Marie Hand RN.

40 The *Telegraph*, 22 June 1987, Press clippings, MAHC.
41 Y Thong, Report on special studies programme, 24 March 1984–21 March 1985; Report dated 8 May 1985, Box 143, SOMCA.
42 *Sunday Sun*, 6 December 1981, the *Courier-Mail*, 3 February 1988, Press clippings, MAHC.
43 The *Courier-Mail*, 24 April 1985, Press clippings, MAHC.
44 The *Courier-Mail*, 13 August 1980, Press clippings, MAHC.
45 P O'Regan, paediatric oncologist, paper at 1981 nurses conference, Golden Jubilee file, Mater Children's Hospital files, Record Store, Mater Health Services; File 9, staff, Mater Children's Hospital, Box 143, SOMCA.
46 The *Catholic Leader*, 3 April 1983, Press clippings, MAHC.
47 The *Catholic Leader*, 12 July 1987, the *Courier-Mail*, 24 August 1987, Press clippings, MAHC.
48 B Riordan, *Chris: A rose with thorns*, Hodder & Stoughton, Sydney, 1987; the *Catholic Leader*, 7 July 1987, 1 May 1988, Press clippings, MAHC.
49 Mater Children's Hospital, Department of Neurosurgery records, MHS; the *Australian*, 14 May 1977, Press clippings, MAHC.
50 The *Courier-Mail*, 19 March 1985, Press clippings, MAHC.
51 Draft of article prepared for 'Spinet' (the spina bifida association newsletter), Spina bifida file, Box 3, Record Store, Mater Children's Hospital records, MHS.
52 Information from Dr Leigh Atkinson, July 2014.
53 Draft of undated article, signed off by Heyworth to appear in 'Spinet' (the spina bifida association newsletter), Spina bifida file, Box 3, Record Store, MHS. The orthopaedic surgeon, Dr Terry McGuire, was 'a most eloquent, persuasive and "aggressive" proponent of the needs of these children and their families'.
54 Jeanece Horne to Superintendent, Mater Children's Hospital, 13 March 1979, Spina bifida file, Box 3, Mater Children's Hospital records, MHS.
55 Barrie Heyworth to Sister Angela Mary Doyle, 19 March 1979, Heyworth to ED O'Callaghan, 19 March 1979, Spina bifida file, Box 3, Mater Children's Hospital records, MHS.
56 Children's Hospital file 1980–84, MAHC; the *Telegraph*, 5 September 1980, Press clippings, MAHC.
57 Children's Hospital file 1980–84, MAHC; the *Courier-Mail*, 21 October 1982, Press clippings, MAHC; *University of Queensland News*, 9 May 1984, Press clippings, MAHC.
58 *Sunday Mail*, 5 May 1985, the *Catholic Leader*, 26 February 1985, Press clippings, MAHC.
59 The *Courier-Mail*, 9 February 1988, Press clippings, MAHC.
60 See, for example, the *Courier-Mail*, 20 March 1981, 23 February 1985, Press clippings, MAHC. The trauma committee of the Royal Australasian College of Surgeons campaigned for seat belts in cars and helmets for cyclists (http://www.surgeons.org/member-services/interest-groups-sections/trauma-committee/road-trauma/).
61 Mater Advisory Board annual reports, 1985, 1987, MAHC; the *Telegraph*, 20 February 1980, the *Courier-Mail*, 21 February 1980, *Daily Sun*, 5 May 1987, the *Courier-Mail*, 25 June 1987, Press clippings, MAHC.

Chapter 9

1 See, e.g., MJ Thearle and H Gregory, 'Child abuse in nineteenth century Queensland', *Child Abuse Negl* 1988;12 (1):91–101.
2 *An act for the more effectual prevention of cruelty to animals*, N.Y. Rev. Stat. Ch. 375, §§ 1–10 (1867); Alister Lamont and Leah Bromfield, History of child protection services, National Child Protection Clearinghouse, October 2010, www.aifs.gov.au, accessed 18 September 2013; Kim Dwyer and Heather Strang, *Violence against children*, Australian Institute of Criminology, Canberra, July 1989, http://www.aic.gov.au/publications, accessed 18 September 2013.
3 J Caffey, 'Multiple fractures in the long bones of infants suffering from chronic subdural hematoma', *AJR Am J Roentgenol.*, 56:163–173. See also American Academy of Pediatrics,

'Diagnostic imaging of child abuse', http://pediatrics.aappublications.org, accessed 18 September 2013.
4   CH Kempe, FN Silverman, BF Steele, W Droegemueller, HK Silver, 'The battered-child syndrome', *JAMA*, Jul 7 1962;181, pp. 17–24.
5   KJ Oates 'Child abuse', *Med J Aust*, Vol. 2, 1977, pp. 28–29; MG Ryan, AA Davis, RK Oates, 'One hundred and eighty seven cases of child abuse and neglect', *Med J Aust*, 1977, pp. 623–628.
6   Entry, 17 October 1968, Sister Mary St Pierre's journal and press clippings, Mater Archives and Heritage Centre (MAHC).
7   Entry, January 1966, Sister Mary St Pierre's journal and press clippings, MAHC; the *Telegraph*, 19 May 1970, Press clippings, MAHC.
8   S Leivesley, 'The police role in child protection in Queensland: an evaluation of the Juvenile Aid bureau's work in child protection 1980–1983', Queensland Police Department, Brisbane, March 1984, p. 14. In 1966, the Police Commissioner stated that, in the ten years between January 1956 and December 1965, police had received reports of 283 neglected children and 29 cases of physical abuse.
9   ED O'Callaghan, memorandum, 10 November 1972, Dr Geoffrey Bourke files, MAHC.
10 The insertion in 1978 of Division 6, Harm to children, in the *Health Act 1937*, which was again amended in 1980. There were active discussions from the late 1970s, following the final report of the Commonwealth Royal Commission on Human Relationships (the Evatt Report) in 1977 and the 1981 Australian Law Reform Commission report *Child Welfare*.
11 Queensland did not enact specific child protection legislation until 1999, relying on amendments to other legislation, e.g., Section 76K of 1980 amendment to *Health Act 1937* entitled 'maltreatment of children'. In 1978, when mandatory reporting was imminent, the Queensland Health Minister's Paediatric Advisory Committee advocated education programs for the community in an effort to prevent child abuse.
12 B Heyworth, 'SCAN teams in Queensland – New legislation to combat child abuse', undated paper, Box 3, Abused Child Trust, Record Store, Mater Health Services (MHS). After 96 hours, an application to extend medical custody had to be referred to a magistrate.
13 Mater Advisory Board Annual Report, 1978, MAHC.
14 ibid.
15 Minutes of Paediatric Advisory Committee, 22 September 1978, Correspondence and minutes files, Paediatric Advisory Committee, MAHC.
16 Alister Lamont and Leah Bromfield, History of child protection services, www.aifs.gov.au, accessed 18 September 2013.
17 The *Courier-Mail*, 22 September 1978, Press clippings, MAHC.
18 *Sunday Sun*, 9 August 1981, Press clippings, MAHC.
19 *Sunday Sun*, 11 February 1979, *Sunday Mail*, 5 April 1981, the *Courier-Mail*, 26 September 1981, 30 November 1984, Press clippings, MAHC. In 1984, the deaths of four children from abuse in the previous year were noted.
20 *Sunday Sun*, 27 February 1983, Press clippings, MAHC.
21 In Ontario, British Columbia and parts of the United States, the same SCAN term was used; the acronym stood for Stop Child Abuse and Neglect; the *Catholic Leader*, 16 January 1983, Press clippings, MAHC. Aide units were established in other parts of the world, e.g., in 1990 in Tucson, Arizona.
22 Janis Hinson to Pat Maguire, 8 April 1988, Abused Child Trust, Box 3, Record Store, MHS.
23 Letters from government ministers affirming funding to Pat Maguire, 30 November 1981, 30 July 1982, 11 August 1982, 3 September 1986, Scan Unit file, Box 2, Mater Children's Hospital various files, Record Store, Mater Health Services; Parent Aide unit history, Abused Child Trust file, Box 3, MHS.
24 *Sunday Sun*, 19 September 1982, the *Telegraph*, 28 January 1983, the *Courier-Mail*, 27 October 1983, Press clippings, MAHC.
25 B Austin, Health Minister, to K Cronin, Chairman, Mater Advisory Board, 20 June 1985, Scan Unit file, Box 2, MCH various files, MHS; the *Courier-Mail* and the *Telegraph*, 20 June 1985, Press clippings, MAHC.
26 Sister Angela Mary to Austin, 24 June 1985, Scan Unit file, Box 2, Mater Children's Hospital various files, MHS.

27 Sister Angela Mary to editors, the *Courier-Mail* and the *Catholic Leader*, 22 June 1985, Scan Unit file, Box 2, Mater Children's Hospital various files, MHS. The Mater's public relations officer, Celestine Doyle, informed the newspapers that there had never been any instruction to refuse admission to a child suspected of having been maltreated and that the SCAN team had never ceased to function and had no intention of doing so. Celestine Doyle to editor, the *Courier-Mail*, 27 June 1985, Sister Angela Mary to editor, the *Courier-Mail*, 28 June 1985, Scan Unit file, Box 2, Mater Children's Hospital various files, MHS.
28 Sister Angela Mary to Austin, 24 June 1985; the *Courier-Mail* and the *Telegraph*, 20 June 1985, Press clippings, MAHC.
29 The *Catholic Leader*, 26 February 1985, Press clippings, MAHC.
30 Cronin to Austin, 8 January 1985, 24 June 1985, Scan Unit file, Box 2, Mater Children's Hospital various files, Record Store, MHS.
31 *Sunday Sun*, 30 July 1985, Press clippings, MAHC; Sister Angela Mary to Toft, 9 July 1985, Scan Unit file, Box 2, Mater Children's Hospital various files, Record Store, MHS.
32 SC Latham to Sister Angela Mary, 28 June 1985, Scan Unit file, Box 2, Mater Children's Hospital various files, MHS.
33 Sister Administrator's Report to Hospital Council, 21 August 1985, Box 147, Sister of Mercy Congregational Archives (SOMCA).
34 Report to Hospital Council, 7 November 1985, Mater Hospital Council meetings 1985, Box 147, SOMCA.
35 See, e.g., the *Telegraph*, 14 June 1982, 1 February 1983, the *Courier-Mail*, 12 July 1984, Hinson letter to editor, the *Courier-Mail*, 20 July 1984, *Daily Sun*, 18 July 1984, Press clippings, MAHC; Janis Hinson to Pat Maguire, 8 April 1988, Abused Child Trust, Box 3, MHS.
36 Gifts, such as the car presented by the Rotary Club of South Brisbane in 1980, were particularly welcome. Maguire to Holden car company, 4 March 1980, Scan Unit file, Box 2, Mater Children's Hospital various files, MHS; *Australian Women's Weekly*, 30 July 1980, Press clippings, MAHC; Janis Hinson to Sister Anne Hetherington at All Hallows' School, 14 September 1988, Scan Unit file, MHS.
37 Parent Aide information booklet, Abused Child Trust, Box 3, MHS.
38 *Sunday Sun*, 29 June 1988, Press clippings, MAHC; Mrs R Harris, Secretary, Parent Aide Auxiliary, 21 July 1988, Box 3, Abused Child Trust, MHS.
39 John McNee to Yvonne Chapman, Minister for Welfare, 5 June 1987, Director-General of Health to Maguire, 11 August 1987, Box 3, Abused Child Trust, MHS.
40 Hinson to ED O'Callaghan, 10 July 1986, Box 3, Abused Child Trust, MHS.
41 *Mater News*, September 2005.
42 The *Sun*, 29 June 1988, p. 12.
43 Child Protection Unit, staffing levels, c.1988, Box 3, Abused Child Trust, MHS.
44 The *Sun*, 29 June 1988, p. 12.
45 ibid.
46 Abused Child Trust, Mater Board Annual Report, 1992, Box 3, Abused Child Trust, MHS.
47 Minutes of Paediatric Advisory Committee, 24 September 1976, MAHC.
48 Peter O'Regan to Stan Walsh, Secretary, Mater Children's Hospital Advisory Committee, 1 November 1977, Dr Geoffrey Bourke's files, MAHC.
49 Irene Apel to Tony McSweeny, 25 October 1977, Dr Geoffrey Bourke's files, MAHC.
50 M Cosgrove, 'Mud Pies in Hospital', paper presented at the Golden Jubilee Nurses Seminar, 1981, MAHC.
51 Heyworth to ED O'Callaghan, Director of Medical Services, 4 June 1980, Dr Geoffrey Bourke's files, MAHC.
52 Connell's survey was based on the methods used by Professor Sir Michael Rutter, often described as the 'father' of child psychiatry, to survey children on the Isle of Wight in the United Kingdom in the mid-1960s. The Isle of Wight report was published as Rutter M, Tizard J, Yule W, Graham P, Whitmore K, 'Research report: Isle of Wight Studies, 1964–1974', *Psychol. Med*, 1976 May;6(2):313–32.
53 Helen Connell to Director-General of Health, enclosing report by the Paediatric Advisory Committee for consideration, 4 April 1979, Dr Geoffrey Bourke's files, MAHC. Connell's

survey of children in one metropolitan school and two on the eastern seaboard was continuing at the time the report on children in isolated areas was written.
54 Child psychiatry, submission for child psychiatry service, Mater Children's Hospital, c.1984, Box 2, Mater Children's Hospital various files, MHS.
55 ibid.
56 Aidene Urquhart cited in a report from the Office of the High Commissioner for Human Rights. See Bob Burton, 'Australia: The daunting task of rebuilding lives', www.ohchr.org/Documents/Issues/Australia.pdf; *Sunday Mail*, 22 October 1989, Press clippings, MAHC.
57 Request for staff for child development unit, 27 December 1984, developmental paediatrics file, Box 2, Mater Children's Hospital various files, MHS.
58 Minutes of Mater Advisory Board, 5 October 1983, MAHC.
59 The *Telegraph*, 11 December 1980, Press clippings, MAHC.
60 O'Callaghan to Sister Angela Mary, 6 March 1985, Sister Angela Mary to O'Callaghan, 14 March 1985, Paediatric Staff Society file, Box 1, Mater Children's Hospital various files, MHS.
61 Under-Secretary, Health Department, enclosing a copy of the Mitchell Report, 25 July 1988, Mater memorandum on Mitchell Report, 19 September 1988, Dr Geoffrey Bourke files, MAHC.

Chapter 10

1 The Commonwealth entered the income taxation field during the Second World War; the states retained the power to levy this unpopular tax, but chose not to do so.
2 S Sax, *A Strife of Interests: Politics and policies in Australian health services*, Allen & Unwin, Sydney, 1984, p. 71; Commonwealth of Australia, Australian Institute of Health and Welfare, *Health expenditure in Australia*, 2008-09, p. ix.
3 Commonwealth of Australia, Department of Health and Ageing, *Health expenditure: Its management and sources*, Occasional Papers, Health Management Series, Vol. 3, 1999, p. 46. The Commonwealth's involvement in health policy grew with its financial contributions.
4 S Sax, *A Strife of Interests*, p. 72.
5 Minutes of Paediatric Advisory Committee, 24 September 1976, Correspondence and Minutes files, Mater Archives and Heritage Centre (MAHC). Dr DP Bowler emphasised that sophisticated research, teaching and preventive health programs, as well as tertiary-level clinical services, were basic requirements of a single children's hospital.
6 The Commonwealth allocated funds in its 1973–74 budget for a capital cities hospital development program, including Mt Gravatt in Brisbane, an idea not welcomed by the Queensland government, which suggested to the Commonwealth in 1975 that $20,000,000 be diverted from the Mt Gravatt project to the Mater, where the adult public hospital badly needed upgrading and expansion. S Sax, *A Strife of Interests*, p. 120; Minutes of Advisory Board, 3 February 1975, MAHC.
7 These were initiatives of the Whitlam Labor government in the 1970s. None of the existing general hospitals were sufficiently close to provide services for the 1982 Commonwealth Games competition centres at Mt Gravatt or Chandler.
8 Professor Eric Saint, Dean of the Faculty of Medicine at University of Queensland, to Sister Angela Mary, 9 July 1975, Blue file, Future of Mater Children's Hospital, MAHC. The AUC had recommended that $850,000 be allocated to a university unit at Mt Gravatt.
9 Saint to Sister Angela Mary Doyle, 9 July 1975, Blue file, Future of Mater Children's Hospital, MAHC.
10 The committee was convened by the Medical Superintendent of the Princess Alexandra Hospital, Dr John Golledge, Interim report on south-side teaching hospitals, presented to Mater Children's Hospital sub-committee of Mater Advisory Board, 19 October 1977, Dr Geoffrey Bourke's files, MAHC. Serious shortages affected all hospitals; dermatology and radiology were frequently mentioned.
11 The committee investigating south-side teaching hospitals estimated that between 150 and 200 acute-care beds in the region were occupied by nursing-home patients.

12 Sister Angela Mary to Dr McSweeny, 2 August 1977, File 143/05, Mater Children's Hospital, Box 143, Sisters of Mercy Congregational Archives (SOMCA). The McSweeny committee examined the hospital shortly after the second wing was opened.
13 McSweeny Report, 'A study of the total function of physical facilities', pp. 15–16, File 143/05 Mater Children's Hospital, Box 143, SOMCA.
14 Sister Angela Mary to Knox, Health Minister, 27 December 1978, enclosing submission dated 27 December 1978 from the Mater, in response to the 'Discussion paper on rationalisation of medical services in the metropolitan area of Brisbane', Box 147, SOMCA.
15 ibid.
16 The appointment of another paediatric plastic surgeon was essential to enable this new field to be developed further.
17 *British Medical Journal*, 19 September 1970, p. 704.
18 B Heyworth, 'Rationalisation of medical services in the metropolitan area of Brisbane', 18 December 1978, Dr Leigh Atkinson collection, Wickham Terrace, Brisbane.
19 'Metropolitan Paediatric Service, A rationalisation plan for 1982', 1983 correspondence, Box 154, SOMCA.
20 Section 20, 'Rationalisation of hospital facilities', AGPS, Canberra, 1979, p. 6.
21 Section 20, 'Rationalisation of hospital facilities', p. 6. The Commonwealth thought that a concentration of specialists on a single site should be encouraged, as specialists needed a regular flow of patients to maintain their skills. The ups and downs of the 1980s economic climate and the condition of state and federal finances precluded the continued rapid escalation of services; Section 167, 'Paying for health care', AGPS, Canberra, February 1979, p. 80.
22 'Metropolitan Paediatric Service, A rationalisation plan for 1982', 1983 correspondence, Box 154, SOMCA.
23 'Promoting health', AGPS, Canberra, 1979.
24 Redcliffe, Wynnum, Beenleigh, Beaudesert and Mt Gravatt were cited as examples.
25 B Heyworth, 'Metropolitan Paediatric Service, A rationalisation plan for 1982', File Golden Jubilee, Box MCH Various files, MHS.
26 At that stage, the specialist full-time staff at the Mater Children's Hospital included Dr B Heyworth, MB ChB, Manchester, DOBTRCOG, DCHRCP (London), RCS Eng, DTMCH Liverpool, MRCP (UK), FRACMA, appointed 28 July 1977; Dr J McNee, Director of Ambulatory Services, MBBS Qld, FRCGP, appointed 1972; Dr M O'Callaghan, staff paediatrician, MBBS Qld, FRACP, appointed 13 August 1979; and Dr A Urquhart, staff psychiatrist, B Sc Otago, MB ChB Otago, MRAZCP, appointed 2 March 1981. Mater Hospital General file 1983, Box 147, SOMCA. The staff of the Institute could be Dr Peter Grant, previous executive director of medical services at the Royal Brisbane Hospital as the superintendent with Dr Barrie Heyworth as his deputy. Dr John McNee could be director of community child health, Dr Simon Latham, Dr P Ong and Dr P de Buse from the Royal Children's Hospital should be directors of medicine, surgery and intensive care respectively. Dr Michael O'Callaghan should be director of developmental paediatrics, as he remained the only person in Australia fully qualified in that field. Dr AJ Board from the Royal Children's Hospital could be director of paediatric anaesthesia and Dr John Masel from the Mater Children's Hospital could be director of paediatric radiology.
27 Minutes of Hospital Council, 10 November 1982, Hospital Council meetings file 1982, Box 147, SOMCA. Sister Angela Mary was a member of the government Standing Committee for Rationalisation of Health Services and chaired the Obstetrics Working Party.
28 Sister Angela Mary to Dr P Livingstone, Director-General of Health, 17 February 1983, Mater Hospital General file 1983, Box 147, SOMCA.
29 Sister Angela Mary to Barrie Heyworth, 14 February 1983, Rationalisation of Hospital Services file, Box 2, MCH various files, MHS.
30 Sister Angela Mary to Heyworth, 22 November 1983, 6 December 1983, Mater Hospital General file 1983, Box 147, SOMCA.
31 Mater Advisory Board Annual Report, 1984, correspondence and minutes, Paediatric Advisory Committee, Geoffrey Bourke collection, MAHC.
32 Ms Kyburz was member for Salisbury. *Sunday Sun*, 23 January 1983, Press clippings, MAHC.

33 SC Latham, acting medical superintendent, Royal Children's Hospital to Des O'Callaghan, 21 November 1985, loose file: discharge surveys and developmental paediatrics, Box MCH various files, MHS.
34 The first meeting of the organising committee of Queensland inter-agency colloquium on child health was held at the University of Queensland Department of Child Health on 26 January 1984. The organisations represented included the Autistic Children's Association, the Foster Parents Association, International Adoptive Families, SPELD, Nursing Mothers, Queensland Parents of the Disabled, the Association for the Welfare of Children in Hospital, Queensland Hyperactivity Association, the Muscular Dystrophy Family Support Association. Apologies from Childbirth Education Association, SIDS Research Foundation, Queensland Arthritis and Rheumatism Foundation, CF Association, Queensland Deaf Society: Minutes and Correspondence 1983–84 file, Paediatric Society, MHS. The St Paul's Centre was attractive and conveniently located next door to the Lady Gowrie kindergarten and childcare centre.
35 SC Latham to Des O'Callaghan, Director of Medical Services, Mater Hospitals, 21 November 1985, Paediatric Society minutes and correspondence, MHS. Such a unit would need a paediatrician, a nurse coordinator, a social worker, a physiotherapist, a psychologist and, possibly, an occupational therapist and a speech pathologist. Eventually, a second centre could be established in Townsville.
36 Report received 22 August 1986. There was also a recommendation for appropriate accommodation for children in adult intensive care units in country and regional areas. The Mater Children's Hospital's intensive care unit was opened in 1979, the *Courier-Mail*, 23 June 1979, Press clippings, MAHC.
37 JCHCC committed itself to greater efforts towards rationalisation and integration and asked the medical superintendents of each hospital to prepare reports on subspecialties, support services, workloads in each specialty and patient numbers. Kevin Cronin to Health Department, 4 February 1988; Minutes of Board, 17 February 1988, MAHC.
38 Dr Michael Williams in Mackay thought the rivalry was 'stupid', particularly as paediatricians in neither hospital were isolated. He asked the Paediatric Society to make greater efforts in post-graduate education. Michael Williams to Simon Latham, President Paediatric Society, 17 June 1982, Latham to Williams, 22 June 1982, Paediatric Society 1982 file, general, Box Paediatric Society minutes and correspondence, MHS.
39 J McNee and David Fraser to Cronin, 8 February 1988, Box Paediatric Society minutes and correspondence, MHS.
40 Proposals forwarded to Chief Executive Officer, Mater, 18 May 1988, Box Paediatric Society minutes and correspondence, MHS.
41 Minutes of JCHCC, 28 June 1989, MAHC.
42 Paediatric Society submission dated 26 April 1990, Pat Maguire to Dr Richard Brown, 14 June 1990, Box Paediatric Society minutes and correspondence, MHS. The Society was also concerned that the new arrangements might not adequately balance the needs of hospitals and community-based health services. PJ Maguire to Ian Robertson, president Queensland committee, Australian College of Paediatrics, 14 Aug 1990, Box Paediatric Society minutes and correspondence, MHS.
43 Minutes of Mater Governing Board, 17 July 1991, Dr James Griffin to Golledge, 26 June 1991, filed with agenda for Mater Board meeting, 17 July 1991, MAHC.
44 Minutes of Board, 14 May 1992, MAHC.
45 Health Minister's press release announcing the feasibility study, 21 May 1992, Box, MCH feasibility studies, steering committee, regional health authority, MHS.
46 S Pechey, oral history interview with Dr John Golledge, 8 December 1999, Diamantina Health Care Museum Inc.
47 ibid.
48 The draft Brisbane South regional strategic plan was considered at the Mater in May 1992, Minutes of Board, 20 May 1992 and 11 June 1992, MAHC.
49 Regional Director to Chief Executive Officer, Mater Health Services, 18 May 1992, Paediatric Society 1982 file, general, Box Paediatric Society minutes and correspondence, MHS.
50 The number of children in the catchment area was 276,983 in 1991 and was expected to be 329,595 – an increase of 19 per cent. 'Demographic transport and hospital flow

analysis', Regional planning team, 18 June 1992, Box Mater Children's Hospital, overview, agreements documents, miscellaneous, MHS.
51 Bernie McKay and Associates, draft report on paediatric services, pp. 71–77, Box Mater Children's Hospital, overview, agreements documents, miscellaneous, MHS.
52 Report on the feasibility study into the relocation of the Mater Children's Hospital Phase 1, Draft 1992, File 4, Box 143, SOMCA. The growth area was described as the Moreton Shire to the south-west of Brisbane, Redland Shire to the south-east and Logan City and the Albert Shire to the south.
53 The greatest population growth was likely to occur in the South Coast region, rather than in Brisbane South, but the South Coast region was included in the Mater catchment. The South Coast increase was predicted to be 26 per cent in the 10-year period of the study, Report on the feasibility study into the relocation of the MCH, Phase 1, Draft 1992, p. 7, File 4, Box 143, SOMCA.
54 Report on the feasibility study, Phase 1, p. 31.
55 Report on the feasibility study, Phase 1, p. 33.
56 The former Boggo Road gaol, close to the Mater, was one possibility.
57 Report on the feasibility study, Phase 1, p. 31.
58 Report on the feasibility study, Phase 1, p. 10.
59 Level 6 support was described as level 6 pathology, pharmacy, X-ray, operating theatres and nuclear medicine and level 5 intensive care and anaesthetics, level 3 coronary care, Report on the feasibility study, Phase 1, p. 16.
60 Report on the feasibility study, Phase 1, pp. 20–22. The QEII had a total full-time equivalent staff of 469.4, including 53.5 medical personnel.
61 Report on the feasibility study, Phase 1, pp. 25–26.
62 Union concern was expressed at the Steering Committee meeting, 11 June 1992. There was no capital works funding to redevelop Mater Children's Hospital on its current site, Minutes of Feasibility Study Steering Committee, 24 July 1992, Box, MCH feasibility studies, steering committee, regional health authority, MHS.
63 Report on the feasibility study, Phase 1, p. 30.
64 Minutes of Steering Committee, 23 Nov 1992, Box, MCH feasibility studies, steering committee, regional health authority, MHS.
65 Report on the feasibility study, Phase 1, pp. 28–29.
66 The architects, Peddle Thorp, analysed current buildings at MCH and QEII and found that, if the Mater Children's moved to QEII, all adult services apart from maternity and dental would be displaced from QEII, generating a public outcry. Some of the QEII workload could be absorbed by Logan, as this was convenient for many patients, Report on the feasibility study, Phase 1, p. 31; See, for example, *Southern Star*, 3 June 1992; the *Satellite*, 10 June 1992, *Quest*, 21 October 1992, p. 6; the *Courier-Mail*, 17 November 1992, p. 5.
67 Option 3 was even more expensive at capital costs of $60,500,000 and annual recurrent costs at $46,200,000.
68 The net present value figures were: QEII redevelopment: $41,100,000; Mater redevelopment: $95,860,000; Logan site: $137,880,000; and new site $138,050,000, Report on the feasibility study, Phase 1, pp. 100, 102.
69 Strategic planning began in 1990 and proceeded through 1991. Minutes of Board, 19 June and 17 July 1991, MAHC. Chris Geckeler succeeded Jenny Speed as Strategic Planning Director in November 1991.
70 C Geckeler, 'The strategic planning process to date', paper dated 24 August 1992 for special board meeting on 8 September 1992, Minutes of Board, 8 September 1992, MAHC.
71 Confidential memorandum, Chris Geckeler to Sister Angela Mary and Pat Maguire, 13 August 1992, Box, MCH feasibility studies, steering committee, regional health authority, MHS.
72 ibid.
73 Dr Robert McCrossin, Queensland Health, to Sister Angela Mary, 22 July 1992, Box, MCH feasibility studies, steering committee, regional health authority, MHS.
74 E.g., Dr Peter McMeniman (26 June) and Professor A Brownlea (8 July), who had been involved with QEII for many years, supported a move to QEII.

75 Dr John Bell, Pathology, to Sister Angela Mary, 12 July 1992, Box, MCH feasibility studies, steering committee, regional health authority, MHS. James King, Mater Mothers' Hospital, wrote to the Brisbane South region on 17 June 1992, pointing out that 'As the organisation of obstetric and neonatal care for the region becomes more coordinated, the Mater sees itself as being the 'hub of the wheel'. The spokes of the wheel would allow a two-way flow.
76 D Tudehope, memorandum to Brisbane South region, 17 June 1992, Box, MCH feasibility studies, steering committee, regional health authority, MHS. In 1987, the reports of the working parties on neonatal services and maternity services to the Standing Committee on Rationalisation of Hospital Services recognised that neonatal and obstetric services should be part of general hospital complexes as they were at the Mater.
77 Some specialists believed that the Mater Children's Hospital might not be accredited to train paediatricians on another site, Report on the feasibility study, Phase 1, pp. 32, 36–37.
78 Dr Aidene Urquhart to Greg Wuth, 7 July 1992, Box, MCH feasibility studies, steering committee, regional health authority, MHS.
79 Report on the feasibility study, Phase 1, p. 40.
80 Chris Geckeler to Sister Angela Mary and Mater Chief Executive Officer Pat Maguire, 30 July 1992, Box, MCH feasibility studies, steering committee, regional health authority, MHS.
81 Critical issues, Sister Angela Mary Doyle file, MAHC. If the Mater Children's Hospital moved, a research centre could be developed in the vacant buildings, perhaps with the public dental hospital relocated from Turbot Street in the city.
82 Michael O'Callaghan, chairman, Mater Paediatric Staff Society, to Golledge, Sister Angela Mary and Mater chief executive officer, 13 November 1992, Box MCH feasibility study, MHS.
83 Wuth to Sister Angela Mary, 8 January 1993, Box MCH feasibility study, MHS.
84 Griffin to Maguire, 19 November 1992, Box MCH feasibility study, MHS.
85 Robert Black, on behalf of ear, nose and throat specialists, to Sister Angela Mary, 1 November 1992, Box MCH feasibility studies, MHS.
86 Wuth to Amanda Smith, 22 December 1992, Box MCH, overview, agreements documents, miscellaneous, MHS.
87 Minutes of Board, 21 October 1992, MAHC.
88 ibid.
89 Maguire to Golledge, 1 October 1992, stating that agreement to take part in stage two of the study was not an acceptance of relocation, merely an undertaking for further study. The second stage would investigate in greater detail the dimension, inclusions and costs for the QEII site and develop an operational plan, Box, MCH feasibility studies, steering committee, regional health authority, MHS.
90 Director, Community and Special Services, to Amanda Smith, 10 November 1992, Box, MCH feasibility study, MHS.
91 Report on the feasibility study into the relocation of the Mater Children's Hospital, Phase 1, 1992, Box 143, SOMCA. The development of a community health centre in the Redlands, managed by the Mater, was a possibility to fill the gap until paediatric facilities became available at Redland Hospital on the eastern edge of the Mater's catchment.
92 Memo, 9 October 1992, to undisclosed recipients, re Phase 2 MCH feasibility study, Box, MCH feasibility studies, steering committee, regional health authority, MHS.
93 Golledge to Stanley, Director-General of Health, 2 October 1992, Box MCH feasibility study, MHS.
94 Wuth to Maguire, 22 December 1992, Box MCH feasibility study, MHS.
95 Wuth to Maguire, 22 December 1992, Box MCH, overview, agreements documents, miscellaneous, MHS.
96 Maguire to Golledge, Brisbane South, 9 December 1992, Box, MCH feasibility studies, steering committee, regional health authority, MHS.
97 Hayward to Maguire, 26 May 1992, Box, MCH feasibility studies, steering committee, regional health authority, MHS.
98 The *Courier-Mail*, 13 October 1992, p. 6.
99 The *Courier-Mail*, 17 November 1992, p. 5.
100 Hayward to Sister Angela Mary, 24 December 1992, Box MCH feasibility study, MHS.

101 Presentation to Mater Health Services Governing Board, *c.* September–October 1992, Feasibility studies, steering committee, regional health authority files, MHS.
102 Minutes of Board, 17 March 1993, MAHC.
103 Chairman of Mater Board to Health Minister, 18 March 1993, file with Minutes of Board, 21 April 1993, 0012/005.3, MAHC; the *Courier-Mail*, 20 March 1993, p. 3.
104 The *Courier-Mail*, 31 March 1993, Press clippings, MAHC. The health department's preferred name was Mater Children's and Women's Hospital, Nathan.
105 The *Courier-Mail*, 22 March 1993, p. 7.
106 The *Courier-Mail*, 4 April 1993, p. 6.
107 Executive Director Medical Services Report, Mater Board Annual Report, 1991–92, MAHC.

Chapter 11

1   Michael O'Callaghan to Wuth, 10 March 1994, Box MCH miscellaneous, Mater Health Services (MHS).
2   Director of Medical Services Report, Mater Board Annual Report, 1981, Mater Archives and Heritage Centre (MAHC). Average length of stay rose slightly in the 1990s.
3   Director of Nursing, Mater Children's Hospital to Chief Executive Officer, 8 August 1994, re Green Paper for organisational review of Brisbane North, p. 11, Box MCH miscellaneous, MHS.
4   Mater Health Services Annual Report, 1997–98, MAHC. In the 1990s and early years of the twenty-first century, there was considerable discussion that nasal spray insulin for high-risk patients could prevent the development of diabetes.
5   Submission for home support funding, Mater Children's Hospital, August 1996, Mater Children's Hospital redevelopment file, Box MCH Quality forum, Reg Leonard units, Mater Hospital special school, MHS.
6   In 2010, that patient, Billie Hamilton-Carswell, was an award winner in a University of Queensland mathematics competition for secondary school students, http://www.maths.uq.edu.au/qamt/results/2010, accessed on 20 September 2013; Mater Health Services Annual Report, 1997–98, MAHC.
7   Dr JS Yeatman to GK Wuth, 3 October 1991, Paediatric Staff Society file, Box MCH various files, MHS. The survey was conducted in April and May 1991.
8   Fourteen of 27 children on ventilators were treated at home, 9 out of 29 children on parenteral nutrition were treated at home, 100 of 134 oxygen-dependent children were at home.
9   The *Catholic Leader*, 2 December 1992, p. 17.
10 Minutes of Board, 27 March 1996, Mater Health Services annual reports, 1990, 1995–96, MAHC.
11 Geoff Hirst and Athol Mackay headed the surgical division at the Mater Children's Hospital, where Peter Borzi was a surgeon, with David Wood and Tony Leslie in charge of medicine. Mater Health Services Annual Report, 1995–96, MAHC.
12 Mater Health Services Annual Report, 1994–95, MAHC.
13 Minutes of Board, 27 March 1996, MAHC. Greg Moloney became the Mater Children's Hospital's third full-time anaesthetist in 1996.
14 The cost was $133.52 in 1980 and $479.09 in 1990; Mater Health Services annual reports, 1981, 1990, MAHC.
15 General practitioners were employed for sessions in accident and emergency and out-patients as up to 80 per cent of casualty patients presented with complaints usually managed in general practice, Mater Health Services Annual Report, 1980, MAHC.
16 The 1985 plan for the future development of the hospital outlined the possibilities for the Potter Building. Stage 2 of the plan was the fit-out of the remaining floors; Stage 3 was to be a new building for pathology, operating theatres, intensive care and central sterilising.
17 Peddle Thorp, Architects, estimate of costs, 26 February 1991, Box Mater Children's Hospital, radiology services, QISPP, child psychiatry, Radio Lollipop, MHS.
18 Mater Health Services Annual Report, 1991–92, MAHC.

19 Program for official opening of babies' ward, 28 July 1994, by Minister Ken Hayward, Box MCH miscellaneous, MHS; Mater Health Services Board Annual Report, 1993–94, MAHC.
20 Minutes of Board, 17 February 1988, MAHC.
21 The *Courier-Mail*, 1 July 1992, Press clippings, MAHC; Mater Health Services Annual Report, 1992–93, MAHC.
22 BA Hills, IB Masters, JF O'Duffy, 'Abnormalities of surfactant in children with recurrent cyanotic episodes', the *Lancet*, 1992; 339: 1323–1324; the *Courier-Mail*, 1 July 1992.
23 Mater Health Services Annual Report, 1997–98, MAHC. Research on surfactant was also examining its possible use in the treatment of asthma and arthritis.
24 Michael O'Callaghan to Wuth, 10 March 1994, Box MCH miscellaneous, MHS.
25 The $1,000,000 sleep studies unit was opened in April 1996. Mater Health Services Annual Report, 1995–96, MAHC.
26 Mater Health Services annual reports, 1993–94, 1994–95, 1995–96, MAHC.
27 IB Masters, J Vance, and BA Hills, 'Surfactant abnormalities in ALTE and SIDS', *Arch Dis Child.*, 1994 December; 71(6): 501–505; Minutes of Board, 17 August 1995, MAHC. Professor Hills's proposal for a study of the role of surfactant in the lung was approved in 1994, Wuth to Avery, 1 November 1994, Box MCH miscellaneous, MHS.
28 Mater Health Services Annual Report, 1996–97, MAHC.
29 Mater Health Services Annual Report, 1995–96, MAHC. The developmental clinic found the Australian Developmental Screening Test to be more accurate than the widely-used Denver Developmental Screening Test: MCH Developmental Clinic file, Annual Report, 1993, Box MCH miscellaneous, MHS.
30 Dr M O'Callaghan to Mater Chief Executive Officer, 12 December 1995, Box Mater Children's Hospital, miscellaneous loose papers, MHS. The clinic's research program included maternal depression and consequent stress on children with developmental problems.
31 Joy Denne to Chief Executive Officer Mark Avery, 19 April 1994, Incentive package pilot study report, File Paediatric rehabilitation/neuromuscular clinic interim report, Box MCH miscellaneous files, MHS. The study began in July 1993 and was compiled by Richard Alexander, Joy Denne and Geoffrey Wallace.
32 Email, Michael O'Callaghan to Helen Gregory, 5 November 2014.
33 The number of children presenting for cardiac investigation increased four-fold in 1996–97. Mater Health Services Annual Report, 1996–97, MAHC. There were only three paediatric cardiologists in the entire state of Queensland.
34 Mater Children's Hospital Report, Mater Health Services Annual Report, 1995–96, MAHC.
35 Minutes of Board, 27 November 1996, MAHC; Mater Health Services Annual Report, 1990–91, MAHC; *Mater News*, Vol. 17, Issue 1, April/May 1997.
36 Ram Suppiah to Peter Steer, Executive Director, Mater Children's Hospital, 3 June 1997, Mater Children's Hospital redevelopment file, Box MCH: Quality forum, Reg Leonard units, Mater Hospital special school, MHS; Mater Health Services Annual Report, 1997–98, MAHC.
37 In the early 1990s, 102 families regularly attended the clinic.
38 J Morris, *Dido has Diabetes*, Greater Glider Productions, Maleny, Queensland, 1992; the *Courier-Mail*, 10 February 1991, p. 5.
39 Mater Health Services Annual Report, 1995–96, MAHC; *Mater News*, Vol. 17, Issue 1, April/May 1997.
40 Minutes of Board, 26 March 1997, MAHC.
41 Mater Health Services Annual Report, 1996–97, MAHC; Lanigan was regarded as 'outstanding'. Professor DR Wilson, Department of Surgery, University of Toronto, to Dr MGF O'Rourke, Brisbane, 28 February 1978; WK Lindsay, Chair, Interhospital Coordinating Committee for Plastic Surgery, to O'Rourke, 24 January 1978, recognised Lanigan's ability for teamwork and team leadership, Doctors file, MAHC.
42 Leigh Atkinson to Sister Angela Mary Doyle, 24 April 1990, Dr RL Atkinson, Private collection; the *Courier-Mail*, 2 September 1991, Press clippings, MAHC. By 2013, Interplast had empowered clinicians in the Asia-Pacific by building their capacity to act independently. More than 70 surgeons and nurses had continued their training in Australia, and more than 600 volunteers had been funded on medical programs, providing more than 32,000 consultations and performing over 21,000 life-changing operations. http://www.

interplast.org.au, viewed 18 September 2013. Interplast paid patients' fares and Rotary International supported some of their accommodation costs. The surgeons donated their time and expertise and the Sisters of Mercy covered any remaining costs.
43 Minutes of Board, 27 March 1996, MAHC; Mater Health Services Annual Report, 1996–97, MAHC. In 2004, Lewandowski was made a Queensland Great for his work for children in developing countries. He was active in research, and was president of The Australian and New Zealand Society of Craniomaxillofacial Surgeons, president of the Plastic and Reconstructive Surgery Society of Qld; Chairman, Royal Australasian College of Surgeons; a member of the Queensland Trauma Committee; and chairman, Queensland Committee, Royal Australasian College of Surgeons.
44 Minutes of craniofacial clinic, 13 February 1991, Dr RL Atkinson, private collection.
45 L Atkinson, 'Paediatric Neurosurgery – The Next Fifty Years', *J. Royal College of Surgeons Edinburgh*, Vol. 27, No. 4, July 1982, pp. 191-4; Minutes of craniofacial clinic, 20 November 1991, Dr RL Atkinson, private collection. Griffin memo to Chief Executive Officer, 1 March 1994. The Mater clinic doctors campaigned for the government to recognise the Mater clinic as Queensland's craniofacial surgery unit.
46 The *Courier-Mail*, 2 March 1991, Press clippings, MAHC. Marie's surgeon in Texas, Dr Ian Munro, was senior surgeon in Toronto where Michael Lanigan trained.
47 Minutes of craniofacial clinic, 13 February 1991, Dr RL Atkinson, private collection.
48 Leigh Atkinson to Pat Maguire, 28 November 1989, Dr RL Atkinson, private collection.
49 Leigh Atkinson and Alayne McDowall to numerous recipients, 9 February 1990, Dr RL Atkinson, private collection. Following the Wu family's large donation to the craniofacial unit, the unit bore the Wu name, surprising the Friends group, which felt that their contribution had been overlooked.
50 The *Courier-Mail*, 20 March 1992, p. 12. Paul D'Urso was then training in neurosurgery.
51 Nursing Report, Mater Children's Hospital, Minutes of Board, 28 February 1996, MAHC.
52 Notes of a discussion with Erica Lee, Executive Manager, Mater Child and Youth Mental Health Service, 12 November 2013, MAHC.
53 Greg Wuth to Griffin, 2 March 1994, citing Aidene Urquhart's recommendations for staff, Box MCH miscellaneous, MHS.
54 Queensland Health, media release, 5 January 1994. The Queensland government responded with additional funding for some regions, but Brisbane South missed out.
55 Minutes of Board, 25 September 1996, 26 February 1997, MAHC; Mater Children's Hospital Report, Minutes of Board, 31 July 1996, MAHC. Beech and Lee also attracted additional funding; Mater Board Annual Report, 1997–98, MAHC.
56 Mater Health Services Annual Report, 1996–97, MAHC.
57 The unit opened on the second floor in October 1996. Minutes of Board, 29 October 1996, MAHC.
58 Notes of a discussion with Erica Lee, 12 November 2013, MAHC. Clinicians attended parent meetings as fellow members of the community of mental health service consumers, rather than as specialists, a structure that avoided uneven power relationships.
59 *Mater News*, Vol. 18, Issue 3, October 1998. The show was coordinated by art therapist Jane Sullivan.
60 There was a clear movement towards day services in all other areas and 'hospital in the home' care. Minutes of Board, 29 May 1996, Mater Board Annual Report, 1996–97, MAHC.
61 Report of orthopaedic team visit to Russia, August 1997, Box MCH Quality forum, Reg Leonard units, Mater Hospital special school, MHS; Chief Executive Officer, Mater Health Services, to G Bentley, Australian ambassador to Russia, 29 September 1997, re sponsorship for Ilia Kitaev to undergo spinal surgery at MCH. Booked for 16 October 1997. The Sisters of Mercy entered into a further funding agreement to support the Russian initiative in the late 1990s. Mater Health Services Board Annual Report, 1998–99, MAHC; information from Dr Terry McGuire.
62 Mater Health Services Board Annual Report, 1996, MAHC. Professor Ian Hardy did the first renal transplant, Minutes of Board, 26 June 1996, MAHC.
63 Mater Children's Hospital Report, Mater Health Services Board Annual Report, 1988, MAHC. The first intensive care unit opened in November 1988. Almost 200 children were treated in its four beds in the first year.

64 Mater Children's Hospital Report, Minutes of Board, 29 May 1996, MAHC. Professor Newth, regarded as very important for the Mater's academic credentials, could not take up the appointment. Dr Bruce Lister was also chairman of the paediatric sub-section of the Australian and New Zealand Intensive Care Society.
65 Australian Association of Paediatric Teaching Centres: survey data 1990/91, Box Mater Children's Hospital, miscellaneous loose papers, MHS.
66 R Pitt, Mater Children's Hospital Emergency Department Annual Report, 1993–94, R Pitt, Box MCH miscellaneous, MHS.
67 ibid.
68 Griffin to Steer, Masel, Livsey, Director of Radiology, Mater Adult Hospital and M Enright, Chief Radiographer, 18 January 1995. Dr John Ratcliffe described the state of the Mater Children's Hospital's equipment as 'disgracefully old'. John Ratcliffe to David Wood, 30 March 1994; David Wood, Chairman, Mater Children's Hospital Senior Staff Society to Health Minister, 9 August 1994, Box Mater Children's Hospital, radiology services, QISPP, child psychiatry, Radio Lollipop, MHS; Griffin to John Ratcliffe, paediatric radiologist, Royal Children's Hospital, 10 May 1994, Box Mater Children's Hospital, radiology services, QISPP, child psychiatry, Radio Lollipop.
69 Director of Medical Services to Chief Executive Officer, 20 April 1995, Box Mater Children's Hospital, radiology services, QISPP, child psychiatry, Radio Lollipop. Without a paediatric radiologist, the Mater Children's Hospital could have ceased to be a children's hospital of any recognition for accreditation. D Wood to Medical Superintendent, 16 September 1994; there was a worldwide shortage of paediatric radiologists, Mater Health Services Board Annual Report, 1991–92, MAHC.
70 MCH submission re paediatric radiology to Queensland Health, 14 April 1994, Box Mater Children's Hospital, radiology services, QISPP, child psychiatry, Radio Lollipop. The child population in 2001 was 278,031 compared with 249,349 in 1996, a considerable growth, which put further strain on radiology.
71 PM Scally to Griffin, 31 January 1995, Box Mater Children's Hospital, radiology services, QISPP, child psychiatry, Radio Lollipop.
72 Mater Health Services Board Annual Report, 1990, MAHC.
73 In two years, $50,000 had been raised for the respiratory group, which allowed the purchase of a spirometer, a computer, a physiotherapy table, baby scales, two percussors and, in 1983, funded the services of a part-time respiratory technician. Mater Board Annual Report, 1983, MAHC.
74 Mater Health Services Board Annual Report, 1996–97, MAHC.
75 Chief Executive Officer to Congregational Leader, 23 March 1987, Box 143/08 Mater Children's Hospital – finance, Sisters of Mercy Congregational Archives (SOMCA). The centre for people with intellectual disabilities was at Holy Cross at Wooloowin.
76 Drs Robertson and O'Regan to Congregational Leader on behalf of Paediatric Staff Society, Mater Children's Hospital, 10 April 1986, File 3 redevelopment project, Box 143, SOMCA.
77 Chairman, Mater Board, to Medical Superintendent, Mater Children's Hospital, 29 May 1986; Report to Sisters of Mercy Hospital Council, 18 November 1986, Mater Hospital Council meetings, Box 143, SOMCA. The decision not to create the foundation was affirmed at the inaugural meeting of the independent Mater Board, 18 March 1987.
78 In 1986–87, the RCH Foundation ran a promotion through Woolworths, Jack the Slasher and BCC stores, raising $211,934. www.workingwonders.com.au/who-we-are/history, accessed 10 July 2013.
79 The *Courier-Mail*, 28 June, 13 September 1991, Press clippings, MAHC.
80 For a definition of casemix funding, see *Med J Aust* 1998 Jun 1;168(11):558–62. The introduction of casemix followed the first review of the Australian hospital system since 1984. An issues paper on the national health strategy was released in September 1991, Mater Health Services Board Annual Report, 1991–92, MAHC.
81 Mater Health Services Board Annual Report, 1994–95, MAHC.
82 DJ Kelly, Chief Operations Officer, 'Resource allocation in a decentralised environment', 13 October 1993, Minutes of Board, 20 October 1993, 31 July 1996, MAHC.
83 Executive Director, Corporate Services Report, Minutes of Board, 28 February 1996; Minutes of Board, 28 February 1996, 27 March 1996, MAHC.

84 Mater Children's Hospital Report, Minutes of Board, 24 April 1997, MAHC; information from Rosalie Lewis.
85 David Kelly, Chief Operations Officer, to Dr J Youngman, Deputy Director-General, 18 April 1997, Mater Children's Hospital redevelopment file, Box MCH – Quality forum, Reg Leonard units, Mater Hospital special school, MHS.
86 Mater Children's Hospital Report, Minutes of Board, 26 March 1997, 24 April 1997, MAHC.
87 Mater Children's Hospital Report, Minutes of Board, 31 July 1996, MAHC.

Chapter 12

1 Linda Bognar held a Dip App Sci Nursing and Unit Management and a Bachelor of Arts degree. She was made a Fellow of the Australian College of Nursing in 1982 and also studied health administration.
2 Mater Children's Hospital Report, Minutes of Board, 27 March 1996, Mater Archives and Heritage Centre (MAHC).
3 Refinements of patient–nurse dependency, Minutes of Board, 25 September 1996, MAHC. Changes in nursing, necessary to manage the budget, were implemented by Linda Bognar. Minutes of Board, 26 February 1997, MAHC.
4 Nursing Report, Minutes of Board, 29 October 1996; Margaret Murphy's report, 24 April 1996, file Mater Children's Hospital redevelopment, Box MCH Quality forum, Reg Leonard units, Mater Hospital special school, Mater Health Services (MHS).
5 Mater Children's Hospital Report, Mater Board Annual Report, 1988, MAHC. The College evolved from earlier links. In 1992, the Australian Confederation of Paediatric Nurses was formed. Its functions expanded to include the teenage age group and, in 2008, the Australian College of Children and Young People's Nurses (ACCYPN) was formed.
6 Minutes of Board, 28 February 1996, MAHC.
7 Mater Health Services Annual Report, 1988, MAHC.
8 Minutes of Board, 28 August, 29 October 1996, MAHC, Mater Health Services Board Annual Report, 1995–96, MAHC. In 1996, for instance, the paediatric endocrinology centre in ward CM2 needed a clinical nurse consultant and two registered nurses.
9 Minutes of Board, 29 October 1996, MAHC. A changeover to a new computerised system of allocating nurses, managed by clinical nurse consultants Barbara Bryan and Judy Perrin, was accomplished in 1997. Minutes of Board, 26 February 1997.
10 Peter Steer's curriculum vita, enclosed in Sister Angela Mary to Mater Chief Executive Officer, 21 February 1997, MAHC. The position was re-named Executive Director in 1997. See also http://fhs.mcmaster.ca/main/news/news_archives/steer.htm, accessed 8 May 2015.
11 Peter Steer to Manager, Industrial Relations, Queensland Health, 24 July 1994, Box MCH miscellaneous, MHS.
12 Mater Health Services Board Annual Report, 1994–95, MAHC.
13 *Sunday Sun*, 21 February 1982, the *Courier-Mail*, 12 January 1983, Press clippings, MAHC.
14 Children's Hospital files 1980–84, 1985–89, MAHC; the *Telegraph*, 4 September 1980, *Daily Sun*, 16 November 1983, the *Telegraph*, 9 December 1985, Press clippings, MAHC.
15 Children's Hospital file 1985–89, MAHC; the *Catholic Leader*, 12 July 1987, Press clippings, MAHC. In 1982, a child needed 14 operations to repair his throat after he ingested dishwasher detergent.
16 J McNee, Medical Superintendent, Mater Children's Hospital to ED O'Callaghan, 22 May 1986, enclosing proposal for pilot study for NISPP, loose files QISPP, Box MCH project control group reports, QISPP, MHS. In the late 1980s, mortality from accidents in Australia was second only to cancer.
17 Memo, Executive Director, Mater Administrative Services, to accountant, 16 September 1987, loose files, QISPP, Box MCH project control group reports, QISPP, MHS.
18 *Sunday Sun*, 26 September 1982, the *Telegraph*, 2 October 1985, *Sunday Sun*, 29 December 1985, Press clippings, MAHC.
19 McNee to Chief Executive Officer, Child Accident Prevention Foundation of Australia, 18 February 1986, enclosing Pitt's system, loose files QISPP, Box MCH project control

group reports, QISPP, MHS. A second Commonwealth grant was announced on 24 July 1989, to allow the project to continue to the end of September 1989.
20 Loose files QISPP, Box MCH project control group reports, QISPP, MHS.
21 NISPP Annual Report, 1989, loose files QISPP, Box MCH project control group reports, QISPP, MHS.
22 QISPP funding submission, 1991–92, loose files QISPP, Box MCH project control group reports, MHS.
23 Dr Rob Pitt quoted in the *Courier-Mail*, 23 February 1990, Press clippings, MAHC.
24 The *Courier-Mail*, 19 and 20 February 1990, 8 September 1990, Press clippings, MAHC. In late February 1990, three children died in three weeks, the *Courier-Mail*, 3 March 1990, Press clippings, MAHC.
25 QISPP funding submission, 1991–92, the *Courier-Mail*, 20 November 1991, Press clippings, MAHC.
26 The *Courier-Mail*, 24 August 1991, Press clippings, MAHC.
27 QISPP funding submission 1991–92, loose files QISPP, MHS.
28 Rob Pitt to Maguire, 18 December 1991, loose files QISPP, MHS. QISPP received $35,000 in state funding on 17 December 1993.
29 'Injury Bulletin', No 25, July 1994.
30 Stan Walsh to Owen McGuinness, 29 January 1991, A Devonshire to Stan Walsh, 5 June 1991, loose files QISPP; *Redlander*, 20 March 1990, published a photo of Matt the Mater Bear and children from Cleveland State School, Press clippings, MAHC.
31 The *Sun*, 26 September 1991, the *Courier-Mail*, 26 September 1991, 17 June 1993, p. 4, Press clippings, MAHC.
32 The *Courier-Mail*, 1 December 1987, Press clippings, MAHC; Ronald McDonald House Committee, notes of meeting with Mater Executive, 24 November 1987, Box MCH – Ronald McDonald House 1980s–1990s, MAHC.
33 The *Courier-Mail*, 9 December 1988, Press clippings, MAHC; Minutes of Ronald McDonald House Management Committee, 10 May 1989, Box MCH – Ronald McDonald House 1980s–1990s, MAHC. The Brisbane City Council issued a development approval in May 1989. Minutes of Ronald McDonald House Management Committee, 14 June 1989, Box MCH – Ronald McDonald House 1980s–1990s, MAHC.
34 The *Courier-Mail*, 11 February 1989, *Bundaberg News-Mail*, 25 June 1990, the *Sun*, 14 February 1991, Press clippings, MAHC; Minutes of Ronald McDonald House Management Committee, 6 December 1989, Box MCH – Ronald McDonald House 1980s–1990s, MAHC.
35 The *Courier-Mail*, 10 October 1989, 13 July 1990, Press clippings, MAHC; Minutes of Ronald McDonald House Management Committee, 22 February 1989, Box MCH – Ronald McDonald House 1980s–1990s, MAHC.
36 Minutes of Ronald McDonald House Management Committee, 11 July 1990, Box MCH – Ronald McDonald House 1980s–1990s, MAHC.
37 *Sunday Mail*, 15 July 1990, Press clippings, MAHC; Mater Board Annual Report, 1990, MAHC.
38 The *Courier-Mail*, 17 November 1990, Press clippings, MAHC.
39 Minutes of Ronald McDonald House Management Committee, 16 May 1990, 6 February 1991, 6 March 1991, Meeting of Ronald McDonald House Management Committee with Assistant Chief Executive Officer, 23 July 1991, Box MCH – Ronald McDonald House 1980s–1990s, MAHC. There were to be 12 volunteers, selected from a large panel of applicants.
40 Mater Children's Hospital Report, Mater Board Annual Report, 1989, MAHC; various documents, Box Mater Children's Hospital, radiology services, QISPP, child psychiatry, Radio Lollipop, MHS.
41 *Sunday Sun*, 4 November 1990, the *Catholic Leader*, 2 December 1990, Press clippings, MAHC.
42 The *Catholic Leader*, 9 December 1990, *Sunday Sun*, 30 June 1991, Press clippings MAHC; Sharon Mickam, senior occupational therapist at the Mater Children's Hospital and the senior physiotherapist, John Gilmour, were the Mater representatives on the Radio Lollipop Committee. Radio Lollipop to Avery, Chief Executive Officer, 23 February 1997,

Box Mater Children's Hospital, radiology services, QISPP, child psychiatry, Radio Lollipop, MHS. The Mater Chief Executive Officer, Mark Avery, and the Medical Director of the Mater Children's Hospital, Peter Steer, visited Radio Lollipop studios in the UK in 1996.
43 Mater Hospital Special School, report for team reviewing hospital schools in Brisbane metropolitan region, October 1992; Vicki Sykes to John Fitzgerald, Executive Director, metropolitan east, 14 September 1992, Box 1 MCH various files, MHS.
44 The *Courier-Mail*, 5 June 1991, Press clippings, MAHC.
45 Mater Hospital Special School, report for team reviewing hospital schools in Brisbane metropolitan region, October 1992, Box 1 MCH various files, MHS.
46 GK Wuth to review panel, 27 October 1992, Box 1 MCH various files, MHS.
47 Mater Hospital Special School, report for team reviewing hospital schools in Brisbane metropolitan region, October 1992, Box 1 MCH various files, MHS. Some students were patients' siblings from the country staying at Ronald McDonald House.
48 GK Wuth to review panel, 27 October 1992, Box 1 MCH various files, MHS.
49 ibid.
50 Aidene Urquhart, Director of Child Psychiatry, to review panel, 29 October 1992, Record Store, Box MCH various files, Box 1, MHS.
51 ibid.
52 GK Wuth to review panel, 27 October 1992; Michael O'Callaghan, Chairman, Paediatric Staff Society, 29 October 1992, Record Store, Box MCH various files, Box 1, MHS.
53 Peter O'Regan to review panel, 27 October 1992, Record Store, Box MCH various files, Box 1, MHS.
54 Rosalie Lewis to Vicki Sykes, 30 October 1992, Record Store, Box MCH various files, Box 1, MHS.
55 Sue L, Jacinta K to Executive Director, Metropolitan East Region, 27 October 1992, V Sykes to Mater Chief Executive Officer, 16 December 1992, Record Store, Box MCH various files, Box 1, MHS.
56 Mater Health Services Annual Report, 1993–94, MAHC.
57 Department of Psychiatry, Report July 1994, Box 2, Mater Children's Hospital TRUSTT files, Mater Health Services. In 1993, for instance, the children of a refugee family from Honduras were treated by TRUSTT to help them adjust to life in Queensland. The hospital school was a very important adjunct to their medical treatment, the *Catholic Leader*, 31 March 1993, p. 3.
58 Aidene Urquhart to Mater Chief Executive Officer, 25 February 1994, Box 1, Mater Children's Hospital TRUSTT files 1994–95, MHS.
59 Aidene Urquhart to Director of Medical Services, Mater Public Hospitals, 17 July 1994, Box 1, Mater Children's Hospital TRUSTT files 1994–95, MHS.
60 A Urquhart, undated report, Mater Children's Hospital TRUSTT files, 1994–95, Box 2, MHS.
61 P Neely, report on review of TRUSTT, 27 February 1995, Mater Children's Hospital TRUSTT files, 1994–95, Box 2, MHS.
62 P Neely to Mater Chief Executive Officer, 28 February 1995, Mater Children's Hospital TRUSTT files, 1994–95, Box 2, MHS; *Sunday Mail*, 5 March 1995, Press clippings, MAHC.
63 Minutes of Board, 24 February 1999, MAHC.
64 Health Minister, Ministerial statement, Queensland Parliament, 16 March 2000.
65 Mater Board Annual Report, 1990, MAHC.
66 Parent Aide Unit file, 1990s, Box MCH, parent aide unit, sleep studies, fit out (level E), MHS.
67 Mater Health Services Annual Report, 1998–99, MAHC.
68 Mater Health Services Annual Report, 2000, MAHC.

Chapter 13

1 The Superintendent of the Mater Children's Hospital, Dr Greg Wuth, energetically promoted the concept of a children's private hospital, a cause embraced by his successor, Dr Peter Steer. Wuth to Maguire, 16 September 1993, Box MCH miscellaneous, Mater Health Services (MHS). Wuth had suggested that a private ward be opened in Mater Children's Hospital in September 1993.

Endnotes

2   Wuth to Avery, 7 January 1994, Box MCH miscellaneous, MHS.
3   Maguire to Wuth, 22 November 1993, Wuth to Avery, 7 February 1994, Box MCH miscellaneous, MHS. Dr Michael O'Callaghan also supported the private hospital proposal. O'Callaghan to Wuth, 10 March 1994, Box MCH miscellaneous, MHS.
4   Wuth to Chief Executive Officer, Mark Avery, 26 July 1994, File Paediatric rehabilitation/neuromuscular clinic interim report, Box MCH miscellaneous, MHS.
5   Wuth to Chief Executive Officer, Mark Avery, 25 November 1994, loose papers in Box MCH miscellaneous, MHS.
6   Wuth to Health Insurance Commission, 25 October 1994, Health Insurance Commission to Wuth, 23 November 1994, loose papers in Box MCH miscellaneous, MHS.
7   Minutes of Board, 31 July 1996, 26 February 1997, Mater Archives and Heritage Centre (MAHC).
8   HMS Consulting Feasibility Report, February 1997, Box MCH project definition plan, MHS; Mater Children's Hospital project definition plan, private paediatric facility, MAHC. The costs were estimated at $1,815,000 in construction, $210,000 in fees and $210,000 for miscellaneous items.
9   HMS Consulting Feasibility Report, February 1997, Box MCH project definition plan, MHS; Mater Children's Hospital project definition plan, private paediatric facility, MAHC. Adolescent wards were becoming more common in hospitals in the southern states and overseas. The first adolescent ward was opened at Canberra Hospital in 1996.
10 Minutes of Board, 28 May 1997, MAHC.
11 Information from Dr Leigh Atkinson, a member of the ACHS survey team in the 1990s, July 2014.
12 Mater Children's Hospital newsletter, July 1997, Mater Children's Hospital redevelopment Box MCH Quality forum, Reg Leonard units, Mater Hospital special school, MHS.
13 Mater Advisory Board Annual Report, 1997–98, MAHC.
14 Minutes of Board, 25 February 1998, 25 March 1998, MAHC.
15 Minutes of Board, 25 March 1998, MAHC.
16 Minutes of Board, 24 June, 29 July 1998, MAHC. Not having a contract with MBF had a big impact on occupancy as MBF had 35–40 per cent of the market in Queensland.
17 Mater Advisory Board Annual Report, 1998–99, MAHC.
18 Health Management Services Pty Ltd, Final report on analysis to support business case for Mater Children's Private Hospital project, 18 August 1998, Sister Angela Mary Doyle collection, MAHC.
19 Acting Chairman, Mater Board, to Health Minister, 11 May 1993, Box MCH – parent aide unit, sleep studies, fit out (level E), MHS.
20 Peddle Thorp, hand-written analysis of space requirements for redevelopment of MCH on current site, 13 July 1992, Box MCH, feasibility study, Regional hospitals, MHS.
21 In July 1995, a team of consultants began preparing the master plan. Strong physical and functional links emerged as a key part of future planning with a new Mater Children's Hospital sited between the Mater Mothers' Hospital and the Mater Adult Hospital, sharing facilities, Mater Health Services Annual Report, 1995–96, MAHC.
22 Special Board Meeting, Master Plan, 15 March 1996, MAHC. The master plan also envisaged that further development of the Mater Private Hospital would improve its functional and physical links with the other Mater hospitals. The new Mater Children's Hospital would be expensive, about $135,000,000.
23 Terence McGuire, orthopaedic surgeon, to Chief Executive Officer, 9 June 1994, Box MCH miscellaneous file, Paediatric rehabilitation/neuromuscular clinic interim report, MHS.
24 David Winkle, urologist, to Mater Chief Executive Officer, 15 April 1994, Greg Wuth to Mater Chief Executive Officer, 15 June 1994, Box MCH miscellaneous loose papers in box, Health Services, Notes of meeting, 13 October 1994, re high-dependency unit, MHS.
25 Dr Bruce Lister to Mater Chief Executive Officer, 3 October 1994, MCH miscellaneous loose papers in box, MHS.
26 Annette McCaul, speech therapist, to Peter Steer, 15 June 1995, MCH miscellaneous loose papers in box, MHS.
27 Michael O'Callaghan to Wuth, 10 March 1994, Box MCH miscellaneous, MHS.

28 Brent Masters, respiratory physician, to Steer, Acting Medical Superintendent, 13 February 1995, MCH miscellaneous loose papers in box, MHS.
29 Report on the feasibility study, Phase 1, p. 19; Partners in Paediatrics, Mater Children's Hospital Newsletter, Issue 1, Volume 1, April 1996, Mater Children's Hospital redevelopment Box – MCH – Quality forum, Reg Leonard units, Mater Hospital special school, MHS.
30 It was not an inexpensive exercise; buying the Stanley Street properties would cost $2,500,000. Minutes of Board, 31 July 1996, MAHC.
31 Mater Children's Hospital Report, Minutes of Board, 28 August 1996, MAHC.
32 Minutes of Board, 25 September 1996, MAHC.
33 ibid.
34 Chairman to Health Minister Horan, 30 September 1996, filed with Minutes of Board, 29 October 1996, MAHC. The Sisters of Mercy had spent some $2,500,000 on property acquisitions.
35 Minutes of Board, 26 February 1997, MAHC.
36 The *Courier-Mail*, 14 January 1997, Press clippings, MAHC.
37 Health Management Services Pty Ltd, Final report on analysis to support business case for Mater Children's Private Hospital project, 18 August 1998, p. 22, Sister Angela Mary Doyle collection, MAHC.
38 Health Management Services Pty Ltd, Final report on analysis to support business case for Mater Children's Private Hospital project, 18 August 1998, p. 11, Sister Angela Mary Doyle collection, MAHC.
39 Health Management Services Pty Ltd, Final report on analysis to support business case for Mater Children's Private Hospital project, 18 August 1998, pp. 16, 18, Sister Angela Mary Doyle collection, MAHC.
40 Health Management Services Pty Ltd, Final report on analysis to support business case for Mater Children's Private Hospital project, 18 August 1998, p.12, Sister Angela Mary Doyle collection, MAHC.
41 Health Management Services Pty Ltd, Final report on analysis to support business case for Mater Children's Private Hospital project, 18 August 1998, Executive Summary, Sister Angela Mary Doyle collection, MAHC.
42 Health Management Services Pty Ltd, Final report on analysis to support business case for Mater Children's Private Hospital project, 18 August 1998, Sister Angela Mary Doyle collection, MAHC.
43 Hasbro, opened in 1994, was a useful model for the new hospital. Avery to B Komiske, Executive Director, Hasbro Children's Hospital, Providence, Rhode Island, 29 January 1996, Mater Children's Hospital redevelopment Box MCH Quality forum, Reg Leonard units, Mater Hospital special school, MHS.
44 Mater Children's Hospital Project Planning Committee, 26 April 1995, Mater Children's Hospital redevelopment, Box MCH Quality forum, Reg Leonard units, Mater Hospital special school, MHS. See also, Kevin Telfer, *The remarkable story of Great Ormond Street Hospital*, Simon & Schuster, London, 2008; Advertising for project manager and architects in 1997, Minutes of Board, 23 April 1997, MAHC.
45 P Steer, Executive Director, Mater Children's Hospital, to all MCH staff, 15 May 1998, Mater Children's Hospital redevelopment, Box MCH Quality forum, Reg Leonard units, Mater Hospital special school, MHS.
46 *The Blessing of our new Mater Children's Hospitals, 16 May 2001*, commemorative booklet, MAHC.
47 Radio Lollipop to Executive Director, Mater Children's Hospital, 7 July 1995, Box Mater Children's Hospital, radiology services, QISPP, child psychiatry, Radio Lollipop, MHS.

Chapter 14

1 M Murphy, 'Mater Children's Hospital birthday, 2001', Sisters of Mercy and staff writings, Mater Archives and Heritage Centre (MAHC).

Endnotes

2   M Murphy, 'Mater Children's Hospital birthday, 2001', Sisters of Mercy and staff writings, MAHC; *The Blessing of our new Mater Children's Hospitals, 16 May 2001*, commemorative booklet, 2001, MAHC.
3   *Sunday Mail*, 20 May 2001, p. 60.
4   R Lewis, Model of care for new Mater Children's Hospital, Transfer of patients, 29 May 2001, MAHC.
5   See, e.g., B Ott, 'Children's hospitals take healing outside', *healthcare design*, http://www.healthcaredesignmagazine.com/article/childrens-hospitals-take-healing-outside; Lucile Packard Children's Hospital, Stanford, USA, http://www.lpch.org, accessed 14 July 2013.
6   *Sunday Mail*, 17 June 2001, Press clippings, MAHC.
7   The *Catholic Leader*, 23 January 2000, p. 1; Patients Anne and Michele, http://www.mater.org.au/Home/Hospitals/Mater-Children-s-Hospital/Farewell-Mater-Children-s-Hospital/MCH-Reflections, accessed 9 October 2014.
8   *Queensland Country Life*, 20 July 2000, p. 80.
9   R Lewis, Model of care for new Mater Children's Hospital, transfer of patients, 29 May 2001, MAHC.
10 Mater Health Services Annual Report, 1998–99, MAHC.
11 Mater Health Services Annual Report, 1999–2000, MAHC.
12 Bruce Charles was the first director of the centre.
13 The lowest level of the service link to the original Mater Mothers' Hospital led from level 6 and was accessible to anyone who needed to access both hospitals.
14 Minutes of Board, 26 July 2001, MAHC.
15 Minutes of Board, 27 August 2001, 29 August 2002, MAHC.
16 Mater Health Services Annual Report, 2001–02, MAHC.
17 For more information on Mark Avery and John O'Donnell, see H Gregory, *Expressions of Mercy: Brisbane's Mater Hospitals, 1906–2006*, UQP, St Lucia, 2006, pp. 289–90, 318, 391.
18 Minutes of Board, 18 December 2001, MAHC.
19 Minutes of Board, 28 February, 27 June 2002, MAHC.
20 Minutes of Board, 27 June 2002, MAHC.
21 There was recognition that cultural differences, particularly between the staffs of the public and private hospitals, would take time to resolve, Minutes of Board, 21 January 2003, MAHC.
22 Minutes of Board, 26 September 2002, MAHC.
23 Minutes of Board, 28 February 2002, MAHC.
24 Mater Health Services Annual Report, 2001–02, MAHC; Minutes of Board, 21 January 2003, MAHC. In the survey, the hospital scored 82.5 per cent for in-patients and 92.4 per cent for day patients and was top in both categories.
25 Minutes of Mater Children's and Mater Children's Private Hospitals operational management team meeting, 17 July 2006, MAHC.
26 Mater Health Services Annual Report, 2003, MAHC. By 2003, the Mater Children's Hospital was treating 15,000 in-patients and 120,000 out-patients annually.
27 Minutes of Board, 26 July 2001, MAHC.
28 Minutes of Board, 28 May 2002, MAHC.
29 Minutes of Board, 26 July 2001, 28 February 2002, MAHC; Mater Health Services Annual Report, 2001–02, MAHC.
30 Mater Health Services Annual Report, 2003, MAHC.
31 ibid.
32 ibid.
33 Minutes of Board, 28 February, 28 May 2002, MAHC. A 2002 proposal to rename it the Cairncross Building was vanquished in favour of Mater Community Services Building.
34 Mater Health Services annual reports, 2001, 2003, MAHC.
35 Mater Health Services Annual Report, 2003, MAHC.
36 *Brisbane News*, June 2004, Press clippings, MAHC.
37 Mater Health Services annual reports, 2001, 2003, MAHC.
38 The *Courier-Mail*, 24 June 2004, Press clippings, MAHC. In the first year of ADAWS, 100 teenagers had passed through the fortnight-long program; 75 per cent of them needed help for heroin or amphetamine addiction.

39 The *Courier-Mail*, 27 April 2004, Press clippings, MAHC.
40 J Woolsey, 'New face and new life', *Mater's 100 stories,* Mater Health Services and Mater Foundation, Brisbane, 2006, pp. 17–18; J Viney, 'The diamond cyst', *Mater's 100 stories*, pp. 31–33.
41 Minutes of Board, 27 February 2003, MAHC. Queensland Department of Education transferred the lease of the existing school to the Mater. In return, the Mater fitted out the new school, Minutes of Board, 28 February 2002.
42 J Pearn, *To Teach the Sick: The hospital schools of Queensland,* Amphion Press, Brisbane [Herston], 2009, pp. 163, 173.
43 Minutes of Board, 18 December 2001, 28 February 2002, 31 July 2003, MAHC.
44 Mater Health Services Annual Report, 2001, MAHC.
45 Chief Executive Officer's Report, Minutes of Board, 28 May 2002, MAHC.
46 Minutes of Mater Children's and Mater Children's Private Hospitals operational management team meeting, 20 February 2005; Minutes of paediatric clinical meeting, 14 February 2006, MAHC.
47 Minutes of Mater Children's and Mater Children's Private Hospitals operational management team meeting, 20 March 2006, MAHC.
48 Queensland Parliament, Question on Notice, No. 40, 18 March 2004, Question on notice, No. 1610, 11 November 2004.
49 The oncology home-care program was launched on 30 October 2000, Minutes of Board, 31 January 2001, MAHC.
50 See www.hithsociety.org.au, accessed 10 October 2014.
51 The specialist respiratory physician, Sadasivam Suresh, emphasised the importance of a commitment to quality and patient-centred care.
52 Mater Health Services Annual Report, 2009, MAHC.
53 Minutes of Mater Children's and Mater Children's Private Hospitals operational management team meeting, 17 July, 21 August 2006, MAHC. See also D Gardiner, 'A second home', *Mater's 100 stories*, pp. 11–12, for the story of the third son of a Mater Mothers' baby who later trained as a nurse at the Mater. Her son with cystic fibrosis used a port-a-cath to deliver his drugs at home, but still needed treatment as an in-patient.
54 In 1998, the Assistant Director of Nursing at the Mater Children's Hospital, Margaret Murphy, identified many of the clinical issues, a study that continued in 1999, when focus groups further highlighted issues for young people. See also Russell M Viner, MB, PhD, 'Do Adolescent Inpatient Wards Make a Difference? Findings from a National Young Patient Survey', *Pediatrics*, Vol. 120, No. 4, 1 October 2007, pp. 749–755; *MailOnline*, 28 October 2012, www.dailymail.co.uk/news, accessed 12 September 2014.
55 For an Australian perspective, see George C Patton, Lena A Sanci and Susan M Sawyer, 'Adolescent medicine', *Med J Aust*, 2002; 176 (1): 3.
56 Notes from discussion with Prof. J Batch, appendix to Mater Misericordiae Hospitals, South Brisbane, Report of the working party chaired by Michael Beech into service for adolescents at the Mater Hospitals prepared for the Mater leadership team, MAHC.
57 The Canberra Hospital opened its adolescent ward for young people between the ages of 12 and 18 in 1996. Westmead Hospital in Sydney had a Department of Adolescent Medicine, a multidisciplinary-team approach.
58 The broader age range was recommended in Britain in 2013, cited in www.dailymail.co.uk/health/article-2430573, accessed 15 September 2014.
59 Mater Misericordiae Hospitals, South Brisbane, Report of the working party chaired by Michael Beech into service for adolescents at the Mater Hospitals prepared for the Mater leadership team, MAHC. Pregnancy was another issue for adolescents and they needed to be treated with respect. Once again, attitude was found to be more important than location.
60 Mater Misericordiae Hospitals, South Brisbane, Report of the working party chaired by Michael Beech into service for adolescents at the Mater Hospitals prepared for the Mater leadership team, MAHC.
61 Minutes of Paediatric Clinical Governance meeting, 15 May 2006, MAHC.
62 Geoff Cleghorn, Chairman, Mater Children's Hospital Paediatric Staff Society, meeting 21 October 1996, re the topic 'A single children's hospital proposal', Mater Children's Hospital redevelopment Box MCH Quality forum, Reg Leonard units, Mater Hospital

special school, MHS. The Royal Children's Hospital was also struggling with its own problems of overcrowding, the *Courier-Mail*, 16 September 1994, Press clippings, MAHC.

Chapter 15

1. J Rendle-Short, short paper dated 26 November 1970, Blue file, Future of MCH, Mater Archives and Heritage Centre (MAHC); See also Chapter 6.
2. Queensland Audit Office (QAO), Hospital infrastructure projects, Report 2: 2014–15, ϖp. 8.
3. QAO, Hospital infrastructure projects, Report 2: 2014–15, p. 8; G Cleghorn, 'A single children's hospital proposal', Papers for meeting, 21 October 1996; Mater Children's Hospital Paediatric Staff Society, 21 October 1996, Mater Children's Hospital redevelopment file, Box MCH Quality forum, Reg Leonard units, Mater Hospital special school, Mater Health Services (MHS); Minutes of Board, 29 October 1996, MAHC.
4. Notes of discussion between Royal Children's Hospital and Mater Children's Hospital, 23 May 1997, Mater Children's Hospital redevelopment file, Box MCH Quality forum, Reg Leonard units, Mater Hospital special school, MHS; Minutes of Paediatric Advisory Committee, 24 September 1976, MAHC.
5. Minutes of Board, 25 July 2002, MAHC. The report also noted that the Mater was the only provider of integrated child and adult metabolic services.
6. Submission to Queensland Parliament, Health and Disabilities Committee regarding Queensland Children's Hospital, 22 October 2011, www.parliament.qld.gov.au/work-of-committees/former-committees/HDC/inquiries/past-inquiries/QldChildHospital, accessed 3 September 2013.
7. P Forster, The Queensland Health Systems Review (Forster Review), September 2005, www.hqcc.qld.gov.au, accessed 17 December 2013, p. 99.
8. Minutes of Board, 30 June 2005, MAHC.
9. The maternity services review was conducted by Dr Cherrell Hirst, Minister for Health, media statement, 10 October 2005.
10. Forster Review, p. 156.
11. Forster Review, p. 157. See particularly recommendation 7.20.
12. The review panel was Professor Craig Mellis (Chair), Professor Tim Cartmill, Professor Annette Dobson, Dr Tom Gentles and Professor Frank Shann. The final review was issued in March 2006.
13. C Mellis, Review of paediatric cardiac services in Queensland (Mellis Review), March 2006, p. 5. Jacinta Kate Robinson died at the Royal Children's Hospital in 2002 from a rare heart complication of central-line therapy, the *Courier-Mail*, 13 June 2009, Press clippings, MAHC. Her inquest was held on 4 May 2005.
14. Mellis Review, p. 4.
15. The *Courier-Mail*, 1 September 2004, Press clippings, MAHC.
16. Mellis Review, p. 5.
17. Minutes of Board, 23 April 2002, MAHC.
18. Mater Children's and Mater Children's Private Hospitals operational management team meeting, 15 May 2006, Minutes, Paediatric Clinical Governance meeting, 11 July 2006, MAHC; the *Courier-Mail*, 21 June 2006, p. 23. Heart to Heart was re-named HeartKids in 2004.
19. Mellis Review, p. 5. The Royal Children's Hospital, Melbourne, a world-famous institution in its quality of clinical care and internationally recognised research, was cited as an appropriate model.
20. The *Courier-Mail*, 30 March 2006, p. 5.
21. Dr Patel's licence had been cancelled in the State of New York and restricted in Oregon. See, for example, the *Courier-Mail*, 13 June 2009, Press clippings, MAHC.
22. Mellis Review, p. 5. The taskforce was established in April 2006 and was chaired by the Director-General of Queensland Health, Uschi Schreiber, and included clinical specialists: Dr Peter Pohlner, Consultant Paediatric Cardiac Surgeon, The Prince Charles Hospital (TPCH); Professor Geoffrey Cleghorn, UQ Professor of Paediatrics & Child Health,

RCH; Dr Susan Moloney, Director of Paediatrics, Gold Coast Hospital; Dr Ross Messer, Director of Paediatrics, Cairns Base Hospital; Dr Cameron Ward, Paediatric Cardiologist, Mater Children's Hospital /TPCH; Dr Tony Slater, Director Paediatric Intensive Care Service, Queensland; Dr Robert Justo, Director Paediatric Cardiac Services, TPCH; Ms Cheryl Burns, Executive Director of Nursing, TPCH; Ms Desley Horn, paediatric nurse, RCH; parent representatives: Ms Nicki Zieth, Brisbane Metro (HeartKids Queensland); Ms Kerri Robertson, Regional Queensland (HeartKids Queensland); and Ms Bernadette Heald, Mackay, Far North Queensland (HeartKids Queensland) (by correspondence); parent and general practitioner Dr Wendy Burton; district managers: Adjunct Professor Alan Isles, RCH, and Dr John O'Donnell, Chief Executive Officer, Mater Health Services; and general manager/area health services: Mr Terry Mehan, Area Health Services, Queensland Health.
23 Mellis Review, p. 37. The Mater had also fostered links with the University of Queensland, Griffith University and Queensland University of Technology.
24 Mellis Review, p. 41.
25 In 2008, on its tenth anniversary, the Mater Children's Private Hospital had grown to 66 beds. Discussions with Queensland Health revealed that access to private beds would be needed so that the new single children's hospital could live within its means, Minutes of Board, 13 December 2007, 24 April 2008, MAHC.
26 Minutes of Board, 26 June 1996, MAHC.
27 Mellis Review, pp. 39, 40.
28 Mellis Review, p. 35.
29 Mellis Review, p. 36.
30 John O'Donnell, Address at the Farewell to the Mater Children's Hospital, 1 November 2014.
31 See Chapter 10.
32 http://www.matermothers.org.au/hospitals. The new Mater Mothers' Hospital opened in 2008.
33 Mellis Review, p. 5.
34 The *Courier-Mail*, 31 March 2006, p. 5.
35 Queensland Children's Hospital, Site Selection Assessment, citing QCH Site Feasibility Report, February 2007, www.amaq.com.au, accessed 21 October 2014.
36 ibid.
37 Queensland Government, media release, 27 August 2006; the *Catholic Leader*, 20 June 2007, the *Courier-Mail*, 13 June 2009, Press clippings, MAHC. The state election was called on 15 August 2006, nine days after the taskforce reported. On 2 July 2007, the Premier wrote to the Mater Board, saying it would be a Queensland Health hospital, 'established and operated in close collaboration with the Mater Board, so that duplication of services could be avoided', Premier to Chairman, Mater Board, 2 July 2007, Minutes of Board, 28 July 2007, MAHC.
38 Peter Beattie interview, the *Australian*, 22 October 2014, Press clippings, MAHC.
39 QAO, Hospital infrastructure projects, Report 2, pp. 3–4, 10–11, 13, 14, 21–24. The health service plan was not completed until 2008.
40 For a summary of the arguments, see CK Davis and H Smith, 'Teaching hospital planning: a case study and the need for reform', *Med J Aust*, 2010; 193: 229–232.
41 Dr Z Hodge, Submission to the Health and Disabilities Committee regarding Queensland Children's Hospital, www.parliament.qld.gov.au/work-of-committees/former-committees/HDC/inquiries/past-inquiries/QldChildHospital, accessed 3 September 2013; CK Davis and H Smith, 'Teaching hospital planning: a case study and the need for reform, *Med J Aust*, 2010; 193: 229–232.
42 Recommendation 11.4, Forster Review, p. ii. All decisions should be supported by full documentation, to enable independent review and ensure accountability and probity of decisions.
43 Chief Executive Officer's Report, Minutes of Board, 29 May 2008, MAHC.
44 Information from Chief Executive Officer, Mater Health Services, 5 September 2014.
45 The car park at the Royal Children's Hospital in Melbourne, for example, is government owned and operated. QAO, Hospital infrastructure projects, Report 2, pp. 30, 32.
46 Construction commenced on 14 April 2008 and the arrangements included another neighbouring school, Somerville House, Minutes of Board, 24 April 2008, MAHC.

47 QAO, Hospital infrastructure projects, Report 2, pp. 29, 31. Acquiring a Telstra telephone exchange and a building occupied by the Leukaemia Foundation added to the government's costs. The AMA Queensland branch asked the Auditor-General to examine these possible 'deals' in February 2009; the *Courier-Mail*, 30 June 2009, Press clippings, MAHC.
48 The *Courier-Mail*, 29 July 2008, Press clippings, MAHC.
49 Information supplied by Mater Health Services, 17 November 2014; Health Minister, statement in second reading debate on Mater Public Health Services Bill, Queensland Parliament, *Debates*, 13 November 2008, p. 3560.
50 *Northside Chronicle*, 5 September 2007, Press clippings, MAHC.
51 Peter Steer, presentation, 'Queensland Children's Hospital, QCH Research Facility', University of Queensland Faculty of Health Sciences Board, 30 November 2012. In 2008, 500 doctors signed a petition pleading that the Royal Children's Hospital should remain; Minutes of Board, 19 June 2008, MAHC.
52 Mellis Review, p. 5.
53 Mellis Review, p. 46.
54 Health Minister's answer to a question without notice, 11 September 2008, Queensland Parliament, *Debates*, 2008, p. 2715. The Queensland Parliament's Health and Disabilities Committee also received dozens of submissions in 2011, www.parliament.qld.gov.au/work-of-committees/former-committees/HDC/inquiries/past-inquiries/QldChildHosp, accessed 3 September 2013.
55 Mellis Review, p. 46.
56 The *Courier-Mail*, 9 March 2009, p. 8.
57 Information from Chief Executive Officer, Mater Health Services, 17 November 2014.
58 Health Minister, reply to question on notice, No. 1698, asked on 12 November 2008, www.parliament.qld.gov.au/work-of-assembly/sitting-dates/dates.
59 Question on notice, No. 426, asked on 11 March 2010, www.parliament.qld.gov.au/work-of-assembly/sitting-dates/dates.
60 The *Courier-Mail*, 30 June 2009, Press clippings, MAHC.
61 Minutes of Board, 28 August 2008, MAHC. The AMA supported the clinicians opposing the project.
62 Minutes of Board, 28 August 2008, MAHC.
63 Minutes of Board, 25 June 2009, MAHC.
64 QAO, Hospital infrastructure projects, Report 2, pp. 14–15; Minutes of Board, 28 August 2008, MAHC.
65 Information from Chief Executive Officer, Mater Health Services, 5 September 2014.
66 Minutes of Board, 20 August 2007, MAHC. Statement by Health Minister, second reading debate, Mater Public Health Services Bill, Queensland Parliament, *Debates*, 11 November 2008, p. 3495.
67 Minutes of Board, 23 April 2008, 27 November 2008, MAHC.
68 Queensland Health investigated buying the original Mater Mothers' Hospital, as it needed additional land for the power plant. The new Mater Mothers' Hospital opened in 2008, Minutes of Board, 28 August 2008, MAHC.
69 The *Courier-Mail*, 9 December 2008, 30 June 2009, Press clippings, MAHC; information from the Chief Executive Officer, MHS.
70 Stephen Robertson, Health Minister, answer to question without notice asked by the Leader of the Opposition, Lawrence Springborg, Queensland Parliament, Legislative Assembly, *Debates*, 11 September 2008, p. 2716; Memo from Alan Isles to all staff, Royal Children's Hospital and Mater Children's Hospital, 15 September 2008, MAHC.
71 The *Courier-Mail*, 10 January 2009, p. 15.
72 The forum was chaired by Professor Jeffrey Braithwaite, Professor of Health Systems Research, University of New South Wales. Stephen Robertson, Health Minister, answer to question without notice asked by the Leader of the Opposition, Lawrence Springborg, Queensland Parliament, Legislative Assembly, *Debates*, 11 September 2008, p. 2715.
73 The *Courier-Mail*, 24 February 2009, Press clippings, MAHC. The Mater Board believed that the furore was continuing to be fuelled by the *Courier-Mail* and the AMA, Minutes of Board, 26 February 2009, MAHC.

74 Queensland Health, SEQ Paediatric planning report, *c*.2009, confirmed these arrangements.
75 Submission to Parliamentary Committee, Queensland Children's Hospital project, 22 October 2010.
76 Des Houghton, 'Opinion: Inside former Premier Anna Bligh's biggest blunder – the Brisbane children's hospital project', the *Courier-Mail*, 25 October 2014, Press clippings, MAHC.
77 Peter Steer, 'Queensland Children's Hospital', 30 November 2012, PowerPoint presentation, MAHC. It was also claimed that in a poll taken shortly after the August 2006 announcement, 78 per cent of the members of the Paediatric Society of Queensland opposed the decision, with limited support coming from doctors who had a vested interest in the Mater site. Richard Slaughter submission, 27 October 2011.
78 Peter Steer began work in his new role on 5 January 2009, the *Courier-Mail*, 9 January 2009, Press clippings, MAHC.
79 The *Courier-Mail*, 21 March 2009, p. 68.
80 Abigroup was appointed to construct the hospital on 28 January 2010.
81 P Steer, memo to all staff, Royal Children's Hospital and Mater Children's Hospital, 17 November 2009, QCH file, MHS. Denisse Best from the Child and Youth Mental Health Service at the Royal Children's Hospital was appointed to the Allied Health Services.
82 The *Courier-Mail*, 10 January 2009, p. 54, 20 October 2010, Press clippings, MAHC; Minutes of Board, 31 July 2008, MAHC; Question on Notice, No. 910, answered 18 June 2010, Queensland Parliament, *Debates*, 19 June 2010, p. 2142, www.parliament.qld.gov.au/documents/tableOffice/questionsAnswers/2010/910-2010.pdf.
83 The research building would accommodate more than 450 scientists, including research partners from the University of Queensland, the Queensland University of Technology and the Translational Research Institute.
84 Mary Parker submission, 31 October 2011; new Ronald McDonald House announced 12 June 2014, http://www.health.qld.gov.au/childrenshospital/html/news.asp, accessed 3 September 2013.
85 Mater Press Release, 1 March 2007, MHS; Mater Health Services Annual Report, 2007, MAHC.
86 The answer to question on notice, No. 1566, asked on 29 October 2008 indicated that 93 staff, or 73.9 full-time equivalents, transferred with the unit, www.parliament.qld.gov.au/work-of-assembly/sitting-dates/dates; Mater Health Services Annual Report, 2008, MAHC.
87 Dr M Waters, report to Mater Board, Minutes of Board, 30 October 2008, MAHC.
88 In responding to question on notice, No. 1250, asked on 11 October 2006, the Health Minister described the additional funding the government would make available to employ additional cardiac specialists and to accomplish renovations at the Mater. See also question on notice, No. 1373, asked on 6 September 2007, www.parliament.qld.gov.au/work-of-assembly/sitting-dates/dates, accessed 11 November 2013.
89 The *Courier-Mail*, 15 August 2008, Press clippings, MAHC.
90 The *Courier-Mail*, 18 May 2009, Press clippings, MAHC.
91 Mater Health Services Annual Report, 2009, MAHC.
92 Mater Health Services Annual Report, 2012, MAHC.
93 *Daily Telegraph*, Sydney, 20 October 2012, Press clippings, MAHC; Mater Health Services Annual Report, 2011, MAHC.
94 Mater Health Services Annual Report, 2007, MAHC. The multifaceted procedure involved breaking the affected bones to allow them to realign; applying a 'halo ring' with screws into the outer cortex of the skull; putting traction with weights of up to 25–30 per cent of her body weight through the halo ring; and finally placing her in a 'wheelie walker', specially designed by GB Orthopaedics to allow her to move while in traction.
95 The *Courier-Mail*, 15 April 2006, Press clippings, MAHC.
96 Mater Health Services Annual Report, 2010, MAHC.
97 Mater Health Services Annual Report, 2009, MAHC.
98 Mater Health Services Annual Report, 2010, MAHC. This was a $16,000 fellowship.
99 The *Courier-Mail*, 17 August 2007, Press clippings, MAHC.
100 Mater Health Services Annual Report, 2011, MAHC. The qualification required a master's degree in speech pathology or audiology, 900 clinical hours using the approach, a written examination and 80 hours of post-graduate study in the field of hearing loss.

101 Mater Health Services Annual Report, 2010, MAHC.
102 ibid.
103 Mater Health Services Annual Report, 2011, MAHC.
104 The *Courier-Mail*, 27 March 2007, Press clippings, MAHC.
105 Mater Health Services Annual Report, 2010, MAHC.
106 Mater Health Services Annual Report, 2011, MAHC.
107 Mater Health Services Annual Report, 2009, MAHC.
108 Mater Health Services Annual Report, 2011, MAHC.
109 Anonymous submission to Health and Disabilities Committee, Queensland Parliament, 5 August 2012, www.parliament.qld.gov.au, accessed 3 September 2013.
110 QAO, Hospital infrastructure projects, Report 2, pp. 2, 17, 19. The Director-General of Health claimed that all 359 beds would be available. QAO, Report 2, Appendix D, p. 36. A further 48 beds could be accommodated on an additional floor.

Chapter 16

1   Jacob's contribution, video presentation, Mercy Day awards, 2014, Mater Marketing, Mater Health Services (MHS).
2   D Martin, 'A wonderful bunch of women', *Mater's 100 stories*, Mater Health Services and Mater Foundation, Brisbane, 2006, pp. 19–20.
3   Michele, http://www.mater.org.au/Home/Hospitals/Mater-Children-s-Hospital/Farewell-Mater-Children-s-Hospital/MCH-Reflections, accessed 18 October 2014. 'Justine', many times a patient at the Mater Children's Hospital, progressed to Mater Adult Hospital care and a treasured position on the Mater staff.
4   Video presentation, Mater Farewell, 1 November 2014.
5   Mary D Mahoney, 'Cilento, Phyllis Dorothy (1894–1987)', *Australian Dictionary of Biography*, National Centre of Biography, Australian National University, http://adb.anu.edu.au/biography/cilento-phyllis-dorothy-12318/text22127, published first in hardcopy 2007, accessed online 11 January 2015.
6   Sister Mary St Pierre McCormack, 'Mater Misericordiae Children's Hospital', Typescript, Sisters of Mercy L–M file, Mater Archives and Heritage Centre; Mater Health Services, Annual Review, 2013, MAHC. Mater Children's out-patient statistics do not include allied health consultations.
7   *Mater News*, 12 September 2014, www.mater.org/home/news.

Vale Mater Children's Hospital

1   J O'Donnell, address at farewell to Mater Children's Hospital, 1 November 2014, Mater Archives and Heritage Centre (MAHC).
2   ibid.
3   The *Brisbane Courier*, 24 May 1926, p. 7.

Brisbane Hospitals

MATER HOSPITALS

1931–29 November 2014	Mater Children's Hospital
1998–present	Mater Children's Private Hospital
2014–present	Mater Hospital Brisbane, *known as:*
1911–2014	Mater Public (Adult) Hospital
1960–present	Mater Mothers' Hospital
1960–present	Mater Mothers' Private Hospital
1906–present	Mater Private Hospital
2000–present	Mater Private Hospital Redland
Scheduled to open end 2015	Mater Private Hospital Springfield

STATE HOSPITALS

29 November 2014–present	Lady Cilento Children's Hospital
1990–present	Logan Hospital
1974–present	The Prince Charles Hospital, *known as:*
1961–1974	Chermside Hospital
1954–1974	Brisbane Chest Hospital
1960–present	Princess Alexandra Hospital, *known as:*
1956–1960	South Brisbane Hospital
1943–1956	South Brisbane Auxiliary Hospital
1901–1943	Diamantina Hospital for Chronic Disease
1980–present	Queen Elizabeth II Jubilee Hospital
2003–present	Royal Brisbane and Women's Hospital, *known as:*
1966–2003	Royal Brisbane Hospital
1867–1966 and	Brisbane Hospital
1938–1966	Brisbane Women's Hospital
1966–2003	Royal Brisbane Women's Hospital
1942–29 November 2014	Royal Children's Hospital, *known as:*
1943–1967	Brisbane Children's Hospital
1878–1943	Hospital for Sick Children

Index

A

ABC *Today Tonight* 62
Aboriginal and Torres Strait Islander communities 133, 167, 176, 182, 212
accidents 23, 24, 35, 60–1, 105, 151–2, 153–4
   analysis of 152–3
Act for Kids (Abused Child Trust) 113–14, 160
Adolescent Drug and Alcohol Withdrawal Service (ADAWS) 159, 167, 182–3, 186
adolescent services 50, 52, 67, 84, 93, 109, 117, 123, 126, 139, 144, 163, 168, 169, 184–7, 192, 209, 213
African Inland Mission volunteer scheme 204
Ahern, Dr ED 3
Ahern, Sister Michaeleen Mary 56
Aikenhead, Mary 7
anaesthetics 31, 37, 47, 58, 86, 129
Anderson, Dr Neville 32, 67
Anderson, Sister Mary Colette (Eileen) 37, 56, 69–70, 174
Anderson, Stan 72
antibiotics 36–7, 62
Apel, Dr Irene 114, 143
Ardill, Len 130
Askin, Dr Geoff 183, 202
asthma 6, 48, 75, 101, 102, 139, 145, 148, 186
Asthma Foundation 102
Atkinson, Dr Leigh 83, 103, 142, 197
Auditory-Verbal Therapy 203
Auer, Rodney 142
Australian Centre for Paediatric Pharmacokinetics 178
Australian College of Children and Young People's Nurses (ACCYPN) 150
Australian College of Emergency Medicine 181
Australian College of Nursing 79
Australian College of Paediatrics 125
Australian Council on Healthcare Standards (ACHS) 163
Australian Medical Association (AMA) 35, 111, 194, 195–6, 199
Australian Nursing Federation 79
Australian Universities Commission (AUC) 47, 51, 120
Avery, Mark 179
AxiliM navigator 202–3

B

'baby boom' 42
Bagley, Cathy 117, 144
Bale, Dr Pat 93
Bateman, Gary 202
'battered baby syndrome' 107
The Battered Child 107
Beattie, Peter 192, 197
Beech, Dr Michael 143–4
Begg, Sister Anne 55
Bell, Dr John 131
Berry, Professor C 93
Best Practice Australia 180

Blair, Sir James 14
Bligh, Anna 144, 197, 199
Bligh Voller Nield 169
Bognar, Linda 149
Boreham, Colleen 142
Borzi, Dr Peter 137
Bourke, Dr Geoffrey Merwin 45, 46, 57, 81, 83, 86, 93, 104, 141
Bowling, Frank 101
brain injuries 61, 117, 140
   ROBIN clinic (Rehabilitation of Children with Acquired Brain Injuries and Neuromuscular Disorders) 140, 178
Brandt, Thelma 24
Brewin-Brown, Fiona 179, 200
Brisbane
   hospitals in 3, 75
   Mater hospitals vii
   population growth 2–3, 11, 42, 66, 67, 98, 123, 128, 133
   Warana Festival 92
Brisbane Courier 10, 12, 14, 15–16, 17 *see also Courier-Mail*
Brisbane Exhibition 62
Brisbane Hospital 4, 9, 10, 24, 44, 51 *see also* Royal Brisbane and Women's Hospital
Brisbane River 2–3, 9, 85
Brisbane and South Coast Hospitals Board 6
Brisbane South Regional Health Authority 127
British Medical Journal 121
Brophy, Professor Tess 68–9, 72
Brosnan, Sister Mary Antonia 10
'bub-hubs' 190
burns unit 60, 121
Bush Children's Health Scheme (BUSHkids) 35
Butler, Mary 92

C

Cadogan, William 46
Caffey, John 107
Cairns Base Hospital 31
Cambodia 100–1, 204
Campbell, Sir Walter 154
Cancer Council Queensland 102
CardioCel® patches 201
Carroll, Dr N 93
Carroll, Dr Tom 20
Case, Mary 35
casemix funding 147–8
Cashen, Sister Pamela 55
casualty 38, 46, 48, 60, 65, 84, 86–7
Catholic Leader 110
Cattoni, Jan 150
cerebral palsy 49, 104, 125, 145
Chadwick, Ailsa 49
Chantler, Dr Cyril 93
Chapman, Harry 70
child abuse 24, 85, 106–17, 159
   first Australian conference on 108
   mandatory reporting 108
   press coverage 109, 111

Index

sexual abuse 109, 110
   statistics 113–14
   Suspected Child Abuse and Neglect Unit (SCAN unit) 109–13, 117, 159–60
child development clinic 116–17, 140
child protection
   legislation and organisations 107, 108, 109
   parent aide support 112–13
Child and Youth Mental Health Service (CYMHS) 143–4, 158, 179
childhood cancers 102, 141 *see also* oncology
   X-ray therapy 11
childhood obesity 182
children
   average length of stay in hospital 136–7
   child development clinic 116–17, 140
   drownings 60, 151–3
   home care 99, 136–7, 141, 181, 184–5, 203
   long-term hospitalisation 6, 23, 62, 102
   psychiatric services for 115–16
   research on injuries 152–3
Children's Health Foundation Queensland 200
Children's Hospitals Appeal 75, 76, 92, 98
Chris: A rose with thorns 102
Christensen, Dr George 38
Churchward, Dr KE 86
Cilento, Lady Phyllis 207
Clark Ryan, Dr Dermot (Steve) 31–2, 66, 86
Clarke, Dr BLW 31
Cleghorn, Dr Geoff 152
Coburn, Amanda 104
Coleridge, Archbishop Mark 212
College of Intensive Care Medicine 165
Commonwealth government
   Commission for Manpower 31
   Health Insurance Commission 162
   health policy involvement 118–19, 122–3, 147
   Hospital Benefits Scheme 31
Conanan, Sister Margaret 56
Congenital Adrenal Hyperplasia (CAH) 204
congenital malformations 23, 61, 202
Connell, Dr Helen 115
Conrad Gargett Riddel 197
Continuous Positive Airway Pressure (CPAP) ventilators 137
Conway, Dr CF 58
Cooper, Dr Lilian 10
Corbett, FJ 14
Corbett, Sister Mary St Gabriel 50, 79
Cotterill, Dr Andrew 141
Courier-Mail 27, 29, 31, 35, 72, 74, 75, 92, 109, 110, 135, 146, 199 *see also Brisbane Courier*
Cowen, Sir Zelman 93
craniofacial clinic 103, 121, 141–3, 183
Crawford, Dr Maree 113
Crimean War 7–8
Croft, Cathy 117
Croft, Dr Grace 149
'cuddle mums' 204
cystic fibrosis 101–2, 186, 208–9
cytogenetics 77

D

Daughters of Charity of St Vincent de Paul 7
David, Dr David 142
Davies, Dr Llewellyn Swiss 37, 57, 59

Deeble, Dr J 93
Deloitte Touche Tohmatsu 147–8
Derevtsov, Vera 144
Dewhurst, Sister Olga 56
diabetes *see* juvenile diabetes
diagnosis related groups (DRGs) 147–8
diphtheria 5, 22, 37
Dittmer, Beth 52
Dods, Robin 10, 14
domiciliary and acute care rehabilitation team (DART) 203
Dommett, Rae 95
Doyle, Sister Angela Mary 54, 62, 64, 70–1, 74, 110, 121, 124, 127
Doyle, Sister Geraldine 83
Dublin Board of Health 7
Ducat, Rex 169
Dugdale, Dr Alan 65–6, 82, 83, 86
Duhig, Archbishop James 11, 13, 16, 23, 33, 213
Dunne, Sister Mary Assissium 10
Dunne, Sister Regis Mary 56, 77
Dunning, Ross 127
D'Urso, Dr Paul 143

E

ear, nose and throat services 22, 57
Earnshaw, Dr Percy Alan 19, 20, 26, 28, 30, 31, 37, 37, 55, 57, 94, 208
Eckert, Dr John 66, 86
Edmond, Wendy 182–3
Edwards, Dr Llew 76, 81, 122
   White Paper 121–2
Egan, Dr PJ 86
emergencies *see* casualty
Emmett, Dr Tony 142
encephalitis 61
Endeavour Foundation 125
England, Sister Mary Chanel 10
English, Dr PB 31
Ewing, Linda 150
Extracorporeal Membrane Oxygenation (ECMO) machine 202

F

family therapy 114
Finch, Kerrin 117
First World War 2, 15, 28
Fishbourne, Sister Madeline 207
Fison, Dr DC 74
Fitzgerald, Sister Francis Mary 10
Fitzgerald, Sister Marie (Mary Rosaire) 24, 37, 50, 56, 68, 79, 80, 100, 104, 174–5
'5Ks for Kids' walk 203–4
Flenady, Peggy 62
Fletcher, Dr PJ 86
Forster Review 189–90, 194
Forster, Rosemary 144
Fothergill, Jordan 203
   Be Brave 203
Frayne, Sister Ursula 8
Friends of the Craniofacial Clinic 142–3

G

Gallagher, Dr Michael 31, 32
gastroenteritis 34, 52
Geckeler, Chris 130–2

Index

Gillies, WN 3
Gilmour, John 144
Golden Jubilee Scientific Week 93
Golledge, Dr John 126–7, 134, 135
Goodwin, Lady 14
Goodwin, Sir John 14, 16
Gorman, Sister Mary Venard (Margaret) 18–19
Goss, Wayne 154
Grace, Grace 127
Grant, Dr Caroline 202
Grant, Gwen 204
Gray, George Wilkie 12
Great Depression vi, 15, 26, 36
Greathead, Sister Germaine 24

H

Hackett, Grant 204
Haeren, Marijke and Leo 155
Hall, Dr DC 86
Hall and Prentice 14, 15
Hall, Francis Richard 14
Hall, Thomas Ramsay 14
Ham, Dr Burnett 6
Hand, Marie 145
Hanlon, Ned 27
Health Services Act 1991 136
HeartKids Queensland 190, 193
Heine, Jacob 5
Heyworth, Dr Barrie 83, 86, 108, 109, 114, 122–4
Hills, Professor Brian 139
Hinson, Janis 109
Hirschfeld, Sister Brigid (Mary Ian) 100
Hirst, Dr Geoff 151
Hoare, Sister Mary Dympna (Mary Ellen) 18–19
Hoge, Robert 103
hookworm 5
Horan, Mike 167
Hosking, Dr Clifford 93
Hospital In The Home (HITH) Society 185
Hospital for Sick Children 3–5, 14, 25 *see also* Royal Children's Hospital
  polio epidemics 6
  school at 49
hospitals
  adolescents and 50
  funding 11, 31
  Queensland pre-First World War 11
  schools in 156–7
  standards of care 9
  visiting hours 24, 50
  voluntary tradition 4, 6–9
Hospitals Act 1923 6
Hospitals Act 1936 36
Howgego, Irene 149
Hudson, Dr Julie 127

I

immunisation 22, 37
Inala 87–8
Infant Life Protection Act 1905 5
infant mortality rates 4–5
International Council of Nursing 43
International Year of Disabled Persons 103
Interplast 142
Ipswich Hospital 95

Ireland 6–8
Isles, Professor Alan 198, 199

J

Jackson, Dr David Clements 32–3, 49, 52, 58, 67, 94
Jackson, Dr Ernest Sandford 9
Jeffs, Professor Robert 102
Jensen, Ailsa and Colin 155
Johnston, Susan 212
Joint Children's Hospitals Coordinating Committee (JCHCC) 124–6
Jolly, Lillie 13
juvenile diabetes 30, 104, 136, 141, 186

K

Kaltenbrunn, Inge 202
Karl, Professor Tom 201
KD Morris & Sons 76
Kearney, Helen 141
Kehoe, Sister Mary Marcelline (Margaret Ellen) 18, 19, 27, 208
Kelly, JP 26, 30, 31, 43, 46, 146
Kelly, Margaret 92
Kelly, Sister Mary Domitilla 29
Kelly, Sister Mary Lea 29, 39, 54–5, 72
Kempe, Dr C Henry 107
Kennedy, Sister Alphonsus (Alfie) 56
Kenny, Grant and Lisa 155
Kenny, Sister Elizabeth 23
Keyte, Cathy 210
Khoo, Dr PPT 86
kidney disease 23, 203
Kids in Mind 182
'Kids Matter' 183
Kirchner, Sister Patricia 101
Koch, Robert 5
Kyburz, Rosemary 124

L

Lady Bowen maternity hospital 7, 36
Lady Cilento Children's Hospital vii, 207–10, 213 *see also* Queensland Children's Hospital
Lahz, John Rudolph Sergius 20–2, 23, 24, 26, 31, 33, 38, 86
Lamont, Dr Tony 146
Lancet 139
Lanigan, Dr Michael 142
Latham, Dr Simon 111, 125
Laycock, Renee 102
lead poisoning 5, 22, 23, 151, 208
Leditschke, Dr Fred 86
Lee, Erica 144
Lennon, Lieutenant-Governor William 13
Leonard, Sir Reginald 75, 92, 96
Leslie, Dr Peter 179
Leslie, Dr Tony 113, 151
Lewandowski, Dr Richard 142
Lewis, Hayley 147, 154
Lewis, Sister Rosalie Mary 79, 84, 99–100, 149, 151, 158, 169, 175
Lions Club 102
Lister, Dr Bruce 145
Logan Hospital 129–30, 131, 134, 140, 199
Loggins, Leroy 147
Lord, Jenny 204

Index

Lucy, Sister Mary Audrey (Hannah Agnes) 18, 19, 54
Lynch, Dr Alban 24, 31
Lynch, Sister Mary Asicus (Margaret Mary) 18–19
Lyons Architecture 197
Lyons, Prime Minister Joe 27

M

McAllister, Helen 95
McAuley, Catherine 6–7, 174, 212
McCarthy, Sister Cathy 100
McCarthy, Sister Libby 100
McCarthy, Sister Mary 100, 102
McConnel, Mary 4
McCormack, Mary Ellen 107
McCormack, Sister Mary St Pierre (Mary Irene) 18–19, 29–30, 38, 43, 54, 56, 57, 60, 61–2, 68, 107
McCrossin, Dr David 200
McCrossin, Dr Robert 131
McDonnell & East 16
McDonnell, Frank 16
McDowall, Alayne 142
McGuckin, Dr Des 57, 72, 86
McGuinness, Dr EJ 37, 59
McGuire, Dr Terry 144, 165
McInerney, Sister Mary Felix 10
Mackay, Dr Athol 137
McKee, Sue 210
Mackinnon, Mary 184
McLeod, Norma 10
McNally, Cecilia 146
McNee, Dr John 97, 98, 105, 146, 152
McSweeny, Dr Anthony (Tony) 32, 34, 83
magnetic resonance imaging (MRI) 203
Maguire, Mother Mary Xavier 8
Maguire, Pat 127
Malcolm, Dr R 26
Malone, Molly 10
Malouf, Anne-Marie 92
Mara, Sister Mary St Aidan (Mary Ellen) 18–19, 28–9
Marchant, George 24
Marriott, Dr Len 58, 61, 86
Martin, Denise 207
Masel, Dr John 142, 146
Masters, Dr Brent 102, 139
Matejic, Marie 142
Mater Adult Hospital 6, 10–11, 25, 26, 27, 31, 37, 39, 54, 67, 71, 95, 120, 123–4, 132, 161, 165, 166, 177, 186, 197, 207, 209, 211
  Golden Jubilee 43
  renaming as Mater Hospital Brisbane 206, 209, 213
Mater balls 14, 53, 60
Mater Children's Hospital
  accommodation for families 85, 96, 154
  accreditation in paediatrics 87
  administration 25–6, 44–5, 166, 180
  Advisory Board 25, 30, 43, 51, 57, 83–4, 111, 127, 146, 162, 189, 190, 192
  age limit 50, 84
  appointments of medical staff 24–6, 30–1, 37
  blessing of 16
  building, original 17

campus development 138–9, 162, 174–9
casemix funding 147–8
casualty 38, 46, 48, 60, 65, 82, 83, 84, 87
changes, challenges of vii, 207–9
child protection unit 109–13, 117, 159
coordination with adult hospital 70–1, 76–7
costs of treatment 138
culture of vi, 213
disease and illness types 22–3, 101, 208
extensions 51–2, 63, 70–1, 75–77, 94
family orientation 98–9, 206–8
farewell ceremony 211–13
fire 71–2, 88
first matron 18, 27
funding of 26–7, 38, 43, 51, 71–3, 98, 111–12
fundraising for 13–14, 15, 27, 52–3, 75, 94, 98, 146–7, 154, 203–4
Golden Jubilee 92–3
home-care programs 185, 203
honorary surgical staff 3, 19, 20, 25–6, 30, 33–4, 37, 51, 58, 86
hospital school 49, 94–6, 155–8
intensive care facilities 48, 52, 65, 67, 74, 75, 76, 94, 125, 145, 165–6, 204
lay nurses 78, 99
McSweeny committee recommendations 83–6, 89, 114, 121
major constructions 1980s 93–8
medical board 24
mercy flights to 35, 105
Model of Care Document 175
modernisation plans 70–6
new hospital Stanley Street 164–70, 174–7
operating theatres 17, 19, 24, 43, 47, 48, 50, 51–2, 57, 94
out-patients department 33, 47–8, 83, 96–7, 96–7, 138
outreach programs 181–2, 192
patient care *see* patient care
patient numbers 22, 35, 39, 44, 52, 60, 87, 207
plans for 12–13
post-war 'baby boom' 42
rationalisation and 73, 85, 119–35, 188–201
relocation feasibility study 127–35
research capacity 46–7, 67, 87, 129, 140
restructure of nursing 149
Royal Children's Hospital, relationship with 188–9
Sisters of Mercy values vi, vii, 175, 176, 206, 213
staff 18–20, 29, 31–3, 46, 49, 54, 55, 57–8, 78–79, 86, 144, 151–2, 208
strategic plan 130–1
subspecialties 81, 82, 86, 87, 122, 127, 128, 132, 140–1
surgery on babies 61
teaching hospital, as 46–7, 59, 83
torture and trauma unit 116, 158
University of Queensland and 46–7, 51, 59, 82, 86, 93–4, 167, 178
volunteers 204
Mater Children's Hospital Honorary Medical Staff Association 66
Mater Children's Hospital Paediatric Staff Society 188

Mater Children's Ladies Auxiliary 52–3
Mater Children's Private Hospital 161–4, 167, 168, 179, 181, 184, 187, 191, 198, 205, 206, 211, 213
Mater Cochlear Implant Clinic 203
Mater Community Services Building 12
Mater Health Services 179, 194, 212
Mater Hospital Brisbane *see* Mater Adult Hospital
Mater Hospital Special School 183
Mater Hospitals' Master Plan Review 165
Mater Little Miracles Easter Appeal 203–4, 209
Mater Medical Research Institute 139, 167, 191
Mater Mothers' Hospital 35–6, 39, 42, 43, 51, 53, 54, 56, 67, 76, 89, 95, 120, 131–3, 165, 166, 177, 180, 184, 189, 193, 197, 199, 204, 205, 206, 207, 211
   New Life Centre 132, 138
Mater Pathology 203, 207
Mater Private Hospital 9–10, 11, 19, 26, 72, 79, 138, 161–2, 164, 165, 167, 179, 206, 207, 211
   Redland 139, 179, 199, 206
   Springfield 206
Mater Trust (Mater Foundation) 147, 203
Mater Volunteer Services 204
Mater Younger Set 53
Mater's Linen Club 16
Mater's Mars Clinic 202
Mater's Ronald McDonald House 154–5, 184
'Matt the Mater Bear Show' 153
Maynard, Ian 212
Medibank Private 205
Medicare 140, 147, 162
Meehan, Arthur Vincent 20, 21, 22, 23, 24, 26, 31
Mellis, Professor Craig 190
Mellis Review 190–1, 196–7, 201
mental health services 143–4, 158–9, 168, 182
   see also psychiatric services
Mexted, Patricia (nee Mahoney) 55
Miracle Max 203
Mitchell, Dr Ken 117
Mohay, Dr Heather 86, 104
Montrose Home 24, 37, 49, 62, 125
MontroseAccess *see* Montrose Home
Moody, Dr Wendy 177
Morris, Jill
   Dido has diabetes 141
MOSHPIT (Mobile Outreach Support and Health Program by Integrated Teams) 182
Mother Teresa of Calcutta 92
multidisciplinary clinics 103–4, 117, 126, 139–40, 143
   child abuse 106, 108–9
   rationalisation and 125
Munn, Lilly 204
Munro, Sister Jennifer 56
Murphy, Annette 113
Murphy, Dr Arthur 22
Murphy, Margaret 149, 150, 169

N

Nadezhda project 144, 181
Nasser, Malcolm 86
National Health and Medical Research Council 140, 182
National Injury Surveillance and Prevention Program (NISPP) 152
National Safe School framework 183
Naughton, William 9
Neylan, Vandra 204
Nightingale, Florence 7–8
Nobilio, Ermanno 127
Nuffield Foundation 34
nursing
   career structures 149–50
   education 79
   overseas 101–2, 204
   shortages 78–80, 150, 181
   standards 68–9
   training 9, 10, 56–7, 80, 149

O

Oates, Professor Kim 107, 199
O'Brien, Dr Jennifer 104
O'Brien, Helen 104
O'Callaghan, Dr Eugene Desmond (Des) 44, 45, 60, 62, 108
O'Callaghan, Dr Michael 89, 116–17, 139, 166, 182
occupational therapy 49, 67, 98, 108, 109, 111, 112, 113, 117, 121, 126, 132, 166
O'Donnell, Dr John 179, 180, 183, 212
O'Duffy, Dr John 139
O'Keeffe, Clem 130
Oley, Christine 142
oncology 141, 150, 200 *see also* childhood cancers
Operation Smile Australia 142, 144, 164
Order of the Visitation of Holy Mary 7
O'Regan, Dr Peter 83, 146
organ transplants 145
orthopaedic services 20, 22, 23, 32, 38, 202
osteomyelitis 23, 62, 65, 207, 208

P

Pabari, Dr Mansu 105, 142
Paediatric Society of Queensland 126
paediatrics 20, 32, 37, 46, 48, 121
   cardiac services review 190–1
   developmental 116–17, 166
   endoscopes 137–8
   paediatric intensive care unit (PICU) 204
   pharmacology 167
   preventative medicine in 80
   rationalisation of services 119–21
   regional centre visits 88
   sleep studies 139, 202
   specialisation in nurse training 80–1
Parry, Trevor 125
Patch, Sister Mary John 54
patient care
   costs of treatment 137–8
   demarcation issues 57–8
   developments in 78–81
   home care 136–7, 141, 181, 184–5
   hospitalisation, reducing 136–8
   specialisation, trend to 58–9, 68
   technology 137
Patterson, Sister Mary Winifrede 55, 61, 104
Pedley, Heath 105
Pepster 208–9
Perkins, Kieren 147

Perrin, Judy 179
Pets As Therapy Scheme (PATS) 177
Phibbs, Dr Roderic 93
physiotherapy 49, 66, 74, 104, 117
Pickering, Alison 204
Pinkerton, Professor Ross 199
Pitt, Dr Rob 145, 152
Pitt, Jennifer 164
pneumonia 23
poliomyelitis 5–6, 23, 34, 38, 49, 65, 208
Pollard, Sister Eileen 80
Post-Acute Care Program 185
Potter, Mother Mary Patrick 9, 11, 13, 15
Pregnancy Help 186
Prentice & Atkinson 36
Prentice, George Gray 14
Preston James Fund 204
The Prince Charles Hospital 67, 82, 120, 190, 199, 201
Prince Henry Hospital, Sydney 43
Princess Alexandra Hospital 51, 53, 68, 82, 85, 95, 96, 119, 120, 121, 192
Protect All Children Today (PACT) 114
psychiatric services 114–16, 125 see also mental health services
Purssey, Dr Brian 44

Q

Quayle, Dr Athol 22
Queen Elizabeth II Jubilee Hospital (QEII) 119, 123, 126–7, 129–30, 133, 134–5, 146, 161
Queensland
  antenatal care and childbirth policies 36
  depression post-First World War 15
  diseases affecting children 5
  Nurses Registration Board 81
  population growth 4
  pre-First World War public hospitals 11
  Second World War, effect of 28–9
Queensland Centre for Adolescent and Young Adult Care 209
Queensland Children's Cancer Centre 200
Queensland Children's Hospital see also Lady Cilento Children's Hospital
  agreement between Mater Board and government 195, 198
  concerns 199–200
  design 197
  governing board 196
  north and south divide 197
  opposition to 194–6
  planning process 194–201, 205
  reviews and discussions 189–94
  senior clinical appointments 200
Queensland Children's Medical Research Institute 200
Queensland government
  Forster Review 189
  Golden Casket lottery 11, 27, 139, 159
  health policies 81–2, 143
  infant mortality rates and 4–5
  public health improvements 5
  rationalisation of health services 119–20, 121–35, 188–201
  review of hospital schools 156–8
  single children's hospital proposal 194–5

Queensland Health 127, 131, 143, 192, 193, 194–5, 199, 212, 213
  Paediatric Advisory Committee 80, 84, 88, 114, 119, 122
Queensland Injury Surveillance and Prevention Program (QISPP) (Queensland Injury Surveillance Unit) 152–3, 182
Queensland Institute of Child Health
  proposals for 123–4, 188
Queensland Institute of Medical Research (QIMR Berghofer Medical Research Institute) 191
Queensland Newspapers 75, 92
Queensland Nurses' Union 102
Queensland Nursing Council 150
Queensland Paediatric Cardiac Service 201–2
Queensland Paediatric Nursing Association (QPNA) 150
Queensland Society for Crippled Children 24
Queenslander 14
Quinn, Bishop James 8

R

Radiation Oncology Mater Centre 177
Radio Lollipop 155, 169, 177, 179
radiology 20, 48, 64, 74, 98, 129, 145–6
Rafter, Pat 170
Ramritu, Prabha 184
Ratcliffe, Dr John 146
rationalisation policies 73, 85, 119–35, 188–201
Read, Peter 127
Red Cross Blood Bank 44
Red Cross Play Scheme 179
Reg Leonard House 96, 154, 184
Rendle-Short, Professor John 46, 58, 122, 123
  recommendations on health services 47–50, 51, 52, 63–5, 70, 81, 188
respiratory medicine 101–2, 166, 202
Reuter, Sister Catherine 212
Riordan, Christine 102
Robertson, Dr Ian 101, 146
Robertson, Stephen 198
ROBIN clinic (Rehabilitation of Children with Acquired Brain Injuries and Neuromuscular Disorders) 140, 178
Robinson, Dr Rae 37
Rodgers, Sydney 24
Rooney, Giaan 204
Rosenberg, Sister Marie Therese 101
Rotary clubs 24, 76
Royal Australasian College of Physicians 45, 82, 86
Royal Brisbane and Women's Hospital 3, 4, 36, 131, 194, 199
Royal Children's Hospital vii, 52, 63, 71, 72, 73, 74, 75, 82, 95, 111, 115, 121, 122, 123, 125, 128, 131, 139, 148, 158, 188, 190, 191, 192–4, 196, 197, 200, 207, 213
  Mater Children's Hospital, relationship 188–9
Russia 144–5
Rutter, Sir Michael 115
Ryan, Dr Bill 144

S

St Helen's Hospital, Brisbane 9
St Kilian's College, Brisbane 9
St Ledger, Dr AW 22, 37

About the Author

Helen Gregory is a professional historian and consultant in Queensland history and cultural heritage conservation. She has written many commissioned histories including *Expressions of Mercy: Brisbane's Mater Hospitals 1906–2006*, *Playing for Keeps: C&K's first century, 1907–2007* for Queensland's Creche and Kindergarten Association and histories of the Endeavour Foundation and MontroseAccess. She has written historical backgrounds for major museum exhibitions, including an exhibition at the State Library of Queensland on Brisbane's nineteenth-century floods. Helen taught at the University of Queensland and was an Adjunct Professor in the Department of History. She was also Director, Cultural Heritage, at Queensland's Environmental Protection Agency, which protects the state's cultural heritage places.

Index

St Mary's Nurses Home 10, 14, 15, 56–7
Saint, Professor Eric 120
St Vincent's Hospital, Dublin 7
St Vincent's Orphanage 8, 15
Salmon, Mother Alban 15, 24–6, 35, 209
Sandy, Uncle Des 212
Sargent, Dr Phil 145
scarlet fever 23
Scott, JES 93
Second World War 28–30, 34, 36
   post-war 'baby boom' 42
Sellars, Susan 109
Shannon, Sister Josephine (Imelda Mary) 56
Sheehan, Sister Mary Dorothea (Yvonne Mary)
   30, 55, 56, 68, 69, 75, 83, 99, 208
Shields, Linda 150
Simone, Dr Joseph 93
Sister Dorothea Jubilee Fund 146
Sisters of Charity 7
Sisters of Mercy, Institute of 6–8, 54, 78, 87, 163,
   167, 192, 208, 212
   arrival in Brisbane 8, 43
   benefactors 9, 12
   Dublin, in 6
   establishment of hospitals in Brisbane 3
   fundraising 10, 13–14, 15, 27
   hospitals in Brisbane, founding 9–11
   Mater buildings 14
   schools established by 8–9
   training for nurses 10
   values and philosophy vi, vii, 175, 176, 206,
   213
Slattery, Sister Mary Mechtilde 'Auntie Moll' 29,
   55, 207
sleep studies 139, 202
Smith, Carmen 95
Smith, Dr Amanda 127
South Brisbane Hospital *see* Princess Alexandra
   Hospital 119
South East Hospital Planning Project 188
Spanish influenza epidemic 15
speech therapy 49, 98, 113, 117, 132
spina bifida 103–4, 125, 186
Springborg, Lawrence 199
Starlight Children's Foundation 170
Starlight Express Room 169–70, 177, 179
Steer, Dr Peter 150, 151, 169, 179, 199
Stillman, Jill 141
Stringer, Dorothy 140
Stringer, Sister Jill (Mary Raymond) 56
Stritch, Sister Mary Edmund 10
sudden infant death syndrome (SIDS) 139
Suggit, Dr Stephen 37, 59
Suggit, Dr Winifred 37
Sullivan, Dr Kerry 86, 108
Sunday Mail 75
Suppiah, Dr Ram 141
Suspected Child Abuse and Neglect Unit (SCAN
   unit) 109–13, 117, 159–60
Sykes, Vicki 95–6, 156

T

Taussig, Professor Lyn 93
Taylor, Dr David 100
technology 137–8, 201–3
Telegraph 72, 75

Thacker, Fay 34–5
Thearle, Dr John 86
Theodore, EG 14
Theodore, Esther 14
Thomsett, Dr Michael 104, 141
Thong, Professor Yee-Hing 86–7, 102
Tiernan, Dr Ray 67
Toakley, Dr Geoff 58, 103
tonsillitis 22
Tooth, Douglas 71, 73
TRUSTT (Treatment and Rehabilitation Unit
   for Survivors of Torture and Trauma) 116,
   158–9
Tudehope, Dr David 89, 131–2
Turner, Dr Alfred Jefferis 4–5, 20
typhoid fever 22

U

Underwood Constructions 76
Underwood, Michael 5
UNICEF 150
United Nations Declaration of the Rights of the
   Child 107, 158
United States National Institutes of Health 140
University of Queensland
   Department of Child Health 56, 65, 82, 86,
   93–4
   Faculty of Health Sciences 192
   Medical School 34, 46, 51, 120, 167
Urquhart, Dr Aidene 115, 116, 132, 157, 159

V

van Leent, John 127
Vance, Dr John 86
Vienna Boys' Choir 61
Viner, Dr Russell 185

W

Wagner, Sister Mary 55
Walker, Dr Rosslyn 199
Wallace, Dr Geoff 207
Ward, Dr Cameron 140, 199
Warrick, Frank 93
Whitty, Mother Mary Vincent 7–9
Williams, Gordon 101
Wilson, Irene 113
Windsor, Dr Harry 'Daddy' 19, 24, 26, 29, 31,
   208
Windsor, Dr Morgan 86
Winkle, Dr David 165, 202
Winnett Orr method 23
Wonga Wonga 8
Wood, Dr David Orme 86, 113, 151, 160, 179,
   199, 210
World Health Organization (WHO) 115, 143
Wright, Bernadette 104
Wuth, Dr Greg 127, 134, 150, 162

X

Xavier Home 32, 37, 125

Y

Yaxley, Dr Ron 104
Yeates, Dr 37